Clinical Cases in Paediatrics: DCH Clinical Examination

Dr Anna Mathew

Dr Poothirikovil Venugopalan

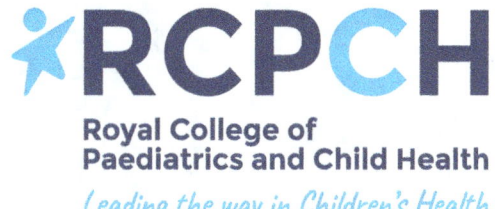

Royal College of
Paediatrics and Child Health

Leading the way in Children's Health

Acknowledgements

We are grateful to all our authors and the Diploma in Child Health (DCH) question-writing group of the UK Royal College of Paediatrics and Child Health (RCPCH), without whom this book would not have been possible. We would like to thank our reviewers, Dr Ashley Reece, Dr Kevin Windebank, Dr Martin Bellman, Mr Mike de la Hunt, Dr Nick Cooper, Dr Peter Saul and Dr Raj Verma, for their advice and insight when reading and reviewing different sections of our book. We would also like to thank Daniel Crane at the RCPCH for his advice and support, and for facilitating this publication.

Foreword

Clinical Cases in Paediatrics: Diploma in Child Health Clinical Examination

I am very pleased to introduce this new textbook from the UK Royal College of Paediatrics and Child Health. It has been written primarily for postgraduate doctors preparing for the UK Diploma in Child Health examination. The editors and contributors are to be congratulated for producing an excellent, up-to-date resource.

Doctors and other professionals contribute to the care of children, and many will not have had the opportunity for postgraduate training in paediatrics. I additionally commend this book as a resource for personal study and continuing professional development.

Professor Neena Modi
President Royal College of Paediatrics and Child Health

February 2016

Preface

This book has been written primarily for postgraduate doctors who are preparing for the UK DCH examination.

With the expansion of RCPCH activities overseas, we do hope that overseas doctors preparing for the DCH clinical examination will also find this book useful.

The DCH examination assesses candidates in all aspects of the doctor–patient interaction. It is recommended that candidates appearing for the examination should have completed a short period of paediatric training, as the scenarios for, and the standards required from, candidates to pass the examination are developed with that in mind. While it is difficult to precisely define the standard against which we are assessing candidates, we do expect them to display a special interest in paediatrics. With that in mind, we hope this book offers insight into the expectations we have of our candidates.

We also recognise that many doctors who work with children in various settings may not have had an opportunity to undergo postgraduate paediatric training. We believe this book could be used as a guide to common doctor–patient interactions alongside established textbooks to enable self-directed study and professional development. We hope the clinical cases approach will help doctors reflect on their daily clinical interactions, and that they will find the 'top tips' provided within the chapters helpful in their clinical practice.

This book would not have been possible without the RCPCH's DCH question-writing group, as all the scenarios used in the book have been lifted out of the RCPCH bank of questions created for the DCH clinical examination. We are grateful for their contributions to the book, both as a group and as individual authors.

We would like to thank Daniel Crane at the RCPCH for his advice and support, and for providing a vital link between the publications team and us.

Thanks to my co-editor Dr P Venugopalan for working so hard towards making this book a reality and for always being responsive with ideas and advice.

Finally, my thanks to Usha Venugopalan, Roy, Rachel and Leah Varughese for their assistance and advice, and for being gracefully accommodating with regard to the time taken away from family during the preparation of this book.

Anna Mathew

Our Contributors

Editors

Anna Mathew, MBBS, DCH, MRCP (UK), FRCPCH, MA (Medical Education)
Consultant Paediatrician
Western Sussex Hospitals NHS Foundation Trust, Worthing, West Sussex, UK

Poothirikovil Venugopalan, MBBS, MD (Paediatrics), MRCP (UK), FRCPCH
Consultant Paediatrician and Honorary Senior Clinical Lecturer
Royal Alexandra Children's Hospital, Brighton, UK

Contributors

Alexandra Rodrigues Da Costa, MRCPCH, MBChB, BSc
Paediatric Specialty Registrar
Kent, Surrey and Sussex Deanery

Amish Chinoy, MBBS, BSc, MRCPCH
Paediatric Specialty Registrar
Kent, Surrey and Sussex Deanery

Anand Kamalanathan, MBBS, DCH, DNB, FRCPCH
Consultant Neonatal Paediatrician
Wirral University Teaching Hospital NHS Foundation Trust, UK

Anna Mathew, MBBS, DCH, MRCP (UK), FRCPCH, MA (Medical Education)
Consultant Paediatrician
Western Sussex Hospitals NHS Foundation Trust, Worthing, West Sussex, UK

Arvind Shah, FRCPCH, MD, DCH
Consultant Paediatrician
North Middlesex University Hospital NHS Trust, London, UK

Asya Al Kharusi, MBBCH, DTCH, FRCPCH
Senior Attending Physician
Doha, Qatar

Benita Morrissey, MBChB, MRCPCH, DTM&H
Paediatric Specialty Registrar
The Royal London Hospital, UK

Caroline Pardy, MBBS, BSc, MRCS
Specialty Registrar in Paediatric Surgery
Royal Alexandra Children's Hospital, Brighton, UK

Ciara Holden, BMBS, BMedSci
Paediatric Specialty Trainee
St Peter's Hospital, Chertsey, Surrey, UK

Daniel Crane
Examinations Manager
Royal College of Paediatrics and Child Health, London, UK

Delair Khider, MBChB, MRCGP, MRCPCH, DCH
GP Trainer
Hillingdon GP Vocational Training Scheme

Duana Cook, MBBS
Paediatric Specialty Trainee
Western Sussex Hospitals NHS Foundation Trust, Worthing, West Sussex, UK

Edward Yates, MBBCH, BaO, MRCPCH
Paediatric Specialty Registrar
Western Sussex Hospitals NHS Foundation Trust, Worthing, West Sussex, UK

Elliott Ridgeon, BA, BMBCh
Foundation Year Trainee
Nottingham University Hospitals NHS Trust, Nottingham, UK

Geetha Fonseka, MBBS, DCH, MRCPCH
Consultant Paediatrician
Royal Alexandra Children's Hospital, Brighton, UK

Geethika Bandaranayake, MBBS, DCH, MD (Paediatrics), MRCPCH
Staff Grade in Paediatrics
Western Sussex Hospitals NHS Foundation Trust, Worthing, West Sussex, UK

Ingran Lingam, MBBS, BSC, MSC, MRCPCH
Neonatal Registrar
King's College Hospital NHS Foundation Trust, London, UK

Jonathan Rabbs, MBChB, MSc, MRCPCH
Consultant Paediatrician
Western Sussex Hospitals NHS Foundation Trust, Worthing, West Sussex, UK

Kate Fisher, MBChB, MSc, MRCPCH
Consultant Community Paediatrician
Western Sussex Hospitals NHS Foundation Trust, Worthing, West Sussex, UK

Lauren Parry, MBBS BSc(Hons), DCH, DRCOG, DFSRH
Lead GP
Queens Road Surgery, London, UK

Lucy Killian, MBBS, MSc, MRCPCH
Paediatric Specialty Registrar
Western Sussex Hospitals NHS Foundation Trust, Worthing, West Sussex, UK

Michael Hii, MRCPCH
Consultant Paediatric Gastroenterologist
Royal Alexandra Children's Hospital, Brighton, UK

Michael N de la Hunt, MS, FRCS
Consultant Paediatric Surgeon
Great North Children's Hospital/Royal Victoria Infirmary, Newcastle upon Tyne, UK

Mwape Thamara Kabole, MBChB, MRCP, FRCPCH, Dip. Allergy
Consultant Paediatrician
Western Sussex Hospitals NHS Foundation Trust, Worthing, West Sussex, UK

Nick Cooper
Associate Professor Clinical Education and Academic Lead, Peninsula Foundation School Health Education South West and Principal General Practice
Plymouth University Peninsula Schools of Medicine and Dentistry, Plymouth and Totnes, Devon, UK

Olive Hayes, MBBCh, FRCPCH
Consultant community paediatrician and Named Doctor for Child Protection
East and North Hertfordshire NHS Trust, QE2 Hospital, Welwyn Garden City, UK

Poothirikovil Venugopalan, MBBS, MD (Paediatrics), MRCP (UK), FRCPCH
Consultant Paediatrician and Honorary Senior Clinical Lecturer
Royal Alexandra Children's Hospital, Brighton, UK

Rachel Varughese, BA, BMBCh
Foundation Year Trainee
Nottingham University Hospitals NHS Trust, Nottingham, UK

Rosemary Jones, BSc, MBChB, DCH, MRCGP, FRCPCH, M.Ed.
Medical Adviser in Adoption and Fostering, Action for Children

Saher Zakai, MBCHB, Bsc, MRCGP, DCH, DRCOG, DFSRH
GP Principal
Boney Hay Surgery, Boney Hay, Burntwood, UK

Salah Mansy, FRCPCH, MRCPI, DCH, Arab Board, MSc (Paediatrics), MBChB
Consultant Paediatrician
Conquest Hospital, Hastings, UK

Satyendra Singh, MBBS, MRCGP, FRCS, DFFP
GP
Clayton Brook Surgery, Bamber Bridge, Preston, UK

Shankar Kanumakala, MRPCH
Consultant Paediatrician (Endocrines and Diabetes)
Royal Alexandra Children's Hospital, Brighton, UK

Sheik Abdul Razak, MBBS, DCH, MRCPCH
Consultant Paediatrician and Honorary Lecturer
Hull York Medical School, York Teaching Hospital NHS Foundation Trust, York, UK

Soluchi Amobi, BSc, MBBS, MRCPCH
Paediatric Specialty Registrar
Kent, Surrey and Sussex Deanery

Thomas Ruffles, BSc, MBBS, MRCPCH
Paediatric Specialty Registrar
Western Sussex Hospitals NHS Foundation Trust, Worthing, West Sussex, UK

Usha Natarajan, MRCPCH
Associate Specialist
Southport and Ormskirk Hospital NHS Trust, UK

Varadarajan Kalidasan, MBBS, MS, MCh, FRCS (Paediatric Surgery), M.A.
Consultant Paediatric Surgeon and Urologist and Director of Medical Education
Royal Alexandra Children's Hospital, Brighton, UK

Contents

Acknowledgements ii
Foreword iii
Preface iv
Our Contributors v

SECTION 1: The DCH Clinical Examination 3
    Chapter 1.1: Introduction 4
    Chapter 1.2: How to Use This Book 9

SECTION 2: The Communication Station 13
    Chapter 2.1: Introduction 14
    Chapter 2.2: Case Study 1: 8 Year Old with Attention Deficit Hyperactivity Disorder 21
    Chapter 2.3: Case Study 2: 13 Year Old with Growth Delay 27
    Chapter 2.4: Case Study 3: 3 Month Old with Scabies 33
    Chapter 2.5: Case Study 4: 15 Year Old Who Had Unprotected Sex 40
    Chapter 2.6: Case Study 5: 2 Week Old with Conjunctivitis 46

SECTION 3: The Data Interpretation Station 51
    Chapter 3.1: Introduction 52
    Chapter 3.2: Case Study 1: 15 Year Old with Abdominal Pain 57
    Chapter 3.3: Case Study 2: 13 Year Old with Palpitations 62
    Chapter 3.4: Case Study 3: 5 Year Old Girl with Dysuria 67
    Chapter 3.5: Case Study 4: 9 Year Old with a Skin Rash 71
    Chapter 3.6: Case Study 5: 2 Month Old with Wheeze 77

SECTION 4: The Structured Oral Station 85
    Chapter 4.1: Introduction 86
    Chapter 4.2: Case Study 1: 7 Month Old with an Abnormal Head Shape 91
    Chapter 4.3: Case Study 2: 8 Year Old with Bed-Wetting 95
    Chapter 4.4: Case Study 3: 8 Month Old with an Inguinal Swelling 100
    Chapter 4.5: Case Study 4: 4 Year Old with a Limp 106
    Chapter 4.6: Case Study 5: 3 Month Old with an Immunisation Reaction 111

SECTION 5: The Clinical Assessment Station 117
    Chapter 5.1: Introduction 118
    Chapter 5.2: Case Study 1: Respiratory: 10 Year Old with Cystic Fibrosis 125
    Chapter 5.3: Case Study 2: Abdomen: 7 Year Old with Intermittent Jaundice 133
    Chapter 5.4: Case Study 3: Cardiovascular: 2 Year Old Post Cardiac Surgery 138
    Chapter 5.5: Case Study 4: Neurology: 12 Year Old with a Limp 146
    Chapter 5.6: Case Study 5: 'Other' System: 10 Year Old with Tall Stature 154

SECTION 6: The Focused History and Management Planning Station 161
    Chapter 6.1: Introduction 162
    Chapter 6.2: Case Study 1: 7 Year Old with Asthma 169
    Chapter 6.3: Case Study 2: 5 Year Old with Chronic Constipation 175
    Chapter 6.4: Case Study 3: 6 Year Old with Communication Problems 183
    Chapter 6.5: Case Study 4: 13 Year Old with Diabetes 189
    Chapter 6.6: Case Study 5: 13 Year Old with Headaches 197

SECTION 7: The Child Development Station 205
- Chapter 7.1: Introduction 206
- Chapter 7.2: Case Study 1: 3 Year Old with Gross Motor Skills Delay 213
- Chapter 7.3: Case Study 2: 4 Year Old with Down's Syndrome/Fine Motor Skills Delay 220
- Chapter 7.4: Case Study 3: 3 Year Old. Language and Communication Skill Difficulties 227

SECTION 8: The Safe Prescribing Station 235
- Chapter 8.1: Introduction 236
- Chapter 8.2: Case Study 1: Hypoglycaemia in a Newly Diagnosed Diabetic 243
- Chapter 8.3: Case Study 2: Anti-Malarial Prophylaxis 249
- Chapter 8.4: Case Study 3: Pain Management in Knee Injury 254
- Chapter 8.5: Case Study 4: Eczema Treatment and Management 261
- Chapter 8.6: Case Study 5: Treatment and Management in Asthma 268

SECTION 9: Problem-Based Learning 275
- Chapter 9.1: Introduction 276
- Chapter 9.2: The Child with a Respiratory/ENT Problem 277
- Chapter 9.3: The Child with a Cardiovascular Problem 279
- Chapter 9.4: The Neonate 280
- Chapter 9.5: The Child with a Neurological Problem 281
- Chapter 9.6: The Child with a Genetic Disorder 283
- Chapter 9.7: The Child with a Gastroenterology or Hepatology Problem 284
- Chapter 9.8: The Child with a Musculoskeletal Problem 285
- Chapter 9.9: The Child with Diabetes or an Endocrine Problem 286
- Chapter 9.10: The Child with a Safeguarding Problem 287
- Chapter 9.11: The Child with an Infection/Immunology/Allergy-Related Problem 288
- Chapter 9.12: The Child with an 'Other' Problem 289

SECTION 10: Clinical Skills Logbook 291
- Chapter 10.1: Introduction 292
- Chapter 10.2: ENT Examination 293
- Chapter 10.3: Cardiovascular Examination 294
- Chapter 10.4: Respiratory Examination 295
- Chapter 10.5: Gastrointestinal Examination 269
- Chapter 10.6: Neurology: Cranial Nerve Examination 297
- Chapter 10.7: Neurology: Peripheral Nervous System Examination 298
- Chapter 10.8: Musculoskeletal System Examination 299
- Chapter 10.9: The Neonatal Examination 300
- Chapter 10.10: Developmental Assessment 301

Index 307

SECTION 1:
THE DCH CLINICAL EXAMINATION

Chapter 1.1: Introduction
Dr Anna Mathew, Dr Nick Cooper, Mr Daniel Crane

The decision to write a textbook for the DCH clinical examination came after close consideration of the views of trainees sitting the examination, and the realisation that there are very few DCH textbooks that accurately reflect the examination in its current format.

The RCPCH's DCH in the UK has evolved over time from a qualification designed to demonstrate competence in the care of children for general practitioners (GPs) and their trainees to its advantages being recognised for doctors who work in specialties allied to paediatrics, such as emergency medicine, anaesthetics, paediatric surgery, psychiatry and dermatology. In countries where primary care paediatrics exists, we believe this qualification would also serve to confirm similar competence in the care of children.

Doctors working in primary care are the initial point of contact for most children, and it is important that these doctors are suitably trained to provide an accurate assessment of the acutely ill child, know how to undertake shared care management of many long-term conditions, recognise the vulnerable child, and understand the steps required to assess and manage these situations. Primary care doctors should also contribute to child health surveillance, healthcare promotion and primary prevention of many conditions that pose an economic burden on healthcare services in both the industrialised and developing world.

In order to keep pace with the changing needs of patients in the UK, medical education, medical training and the delivery of services in the UK will need to evolve over time. Patients (including children with chronic illnesses) are living longer and, as a result, frequently develop multiple comorbidities. Several reviews commissioned by the government have been undertaken to look at these specific issues over the last decade. Recommendations arising from these reviews include an emphasis on the need for shorter postgraduate training programmes and a future workforce of generalist doctors more broadly trained and who can deliver care to patients with chronic illness. Many of these doctors would need to work closer to the home, both in primary care and other community settings. As such, the delivery of care will be primarily determined by the needs of patients. Paediatrics will be affected by these changes when they are implemented, and doctors who are able to demonstrate competence in several areas of medical practice will be more sought after when seeking employment. As such, obtaining the DCH and demonstrating competence in the care of children would be beneficial to those choosing to undergo such training and subsequent medical practice.

In 2014, more than 3,000 GP trainees were recruited across the UK. Currently, the number of GP trainees completing their training without undertaking a paediatric rotation is steadily increasing, and it is estimated that up to 50% of GP trainees do not receive postgraduate paediatric training. This concern has been noted by both the RCPCH and the Royal College of General Practitioners (RCGP) in relation to estimates that approximately 25–30% of the daily work of a GP commonly entails some aspect of paediatrics. Recent reviews have suggested a number of possible changes to early postgraduate training, including increasing the length of GP training to 4 years, developing models of broad-based training post-foundation programmes, and enhancing more diversity in Foundation Programme Year 2, including increasing opportunities for general practice and paediatric placements. The RCGP also encourages the development of GP skills in the first 5 years after MRCGP, in the early years of independent practice.

Aim of the DCH clinical examination

The aim of the examination is to assess whether candidates have reached the standard in clinical skills expected of a newly appointed GP who has completed a short period of training in paediatrics. The clinical examination assesses every aspect of the doctor–patient interaction, including the ability to communicate clearly and effectively, undertake comprehensive clinical assessments, integrate the information received to formulate a diagnosis and management plan, and finally translate the information into effective care for the patient.

Scenarios are generally written with reference to the candidate being a GP.

Candidates are expected to demonstrate proficiency in:

- Child development
- Clinical judgement
- Communication
- Establishing rapport with both parents and children
- Ethical practice
- History taking and management planning of chronic conditions
- Interpretation of data
- Knowledge and understanding of common problems in child health
- Organisation of thoughts and actions.
- Physical examination
- Professional behaviour
- Safe prescribing

The DCH clinical examination is held twice a year in the UK and at varying frequencies overseas.

The DCH examination

The DCH examination consists of both a theory and a clinical examination.

The theory examination

The *Foundation of Practice* paper is the theory component for the DCH examination. This paper also serves as one of the theory components for the MRCPCH examination. The Foundation of Practice paper consists of a combination of extended matching, multiple choice and best-of-5 questions.

A DCH syllabus is available on the RCPCH website to support candidates sitting this examination. Specimen papers and answers are also available for candidates to familiarise themselves with the format of the examination.

Candidates need to have passed this paper before they can progress to the DCH clinical examination.

The RCPCH moved from paper-based examinations to computer-based testing in January 2015. The RCPCH does not expect to run any further paper-based testing from this point onwards.

Candidates may apply to sit both the theory and clinical examinations at the same time, or complete the Foundation of Practice examination first and then move on to the DCH clinical examination during another application period. All theory and clinical examination applications are completed online.

The clinical examination

The current format of the DCH clinical examination was introduced in 2011. This examination runs on an Objective Structured Clinical Examination (OSCE) format and consists of 8 stations containing 'talking' and 'clinical' stations. Three new stations were introduced into the circuit in 2011, including 'safe prescribing', 'structured oral' and 'data interpretation' stations. As 'communication' with the child and family is the cornerstone of all paediatric consultations, it features twice in the DCH clinical examination circuit.

The 8 stations are divided into 2 circuits that candidates need to pass through to complete the examination. A different examiner will be present at each station to assess the candidate. All stations in Circuit A last 6 minutes and, in each of these stations, the candidate is faced with 1 task. Each of these tasks will earn a mark. All stations in Circuit B last 9 minutes and, in each of these stations, the candidate is faced with 2 tasks, usually an interaction followed by a discussion. Each of these tasks will earn a mark. There is a 3-minute interval between all of the stations to allow candidates to move between stations.

The 8 stations are:

Circuit A:
- Communication skills 1
- Structured oral
- Communication skills 2
- Data interpretation

Circuit B:
- Focused history and management
- Child development
- Clinical assessment
- Safe prescribing

Marking scheme and the pass mark

One mark is awarded for each of the stations in Circuit A. 2 marks are awarded for each of the stations in Circuit B, as each of these stations has 2 tasks for the candidate to complete the assessment. Altogether, the candidate is assessed 12 times over 8 stations.

The following marks are awarded for each of the station judgements:

Clear pass	12 points
Pass	10 points
Bare fail	8 points
Clear fail	4 points
Unacceptable	0 points

Candidates must score a total of 120 points in order to pass the examination. It is possible to compensate for poor performance in some stations by performing better in other stations.

Circuit layout

'Talking stations': 6-minute stations

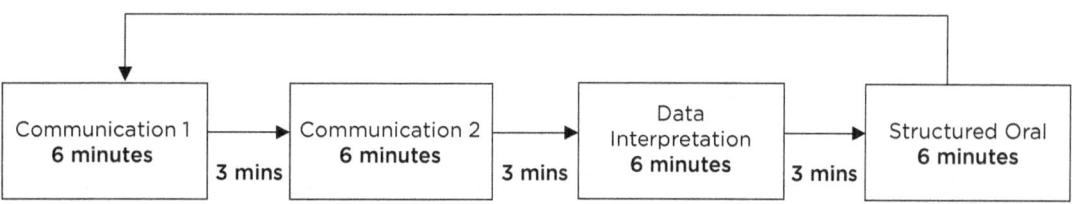

'Clinical stations': 9-minute stations

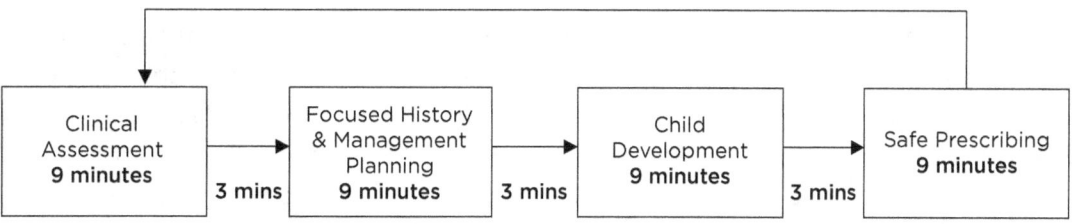

What to expect on the day

Candidates are asked to arrive early to the examination centre so that the host centre can conduct registration and identification formalities. As the circuits are run repeatedly over the day, candidates will be asked to arrive at different times during the day. Once the initial formalities are completed, candidates usually wait in the candidate waiting room along with colleagues allocated to the same circuit.

Prior to the beginning of the examination, the 'Senior Examiner' will greet all candidates and explain the important points for the day. A 'walk around' the circuit will also be conducted prior to the start of the examination. Candidates should expect further waiting periods, as the circuits swap over and the examiners conduct 'standard settings' for the patients attending the clinical assessment stations later in the day. Inevitably, there will be times when candidates from different circuits are simultaneously present at the examination centre, and it is important that no information should pass from one candidate to the next.

Role of the examiner

The RCPCH welcomes paediatricians and those who work in allied specialties to examine for the DCH clinical examination. Many GPs, psychiatrists, paediatric surgeons and community paediatricians examine for the DCH.

All examiners receive training from the RCPCH prior to becoming a DCH examiner and are therefore familiar in their roles for the day. They will be there to help facilitate the examination and provide as much support to the candidate as is necessary at each station. At some stations, examiners are asked not to interact with the candidate other than providing the initial introduction. This should not put off candidates. At other stations, examiners will interact as the station allows. A 'good' candidate will be open and receptive during these periods and listen carefully to what the examiner is saying, as it frequently guides the candidates with the task in front of them.

It is important to note that, in some exceptional cases, if a candidate's behaviour is unprofessional, the Senior Examiner may stop them from continuing with the examination. Unprofessional behaviour (e.g. rough handling of a child) **is extremely likely to result in the automatic awarding of an unacceptable mark.**

Recommended training

The RCPCH recommends that all potential DCH candidates should have completed a short period of paediatric training prior to sitting the clinical exam in order to be able to demonstrate added competence in paediatrics.

It is strongly recommended that all candidates read the RCPCH DCH syllabus in full, alongside common paediatric textbooks, when preparing for the examination. On the job, daily practice cannot be more highly emphasised. Candidates should undertake self-directed learning, but also use opportunities in the workplace to practise in small groups, as the ability to receive feedback from colleagues and seniors can be very valuable for honing clinical examination and communication skills. Utilising opportunities during outpatient clinic sessions and ward rounds by offering to undertake assessments of the patient with supervision are also recommended. We hope this book will provide insight into the different stations in the examination, and will provide guidance into the type of preparation required for the examination.

Further reading and references

1. Cooper N. Primary care for children: Back to the future. *Education for Primary Care* 2011; 22: 148–51
2. General Medical Council. Securing the future of excellent patient care. 2013. http://www.gmc-uk.org/Shape_of_training_FINAL_Report.pdf_53977887.pdf (accessed July 2015).
3. RCGP. *Business Case for the Extension of GP Training.* London, 2010.
4. Taylor C et al. The First5 Concept. *British Journal of General Practice* 2011; 61: 72–3
5. Wolfe I, Cass H, Thompson MJ et al. Improving child health services in the UK: Insights from Europe and their implications for NHS reforms. *BMJ* 2011; 342: d1277
6. Web links:

    DCH clinical syllabus:
    http://www.rcpch.ac.uk/training-examinations-professional-development/assessment-and-examinations/examinations/dch-clinical#syllabus

    Register for an RCPCH examination account:
    http://www.rcpch.ac.uk/training-examinations-professional-development/assessment-and-examinations/examinations/register-exa

    Apply for the RCPCH theory examination:
    http://www.rcpch.ac.uk/training-examinations-professional-development/assessment-and-examinations/examinations/theory-exa-4

    Apply for the DCH clinical examination:
    http://www.rcpch.ac.uk/training-examinations-professional-development/assessment-and-examinations/examinations/dch-clinic-0

Chapter 1.2: How to Use This Book
Dr P Venugopalan

This DCH clinical cases book has been written to help candidates prepare for the DCH clinical examination. It reviews each station in the examination circuit, presents possible clinical cases, and goes on to suggest answers to questions that candidates may face during the examination. Additional information on the relevant topic is provided to encourage candidates to develop a broader knowledge around the subject.

This book is the first of its kind, in that all scenarios in this book have been used in previous DCH clinical examinations and have therefore been lifted from the 'bank' of questions in the RCPCH. When choosing these scenarios, the editors mapped them onto the current DCH curriculum, in order to provide a broad coverage of the curriculum and, in doing so, give the candidate a real flavour of the type of scenarios that could appear in the examination.

This book is also unique in that most of the authors are current or past examiners for the DCH clinical examination. They have provided 'top tips' on answering questions to enable candidates to be well prepared for the examination. The practical focus of examination preparation has been maintained with an interactive style that encourages candidates to think about their own clinical practice.

We would like to emphasise that this book should be used alongside recommended paediatric textbooks during preparation for the examination. Competence can be further developed by supervised clinical examination of children, bedside teaching and tutorials.

Overview of the structure and layout of this book

This book is organised into 10 sections. Section 1 is an introductory overview of the DCH clinical examination. Sections 2 to 8 deal with the different stations in the examination circuit, and sections 9 and 10 offer guidance on self-directed learning.

Section 1 describes the DCH clinical examination and the circuit, and addresses the requirements needed in order to be able to sit the examination.

Sections 2, 3 and 4 deal with the 'talking stations', consisting of chapters on communication, data interpretation and the structured oral stations. In the DCH clinical circuit, there are 2 communication stations, which have been condensed into section 2 of this book. Sections 5 to 8 discuss the 'clinical stations', consisting of chapters on focused history and management, clinical assessment, developmental assessment and safe prescribing.

Each of the sections from 2 to 8 starts with an introductory chapter, followed by 5 scenarios, each formatted as a separate chapter (chapters 2 to 6). The introductory chapter explains what to expect in the station and how to manage your time, and provides tips on performing well in these stations. There is also a brief mention of the steps taken by the RCPCH to ensure consistency and a uniform and fair scoring system for each station. In addition, sample anchor statements (on which the examination scores are based) and a copy of the relevant mark sheet are attached. Each of the chapters from 2 to 6 deals with a specific scenario that can appear in the examination, and begins with candidate instructions that would be given in the real exam. Subsequent discussion focuses on the possible questions that could be asked of each candidate and sample responses. These answers are deliberately long and contain more information than a candidate would be able to realistically give, but do explain underlying principles in a way that will help cement understanding and knowledge. 'Additional information' has also been provided as an educational resource. 'Top tips' in each chapter reflect the experience of the authors as examiners, and we hope prospective candidates will find these useful.

Sections 9 and 10 offer guidance on self-directed learning, which if undertaken forms the backbone of sound clinical knowledge and skills. Section 9 helps to establish a good knowledge base with the help of problem-orientated, open-ended clinical scenarios. These scenarios, mapped onto the DCH curriculum, provide a framework for learning and discussions. We hope that candidates will work in groups, preparing answers to each question on their own at their convenience and then actively participating in a group discussion facilitated by a senior colleague/tutor. Section 10 promotes clinical examination skills, which are best learnt at the bedside. Again, this is optimally achieved by working in groups, supervised by a senior colleague/tutor.

Best use of this book

This book serves to provide a definitive, one-stop revision resource for candidates appearing for the DCH clinical examination. The introductory chapters help to familiarise candidates with the format and scoring systems, and should be read at the start.

Candidates may read this book at leisure, in which case they are likely to read through each chapter in full. However, it would be useful to read the specific questions in the context of clinical exposure to a particular clinical case or clinical query. The different chapters address some aspects of daily clinical interaction with patients, which would involve history taking, physical examination, diagnosis and differential diagnosis, developmental assessment, data interpretation, prescription writing and, above all, communicating with patients, carers and colleagues. Therefore, it is possible to review a chapter that relates to that day's clinical experience. The index at the end of the book provides a guide as to where the topic is discussed in the book.

After reading through an individual scenario and the questions that follow, we would recommend careful consideration of the possible answers. Ideally, a candidate would commit these thoughts to paper, prior to looking at the answers provided in the book. Working in a group during preparing for the examination would require a discussion before reviewing the suggested answers in the book. The authors and editors have ensured that the contents of the book reflect current practice and guidelines at the time of writing. However, it is possible that there could be variations in the practice of specific aspects of the management of individual clinical problems. Where in doubt, we recommend following local guidelines and the British National Formulary for Children (BNFC).

Sections 9 and 10 can be beneficially applied to day-to-day teaching and discussions in the workplace to ensure that performance in the examination is structured and systematic, and that interaction with the children and carers reflects a honed approach based on regular practice. Every examiner is able to identify a candidate who has had limited clinical exposure to children and families in their daily practice. It is also important, while working through these 2 chapters, for candidates to work in groups and receive feedback from each other to facilitate the adult learning process.

Although directed at DCH candidates, this book will also be a useful resource for paediatric trainees in their day-to-day clinical practice. During short paediatric attachments, with decreasing hours of work for junior doctors, we hope this book will provide exposure and insight to a diverse range of paediatric conditions.

Further reading and references

This is book is not designed to be a comprehensive textbook, and hence needs to be complemented by recommended textbooks (listed below in alphabetical order). Advice on further reading is also provided at the end of each chapter in the book.

1. *British National Formulary for Children* (BNFC). London: RCPCH Publications Ltd, 2014. ISBN 978 0 85711 136 4 (and subsequent updates)
2. Kliegman RM, Stanton BF, St Geme JW et al. *Nelson Textbook of Pediatrics*, 20th edition. Philadelphia: Elsevier, 2015. ISBN 978-1-4557-7566-8
3. Lissauer T, Clayden G. *Illustrated Textbook of Paediatrics*, 4th edition. Edinburgh: Mosby, 2012. ISBN 978-0-7234-3565-5
4. McIntosh N, Helms P, Smyth R et al. *Forfar and Arneil's Textbook of Pediatrics*, 7th edition. Edinburgh: Churchill Livingstone, 2008. ISBN 978-0-443-10396-4
5. Rudolf M, Lee T, Levene M. *Paediatrics and Child Health*, 3rd edition. Chichester: Wiley-Blackwell, 2011. ISBN 978-1-4051-9474-7

PAGE INTENTIONALLY BLANK

SECTION 2:
THE COMMUNICATION STATION

Chapter 2.1: Introduction
Dr P Venugopalan, Dr Lauren Parry

Communication with children and their parents or caregivers makes up a large proportion of the day-to-day life of most health professionals, especially in general practice. This station assesses your discussion with a role player. Communication is the key skill addressed, but clinical knowledge and the manner in which information is shared is also assessed.

The role player will usually play the role of a parent who comes with a health-related problem or concern related to the diagnosis or management of their child. On occasion, the role played may be that of a medical student or another health professional who is seeking information.

In this station, you are likely to be asked to communicate with the role player based on one of the following situations:

- Information giving (e.g. "please discuss the diagnosis with the parent").
- Consent (e.g. "please explain why you need to do a lumbar puncture with a view to obtaining consent").
- Critical incident (e.g. "please talk to the parent of the child who has been given the wrong drug").
- Ethics (e.g. "please discuss the problem as Chloe has refused to have any blood tests").
- Education (e.g. "please explain to the healthcare professional so that she can deal with the situation").

You may also be asked to explain the use of common medical devices. A manikin or model may be used in the station.

The examiner observes your interaction with the role player and scores your performance. There is no discussion directly with the examiner.

What to expect

In the communication station, you will be provided with background information stating the parent's or health professional's concern and the task required. This is clearly written on an information sheet. You will have 2 minutes to prepare yourself while waiting outside the station. During this time, also enter your identification details on the appropriate mark sheet.

When you enter the station, the examiner will greet you and request the appropriate mark sheet. The examiner will then introduce you to the role player. You will have 6 minutes to complete your task while the examiner observes and scores your performance.

It is an advantage to have a consistent approach in this station. You should:

- Undertake a polite and friendly greeting, with full introduction.
- Confirm the reason for attendance and explore the parent's or health professional's ideas, concerns and expectations.

- Identify the parent's or health professional's existing knowledge.
- Check understanding and encourage questions, which should be answered accurately and honestly.
- Respond and adapt to the emotional context of the station.
- Explain issues in an appropriate manner without jargon.
- Explore any further concerns and address them accordingly.
- Discuss the option of further meetings.
- Offer any information leaflets or websites that may help to reinforce the information shared.
- Summarise the discussion in the final minute of the station, and agree on further management if needed.
- Offer further appointments if appropriate.

Managing time in the communication station

Timing: This is a 6-minute station. A knock at 5 minutes will warn you that 1 minute remains. The final minute should be dedicated to summarising key points in the discussion, confirming that the role player has understood your information, offering further information (such as patient leaflets or links to websites) and offering further appointments where appropriate. Remember to thank the role player before you leave the station.

As this station lasts only 6 minutes, it is important to complete the task in the allocated time. Failure to complete the task will lead to you being marked down.

How consistency is ensured

Scenarios and the expected standards for this station are set centrally by the RCPCH well ahead of the examination. Host examiners receive these scenarios 3 to 4 weeks before the examination in order to identify and adequately prepare role players to ensure consistent standards in role players' performances on the day of the examination. On the day of the examination, examiners work in pairs to review these scenarios and standards. They review the 'standard setting', and, where necessary, make final changes.

'Mark sheets', individualised for each station, help guide examiners in their assessment. Mark sheets can inform you of the different areas examiners consider when awarding marks and, more importantly, areas where marks will be deducted (Appendix 2.11).

The RCPCH has developed 'anchor statements' that examiners refer to when deciding on pass/fail criteria. They use these as further guidance during standard setting and marking. You should review these documents to familiarise yourself with the scoring criteria explained in the anchor statements (Appendix 2.12).

Technique

This station is about communication. The manner in which a doctor communicates information is as important as the information being communicated. Therefore, marks will be given to what is said, the rapport created, and the manner in which things are said. Consideration will be given to how the role player feels at the end of the conversation – for example, empowered and clear, or confused and upset.

The examiner will observe how you communicate with the role player, especially if they ask you questions, or appear to be upset or dissatisfied with your explanations. Remain calm, considerate and polite while responding to these situations and remember to consider seeking advice or help from colleagues or senior members of staff if you are unable to satisfy the role player.

Being able to demonstrate fluid, systematic and structured communication in a short period of time requires confidence and good communication skills, both verbal and non-verbal. To prepare for this station, it is imperative to practise with colleagues, and have someone purely watch and critique the manner in which you communicate. It is often helpful to use a friend or family member who is not medical. Get them to mark you on the areas listed below. Encourage them to comment on any annoying habits you may have, such as fiddling or interrupting the role player.

Everyone has their own style of communicating, but you may like to reflect on these suggestions:

- **Elicit information using effective questioning skills.** Begin with open-ended questions, but direct the answers to the area of the expected discussion. Generally, the role player is expected to answer the questions that you put forth, but occasionally, they may ask a question, and it would be appropriate for you to answer this.

- **Listen carefully and effectively.** Pay attention to verbal and non-verbal clues and act on them. If you need to make notes, do not let this hinder your listening.

- **Provide information effectively.** Avoid jargon, or explain necessary terms. Small bite-sized information is better than a long monologue.

- **Assess what the role player already knows** and pitch your information at the right level. Clarify or carefully challenge myths or inaccuracies.

- **Assess what the role player wants to know.** Some people want to know lots of detail. For others, too much information is confusing and can create anxiety. Tailor this.

- **Check the role player's understanding of the information.** Be alert to the nature of their questions. Are they still seeking clarification, showing some confusion, or are they probing for more detail? *Let their questions guide the information you provide.*

- **Be empathic.** Think about reassuring sounds and phrases to encourage communication. Be aware that some subject areas may be sensitive. Probe sensitively if more information is required.

- **Think about the use of silence and slow down when you speak.** Pauses can be a powerful method of encouraging communication and also provides time for you to reflect on what has been said and what is still needed.

In summary, think about your words, information depth, speech patterns, body position and facial expressions. If you practise, these will become second nature.

Syllabus mapping

Knowledge

The candidate must:

- Understand and follow the principle that all decisions are to be made in the best interests of the child or young person.
- Be able to undertake teaching and learning in clinical contexts.
- Know the appropriate use of clinical guidelines to support evidence-based practice.
- Understand the issues relating to consent and confidentiality, including Fraser competence.
- Be aware of religious and cultural beliefs that parents may hold.
- Demonstrate the ability to seek help when required.
- Be able to recognise and respond to psychological effects of illness.
- Be able to recognise the benefits of multidisciplinary teams in the care of children.

Skills

The candidate must:

- Be able to explain, and counsel children and the family on, the conclusions reached.
- Demonstrate good generic communication skills when dealing with children and adolescents.
- Recognise the special needs of adolescents during consultation.
- Be able to maintain appropriate interaction with special needs children.

Further reading and references

RCPCH (2015) 'DCH Clinical Examination 2013 Syllabus': http://www.rcpch.ac.uk/training-examinations-professional-development/assessment-and-examinations/examinations/dch-clinical (accessed August 2015).

Appendix 2.11: Mark Sheet (Front and Back): Communication Stations

Royal College of Paediatrics and Child Health
DCH Clinical Examination

Communication Skills Station 1

Date: Time: Age of child:

Occasion used (1st, 2nd etc.):

CANDIDATE NUMBER CANDIDATE NAME EXAMINER NUMBER Scenario

Please enter candidate number in the grid to the left and print name below

EXAMINER NAME

Please enter examiner number in the grid to the right and print name below

Do not write in this shaded area

Description of case

Rapport

Full greeting and introduction.
Clarifies role and agree aims and objectives.
Good eye contact and posture.
Perceived to be actively listening (nod etc) with verbal and non verbal cues.
Appropriate level of confidence.
Empathetic nature. Putting parent/child at ease.

Information Gathering

Asks clear questions. Patient and examiner can hear and understand fully.
Mixture of open and closed style. Avoids jargon.
Allows parent/child sufficient time to speak.
Picks up verbal and non verbal cues.
Verifies and summarises parent/child history.

Information Giving

Information given is accurate.
Language is understandable to parent/child.
Knowledge base is appropriate.

Please record your overall judgement of the candidate's performance

MARK FINAL GRADE HERE ➤

Clear Pass | Pass | Bare Fail | Clear Fail | Un-acceptable

In order that proper feedback is available for the candidate please print your comments on their overall performance on the reverse of this document.

© Speedwell Computing Services +44 (0)1223 815210 enquiries@speedwell.co.uk www.speedwell.co.uk

☐ Poor approach - Unstructured (please add additional comments)

☐ Failure to deal with the set task (please add additional comments)

☐ Lacking in empathy - failure to respond to verbal & non-verbal cues (please add additional comments)

☐ Factual inaccuracy (please add additional comments)

Please add any additional comments here:

Appendix 2.12: Anchor Statement: Communication Stations

	Expected Standard/ CLEAR PASS	PASS	BARE FAIL	CLEAR FAIL	UNACCEPTABLE
RAPPORT	Full greeting and introduction. Clarifies role and agrees aims and objectives. Good eye contact and posture. Perceived to be actively listening (nod etc) with verbal and non-verbal cues. Appropriate level of confidence. Empathetic nature. Putting parent/child at ease.	Adequately performed but not fully fluent in conducting interview.	Incomplete or hesitant greeting and introduction. Inadequate identification of role, aims and objectives. Poor eye contact and posture. Not perceived to be actively listening (nod etc) with verbal and non-verbal cues. Does not show appropriate level of confidence, empathetic nature or putting parent/child at ease.	Significant components omitted or not achieved.	Dismissive of parent/child concerns. Fails to put parent or child at ease. Lack of civility or politeness. Inappropriate manner including flippancy.
INFORMATION GATHERING	Asks clear questions. Patient & examiner can hear & understand fully. Mixture of open & closed style. Avoids jargon. Allows parent/child sufficient time to speak. Picks up verbal & non-verbal cues. Verifies & summarises parent/child history.	Questions reasonable and cover all essential issues but may omit occasional relevant but less important points. Overall approach structured. Appropriate style of questioning responsive to parent/child. Summarises history.	Misses relevant information which if known would make a difference to the management of the problem. Excessive use of closed instead of open questions. Uses medical jargon occasionally. Misses verbal or non-verbal cues. Summary inaccurate/incomplete.	Asks closed questions instead of open questions. Questions poorly comprehended by parent/child. Inappropriate use of medical jargon. Inappropriately interrupts parent/child. Hasty approach. Does not seek views of parent or child. Poorly structured interview.	Shows no regard for parent or child's feelings. Rudeness or arrogance. No verification or summarising.
INFORMATION GIVING	Information given is accurate. Language is understandable to parent/child. Knowledge base for information is appropriate for F2 doctor (or equivalent) with paediatric training.	Accurate information except in minor detail. Language is generally appropriate for parent/child's level of understanding. Knowledge base poor in minor areas.	Some inaccurate information given. Language difficult for parent/child to understand. Knowledge base poor in major areas.	Much information inaccurate but not dangerous. Language inappropriate for parent/child to understand. Knowledge base generally poor.	Dangerous or grossly inaccurate information. Language impossible for parent/child to understand. Knowledge base below that expected for any qualified doctor.

Chapter 2.2: Case Study 1: 8 Year Old with Attention Deficit Hyperactivity Disorder

Dr Rosemary Jones, Dr Lucy Killian

This station assesses your ability to share information effectively with a patient or parent. You will not be assessed on the speed at which you communicate; however, the content and manner in which the consultation is held is important.

Logistics:

Timing: This is a 6-minute station. A knock at 5 minutes will indicate that 1 minute remains before the end of the station. You will have 2 minutes beforehand to read the candidate information provided to prepare yourself.

When the bell rings: On entering the room, the examiner will greet you and take your mark sheet. The examiner will then introduce you to the role player. In this station, you do not have any discussion with the examiner, who will be observing you and scoring your performance.

If you complete your discussion with the role player early, you will be asked to remain in the room until the session has ended.

Candidate role and task:

You are a GP working in a GP practice.

You will be talking to Andrea, mother of 8 year old James.

Andrea is concerned about James, as his school performance has deteriorated recently. The class teacher has told her that James is disruptive and easily distracted. The teacher has mentioned Attention Deficit Hyperactivity Disorder (ADHD) and so Andrea has come to the surgery to request a referral to a specialist. She feels that the school has not looked into James's problems properly, and is also worried as she has heard there is a long waiting list for assessment. Andrea is concerned about much of the information she has read on the internet about ADHD, particularly about the side effects of drugs used to manage ADHD.

Task: Discuss Andrea's concerns and explain why you think that James may not have ADHD.

You are not expected to gather any further medical history during the consultation.

Information given to role player:

You are Andrea, mother of 8 year old James. You are concerned that his teacher has suggested that James may have ADHD.

James had been doing well at school, but halfway through Year 3, you moved house, so he had to change school. James has taken a while to settle in at this new school, and his school performance has deteriorated. The teacher has told you that James is not interested and is disruptive during lessons. He is very distractible and cannot focus his attention on any task. James has told you that he is not happy at the new school, and does not like some of his classmates.

> You have gone to the school to discuss your concerns about James, and the teacher has mentioned possible ADHD. You have looked briefly on the internet and have found that lots of people are worried about the powerful drugs being prescribed for ADHD. You would be relieved if James does not have ADHD, but you want to discuss whether a specialist in the hospital should assess this.

> **Recommended candidate approach:**
>
> Once you realise that James was doing well at school and this deterioration has been only since moving home (which necessitated a new school), you should reassure Andrea that James is unlikely to have ADHD and should suggest other possible reasons behind his behaviour change.
>
> You should be able to:
>
> - Explore the mother's concerns with open-ended questions.
> - Display empathy.
> - Display confidence in discussing the features of ADHD, its diagnosis and management.
> - Display confidence in discussing the range of causes of attention difficulties and exploring key events around the timing of the onset of difficulties, e.g. environmental changes.
> - Share awareness that pathways exist in the community in relation to diagnosis and management of ADHD, and that ADHD may coexist with other comorbidities.
> - Suggest how Andrea and James may access further help and educational support.

Possible questions from the role player

■ *What is ADHD?*

ADHD is a behavioural disorder that affects approximately 2.4% of children in the UK (NICE 2014). It is more common in boys than in girls. For a diagnosis to be made, there should be evidence of symptoms occurring before the age of 7 years and for longer than 6 months. The symptoms should be present in more than 1 setting (e.g. home, school) and situation (e.g. school work, friendships, play, self-care). These difficulties should lead to significant impairment in social, psychological or educational functioning.

Children with ADHD present with symptoms in the 3 key areas of:

- **Impulsivity**
- **Inattention**
- **Hyperactivity**

These symptoms must be assessed against skills expected for the child's developmental age.

> *Top tip!*
> You should be able to pick out the key points in the history. A previously well child has developed emotional difficulties related to 2 significant environmental changes, and he has communicated his emotional difficulties. This helps you to explain why his behaviour and school performance may have changed, and why this is unlikely to fit the criteria for a diagnosis of ADHD.

■ What would happen if James were referred for an assessment?

The process for ADHD diagnosis varies around the country, and referral will be made to either the community paediatric team or child and adolescent mental health services (CAMHS). The first stage of the diagnosis is to investigate the severity of the child's symptoms and the impact on their functioning. This is usually done by screening questionnaires that are sent to more than 1 setting. The most commonly used are Connor's questionnaires.

Diagnosis will involve information gathering with a detailed medical and developmental history, followed by observation of the child in a clinic and, in some cases, at school. If a diagnosis is made, the clinician should provide information resources to the school and family regarding behavioural management strategies. A review will be arranged to discuss progress and further treatment options if required.

Top tip!
It is important to recognise the role of reassurance in this scenario. James is likely to respond well to behavioural management strategies and will rely on supportive and consistent role models.

■ What else might be causing the change in his behaviour and performance?

Other causes of attention difficulty and behaviour problems in children and young people should be considered. These include:

- Ongoing medical problems
- Environmental influences
- Emotional events
- Learning difficulties
- Other behavioural disorders (Table 2.21)

It is also important to ask about sleep and diet. Sleep deprivation is increasingly a problem in school-aged children. At the age of 7, children need around 10 hours sleep per night. There is increasing evidence that screen use (computers, phones, etc.) within 1½ hours of bedtime increases the time taken to go to sleep and can reduce sleep quality. There is no evidence for any dietary causes of ADHD; however, history may link certain foods and drinks to hyperactivity and it is important to address this and encourage healthy eating.

Table 2.21: Possible causes for attention difficulties	
Presenting problem	**Causes**
Ongoing medical problems	Genetic syndromes Prematurity Acquired brain injury Hearing or vision impairment Chronic pain or illness Depression
Environmental influences	Toxin exposure (e.g. alcohol) Domestic changes Family dysfunction Neglect Distractions within the school environment School work at an incorrect level for the child's abilities
Emotional events	Attachment disorder Psychological trauma
Learning difficulties	General (IQ <70) Specific (dyslexia) The child may require an educational psychology assessment.
Behavioural disorders	Autistic spectrum disorder (a child may seem inattentive) ADHD Conduct disorder Anxiety

■ *What alternate steps could improve James's school performance?*

In this situation, providing reassurance to the family by offering behavioural advice and follow-up would be the first stage of management. Families should be encouraged to discuss difficulties with their child's teacher or a Special Educational Needs Coordinator (SENCO). Areas for discussion could include friendships as well as academic progress. The mother could take James's previous school reports to show how he was progressing before the move. Helpful advice to give to the class teacher would be to sit the child near the front of the class, away from distractions, and to increase the child's self-esteem by using short instructions with positive reinforcement. At home, parents should be encouraged to provide the child with consistency and a regular routine.

Top tip!
You should reassure James's mother that, with support, his difficulties are likely to improve. It is important to encourage James's mother to meet with his schoolteacher and discuss possible behavioural strategies together. She should be encouraged to discuss support that the school may be able to provide for James to help him form new peer relationships.

Additional information

Treatment options for ADHD

Behavioural support at home and at school

Training sessions help parents and carers use positive behavioural strategies to manage their child's difficulties, as well as to increase parental confidence and competence. The information and support programmes offered vary across the country, but are generally a 6-week programme coordinated by CAMHS/school nursing service. Schools may offer teacher training in classroom management of challenging behaviours. Parent information leaflets are available at the Royal College of Psychiatry website and Young Minds website.

Role of medication

Consider the use of medication if a trial of behavioural support does not prove effective. Methylphenidate is the most commonly prescribed drug in the UK for the management of ADHD. It does not have a product licence for children less than 6 years, but some paediatricians use it from the age of 5 years with careful monitoring. The dose is titrated to achieve control of symptoms without significant side effects. The most common side effect is appetite reduction, which may lead to poor weight gain. Rarely, it can cause tachycardia and hypertension. Dexamphetamine and atomoxetine are other medications that can be tried.

Medication should be initiated by a specialist (CAMHS or community paediatrician) and managed as part of local, shared care agreements with GP.

Syllabus mapping

General competence

The candidate must:

- Demonstrate good generic communication skills when dealing with children and adolescents.
- Be able to explain, and counsel children and the family on, the conclusions reached.

Behavioural problems

Knowledge

The candidate must:

- Be able to demonstrate skills to support and engage parents of children with emotional or mental health difficulties.
- Know about the role of CAMHS.
- Be aware of the signs and symptoms of ADHD, autistic spectrum disorders and *depression*.

Skills

The candidate must:

- Be able to look at behaviour as a form of communication and to take this into account when interviewing, examining and assessing children.

Further reading and references

1. Attention-deficit hyperactivity disorder and hyperkinetic disorder: information for parents, carers and anyone working with young people. Royal College of Psychiatrists. http://www.rcpsych.ac.uk/healthadvice/parentsandyouthinfo/parentscarers/adhdhyperkineticdisorder.aspx (accessed August 2015).
2. Conners CK. Development of the CRS-R. In: Conners CK, ed. *Conners' Rating Scales-Revised*. North Tonawanda, NY: Multi-Health Systems, 2001: 83–98
3. Green C, Chee K. *Understanding ADHD. A parent's guide to Attention Deficit Hyperactivity Disorder in children*, 2nd edition. Vermillion: London, 1997.
4. National Institute for Health and Clinical Excellence. Clinical Knowledge Summary – Attention deficithyperactivitydisorder.London,2014.http://cks.nice.org.uk/attention-deficit-hyperactivity-disorder (accessed August 2015).
5. National Institute for Health and Clinical Excellence. (CG72) – Attention deficit hyperactivity disorder. Diagnosis and management of ADHD in children, young people and adults. London, 2008. http://guidance.nice.org.uk/cg72 (accessed August 2015).
6. Young Minds. Parents Survival Guide. http://www.youngminds.org.uk/for_parents/parents_guide (accessed August 2015).

Chapter 2.3: Case Study 2: 13 Year Old with Growth Delay
Dr Amish Chinoy, Dr P Venugopalan

This station assesses your ability to share information effectively with a patient or parent. You will not be assessed on the speed at which you communicate; however, the content and manner in which the consultation is held is important.

Logistics:

Timing: This is a 6-minute station. A knock at 5 minutes will indicate that 1 minute remains before the end of the station. You will have 2 minutes beforehand to read the candidate information provided to prepare yourself.

When the bell rings: On entering the room, the examiner will greet you and take your mark sheet. The examiner will then introduce you to the role player. In this station, you do not have any discussion with the examiner, who will be observing you and scoring your performance.

If you complete your discussion with the role player early, you will be asked to remain in the room until the session has ended.

Candidate role and task:

You are an ST3 GP trainee working in a GP practice.

You will be talking to Joanne Davies, mother of Andy aged 13 years.

You had referred Andy to the local hospital for short stature, and they have diagnosed constitutional delay in growth and puberty (CDGP).

Andy's height is on the 0.4th centile and his weight is on the 9th centile. Andy is otherwise well, with no significant past medical history. He is pre-pubertal, and his target height, based on parental height, is predicted to be on the 25th centile. The only family history of note is that his father was also late in achieving his growth spurt and going into puberty. Andy's basic blood tests at the hospital are normal and his bone age is delayed.

Joanne has received a clinic letter from the hospital paediatrician, and is confused by the terminology used in the letter.

Task: Explain to Joanne what CDGP is, and answer any questions she may have.

You are not expected to gather any further medical history during this consultation.

Information given to role player:

You are Joanne Davies, a 45 year old housewife and mother of Andy, aged 13 years. You are concerned that Andy is considerably shorter than his friends.

Andy has always been a well child, and has excelled in school academically. Both you and Andy's father, Charlie, are a reasonable height, although Charlie has mentioned that he only achieved a growth spurt late in his teenage years.

> When you had gone to the hospital for Andy's first appointment, the doctor did not seem too concerned about Andy's height and had performed some 'basic' tests. The next time you saw the doctor at the hospital, 6 months later, the doctor was satisfied with the test results and told you that "Andy's height will catch up to his friends later on as a teenager".
>
> Last week, you received a letter from the last clinic appointment that says he has "constitutional delay in growth and puberty", which you feel had not been mentioned at the hospital. You have no idea what this diagnosis means. You make an appointment with the GP to discuss this diagnosis and what this means for Andy, as well as ongoing concerns about his height. Andy is at school during this appointment.

> **Recommended candidate approach:**
>
> You should reassure Joanne that Andy will reach his predicted height range with no adverse consequences, and offer further reviews to monitor growth and progress towards puberty.
>
> You should be able to:
>
> - Explore Joanne's concerns with open-ended questions.
> - Display empathy.
> - Display confidence in discussing the features of CDGP, and how the clinical features and tests performed so far helped to arrive at the diagnosis. You should do this without using medical jargon.
> - Inform Joanne that, at present, no treatment is required for his short stature or delayed puberty.
> - Display confidence in assuring her of a good outcome, sharing the fact that his growth will continue for longer than his peers.
> - Summarise towards the end of the discussion, offer steps for continued monitoring of growth and onset of puberty, and offer patient information leaflets or a source containing similar information.

Possible questions from the role player

■ What is CDGP?

CDGP is one of the most common causes of short stature, so you should have a good knowledge of this condition and convey the salient points while avoiding medical jargon. CDGP is one of the variants of normal growth and development, along with familial short stature. When assessing children in primary care, it is important to differentiate these patterns from pathological causes of short stature.

CDGP is characterised by relatively short stature in childhood, but with a normal adult height. Affected children tend to have a low-normal growth velocity during their pre-pubertal years, with delayed pubertal development, leading to further height discrepancies when compared to their peers. However, once they enter puberty, these children display catch-up growth and their growth continues for longer than their peers. There is often a family history of delayed growth and puberty that point towards the diagnosis. The key diagnostic aid in these children is a delayed bone age, although a delayed bone age is seen in many pathological causes as well.

Familial short stature is largely genetic in nature, with both parents often being short. The child's height and growth will follow the target centile range based on parental heights. These children tend to have low-normal growth velocities and a normal bone age (i.e. consistent with their chronological age). Ultimate height would be consistent with parents' heights and, therefore, tend to be below average.

> *Top tip!*
> The key points to cover are that this is a variant of normal, often runs in families, and is characterised by a delay in both growth and puberty, which means that the child's growth spurt occurs later than his peers.

■ Will Andy be the same height as his friends eventually?

Yes, children with CDGP have a delayed onset of puberty and their growth continues longer, as their bones continue to grow until a later age. His predicted height, based on parental heights, is on the 25th centile and there is no reason to believe he will not achieve this height.

> *Top tip!*
> Reassurance is the mainstay of this scenario and it is important to convey that, once Andy has his pubertal growth spurt, his final height should be within his target height range and roughly comparable to his peers.

■ How can we be sure there are no underlying problems making him short?

Children with pathological causes of short stature typically have heights that are falling down across the centiles, with markedly reduced growth velocities. They will often have other symptoms and signs.

The pathological causes can be divided into:

- Malnutrition – Poor intake from poverty or neglect
- Chronic disease – Chronic renal failure, juvenile idiopathic arthritis, malignancy, coeliac disease, inflammatory bowel disease, severe heart disease, cystic fibrosis, etc.
- Endocrine – Hypothyroidism, growth hormone deficiency, glucocorticoid excess (usually iatrogenic)
- Genetic syndromes – Turner, Noonan, Russell-Silver, Prader-Willi
- Skeletal dysplasias – Achondroplasia, hypochondroplasia

Andy has been reviewed by the paediatrician, and his baseline bloods are also normal. There is a positive family history and his bone age is delayed. All these factors are consistent with the diagnosis of CDGP and help to exclude pathological causes.

However, follow-up and monitoring of growth are important, and a small minority of these children may require endocrine evaluation and hormone therapy to 'kick-start' their pubertal development, under guidance from the paediatric endocrinologist.

> *Top tip!*
> As well as reassurance, examiners expect you to provide the safety net of future reviews to enable monitoring of growth and pubertal development to confirm the diagnosis and ensure an appropriate outcome.

Additional information

Normal growth

There are 3 phases of growth in childhood. Rapid growth occurs in the first 2 years of life, influenced largely by nutrition. From this point until puberty, growth is slow but constant and determined mainly by the growth hormone. A second growth spurt occurs during puberty, effected mainly by gonadal steroid hormones.

Definition and causes of short stature

Short stature is defined as the height of a child that is 2 standard deviations or more below the mean for children of that sex and chronological age. On a growth chart, this is the equivalent to being below the 2nd centile. Table 2.31 lists the main causes of short stature.

Table 2.31: Clinical approach to short stature			
Category	Features	Investigations	Treatment
Normal variant	Family history Low-normal growth velocity	Usually nil Can test bone age	Usually just reassurance and observation Occasionally, CDGP requires gonadal steroids
Malnutrition	Poor socioeconomic background Behaviours typical of neglect Cachectic	History and examination usually sufficient Admission to demonstrate improvement in growth	Social support Social support Social support
Chronic disease	Poor weight gain Signs and symptoms specific to disease	Dependent on specific possible diseases E.g. urea and electrolytes (U+E), coeliac screen, inflammatory markers	Treating the specific disease
Endocrine	Often overweight	Hormonal tests, including dynamic testing	Addressing specific hormonal imbalance
Syndromes	Dysmorphic features	Genetics	Multidisciplinary team approach
Skeletal dysplasia	Disproportion between limb length and axial length	Usually clinical	Supportive

Evaluation of children with short stature

A thorough history and physical examination is crucial in the initial assessment of these children. Accurate measurement of height and weight and plotting these on a growth chart, along with previous measurements, is the next step. The pattern of growth and growth velocity are important in distinguishing between normal variants of growth and pathological causes; therefore, children should have their height measured on at least 2 occasions, ideally at least 6 months apart.

Growth velocity (cm/yr) = Increase in height over 6 months (cm) × 2

Another useful measure is to obtain parental heights and to calculate the child's target height and centile range.

Boys: Predicted adult height (cm) = $\dfrac{\text{Mother's height (cm)} + \text{Father's height (cm)} + 14 \text{ cm}}{2}$

Girls: Predicted adult height (cm) = $\dfrac{\text{Mother's height (cm)} + \text{Father's height (cm)} - 14 \text{ cm}}{2}$

Target height range (cm) = Predicted adult height (cm) +/- 2 centile ranges

The most useful first-line investigation for short stature is bone age. Blood tests may be indicated depending on signs and symptoms, as well as growth patterns and growth velocity. Baseline bloods (urea and electrolytes, bone profile, full blood count, ESR, coeliac screen, thyroid function test) help to exclude pathologic causes.

Additional tests that may be indicated in selected children include karyotype and insulin-like growth factors (IGF-1/IGFBP-3).

Syllabus mapping

Growth and development/general competence

Knowledge

The candidate must:

- Understand normal growth and development, including puberty.
- Know the causes of short stature and the clinical features of these conditions.
- Know when short stature needs to be investigated, and be able to discuss appropriate investigations and treatment.

Skills

The candidate must:

- Be able to demonstrate good generic communication skills when dealing with children and adolescents.

Further reading and references

1. Garganta MD, Bremer AA. Clinical dilemmas in evaluating the short child. *Pediatr Ann* 2014; 43: 321-327. doi: 10.3928/00904481-20140723-11
2. Rogol AD, Hayden GF. Etiologies and early diagnosis of short stature and growth failure in children and adolescents. *J Pediatr* 2014; 164: S1-14. doi: 10.1016/j.jpeds.2014.02.027
3. Song KC, Jin SL, Kwon AR et al. Etiologies and characteristics of children with chief complaint of short stature. *Ann Pediatr Endocrinol Metab* 2015; 20: 34-9. doi: 10.6065/apem.2015.20.1.34
4. Spadoni GL, Cianfarani S. Bone age assessment in the workup of children with endocrine disorders. *Horm Res Paediatr* 2010; 73: 2-5. doi: 10.1159/000271910
5. Villanueva C, Argente J. Pathology or normal variant: what constitutes a delay in puberty? *Horm Res Paediatr* 2014; 82: 213-21. doi: 10.1159/000362600

Chapter 2.4: Case Study 3: 3 Month Old with Scabies
Dr Olive Hayes

This station assesses your ability to share information with a patient or parent. You will not be assessed on the speed at which you communicate; however, the content and manner in which the consultation is held is important.

> **Logistics:**
>
> *Timing:* This is a 6-minute station. A knock at 5 minutes will indicate that 1 minute remains before the end of the station. You will have 2 minutes beforehand to read the candidate information provided to prepare yourself.
>
> *When the bell rings:* On entering the room, the examiner will greet you and take your mark sheet. The examiner will then introduce you to the role player. In this station, you do not have any discussion with the examiner, who will be observing you and scoring your performance.
>
> If you complete your discussion with the role player early, you will be asked to remain in the room until the session has ended.

> **Candidate role and task:**
>
> **You are an** ST3 GP trainee working in a GP practice.
>
> You will be talking to Samantha Collins, mother of Leona aged 3 months.
>
> Samantha brought Leona to the surgery with persistent crying and a rash. She visited the Emergency Department 6 weeks ago and was given some creams, which are not helping. She recently obtained a different cream from her neighbour, but that has not helped either.
>
> On examination, you notice that Leona is dirty and unkempt. She has a widespread rash suggestive of scabies. She has severe cradle cap and is miserable when you examine her.
>
> This family is known to social services, as Samantha has moderate learning difficulties. She has 2 other children. Leona is Samantha's third child and they all live with Samantha's mother. Samantha attended a special needs school and has a designated social worker whom she has not seen for a long time. She cannot remember her name.
>
> **Task: Explain to Samantha your concerns about Leona and outline your management plan.**
>
> You are not expected to gather any further medical history during this consultation.

> **Information given to role player:**
>
> You are Samantha Collins, 19 years old and have 2 other children by a different partner. Leona is your third child, and you are finding it difficult to cope with the demands of looking after her. You live with your mother, who is out of the house working most of the time.

> Leona has had a rash for a number of weeks and you have been using a cream that a neighbour gave you, but this is not working. Leona's rash is worse and she is crying most of the time and not really feeding. You have come to the end of your tether and have taken her to the GP.
>
> As a child, you had attended a special school for children with moderate learning difficulties. You have a social worker who you feel interferes in your life and whom you haven't seen for a long time.
>
> Your friend recently had a child taken into care and you are worried that this might happen to Leona. You are reluctant to involve the social worker.

> **Recommended candidate approach:**
>
> You should communicate your concerns in relation to Leona's welfare with openness and sensitivity, after allowing Samantha to discuss the reasons for her seeking medical advice.
>
> You should be able to:
>
> - Explore Samantha's concerns about Leona with open-ended questions.
> - Display empathy.
> - Recognise that there is both a medical and social need that have to be addressed.
> - Be confident in discussing the features of scabies, and why this is a cause for concern from a safeguarding perspective.
> - Recognise that this is a family in need and offer support to the family.
> - Communicate with the understanding that Samantha has learning difficulties.
> - Demonstrate an understanding of safeguarding procedures.
> - Formulate a clear management plan, including discussion with the existing social worker, involvement of a health visitor and treatment of scabies for all of the family, and ensure a follow-up is in place.

Top tip!
Effective and sensitive communication of safeguarding concerns is the mainstay of this scenario. You should identify the poor hygiene and difficulties that Samantha is experiencing in managing as a single parent with 3 children. At the same time, do not forget to adequately address the medical concern.

Possible questions from the role player

■ **Why don't you just give me different creams to try?**

Leona appears to have scabies. Reinfestation is common unless all other household members are treated, even if they are asymptomatic. Therefore, using another cream will not help. Scabies is the result of infestation by the mite *Sarcoptes scabiei*. The main mode of transmission is through skin-to-skin contact. Scabies typically presents with intensely itchy, small, erythematous papules. The classic finger-web burrow (which appears as a short, linear, scaly lesion between the fingers) is often absent in young children. Scabies in infants is often more widespread and eczematous than in adults. The face, scalp and feet may be involved.

Anti-scabietic treatment is required. Permethrin is the treatment of choice for children over 2 months of age. This is applied all over the body, from the neck downwards, in addition to any affected areas on the head. The treatment should also be applied to the skin folds and under fingers and toenails. It needs to be left on for 8 to 10 hours (usually overnight) and then washed off. This should usually be repeated in 5 to 7 days.

It is important that all household members are simultaneously treated, whether symptomatic or not. Bed linen and towels should be washed and dried at a high temperature to eradicate the mite from clothing.

Symptomatic treatment for the itching may also be offered.

It is important to ensure that Samantha fully understands the treatment regime.

Top tip!
You should be able to recognise that Samantha has learning difficulties. Therefore, talk slowly and clearly, use simple words and check her understanding of what you have conveyed to her. You should offer to *write* the treatment plan down for her.

Are you going to take my baby away?

Samantha is understandably anxious, especially as she has a friend whose baby was removed by social services. A common misconception among families is that a referral to social services equates to the removal of the child from the home. This is usually not the case. Samantha herself admits to finding things difficult. She is failing to meet Leona's physical needs, as Leona is observed as being unkempt and dirty. On the other hand, she has attempted to treat the condition and has sought medical advice from the Emergency Department and the GP.

Samantha should be referred for a 'child in need' assessment. Multiagency frameworks such as the Common Assessment Framework (CAF) and child neglect practitioner toolkits such as Graded Care Profiles may be used as part of the process. The aim is to identify the areas of difficulty and to put processes in place that support Samantha in meeting her children's physical, emotional and developmental needs. It is important that Samantha engages in the process and works with social care, as a persisting failure to meet Leona's needs, despite support, will lead to an escalation to child protection procedures.

Top tip!
Reassurance is important. Samantha needs to be encouraged to accept the support of social services in order to achieve the best outcome for Leona and her siblings.

I've got my mother to help me – why can't you just let me go home?

All NHS staff have a statutory duty outlined in Section 11 of the Children Act to safeguard and promote the welfare of children and young people. The General Medical Council has also issued guidance that states: "All doctors must act on any concerns they have about the safety or welfare of a child". In this case, it is important to place Leona's needs over her mother's discomfort, and emphasise the need for input from social services. Although Samantha's mother is involved, she does not appear to be at home much and Samantha herself is now struggling to cope. It is apparent that Samantha is struggling with her parenting skills and would benefit from additional support. Leona would currently fall within a 'child in need' category.

> *Top tip!*
> The needs of the child are paramount. In any safeguarding discussion, always return to the welfare of the child. It is easy to get distracted by the parent's needs and requests.

A child in need is defined in Section 17 of the Children Act when:

a) The child is unlikely to achieve or maintain, or have the opportunity of maintaining, a reasonable standard of health or development without the provision of supportive services.
b) The child's health or development is likely to be significantly impaired without the provision of such services.
c) The child is disabled.

Although Samantha has a social worker, they do not appear to be currently involved in the case. It is important that a discussion occurs with this worker to understand the current level of support. Persistent failure to meet Leona's hygiene, health or developmental needs despite support may lead to an escalation to child protection due to neglect.

> *Top tip!*
> Always consider the siblings in safeguarding situations. It would be advisable to contact the school nurse to identify any concerns in relation to their wellbeing.

Additional information

■ *What is the difference between safeguarding and child protection?*

'Safeguarding' is an umbrella term that includes child protection along with other aspects of child welfare promotion.

Safeguarding involves:

- Protecting children from maltreatment
- Preventing impairment of a child's growth or development
- Ensuring that children are growing up in circumstances consistent with the provision of safe and effective care
- Taking action to enable all children to have the best life chances

Child protection refers to the steps taken when a child is suffering, or is likely to suffer, significant harm.

Parental risk factors contributing to child abuse

When considering safeguarding for children, it is important to assess all parental risk factors and recognise when adult behaviour has an adverse impact on their children. The **"toxic trio"** refers to the risk factors of domestic violence (DV), substance misuse and mental health difficulties. The combination of these 3 factors increases the vulnerability of a child to abuse and neglect.

Domestic Violence (DV)

DV is any incident or pattern of incidents that involves controlling, coercive or threatening behaviour, violence or abuse between people aged 16 years or over who are, or have been, intimate partners or family members. It is a common occurrence with at least 750,000 children a year witnessing DV, and is a risk factor in almost two thirds of serious case reviews. Pregnancy is usually when there is an increased risk for violence to start or escalate.

DV can harm children in a number of ways. Witnessing violent events can have adverse effects on a child's mental health. There is increasing evidence that early exposure to DV adversely impacts development, with an increased prevalence of anxiety, distractibility and impulsivity noted in affected children. These children are also at increased risk of physical injury from getting 'caught in the crossfire' or attempting to defend a parent. In addition, there may be associated neglect due to the presence of a traumatised or depressed mother. Continuity of medical care can be difficult for families fleeing DV.

Substance and alcohol misuse

Parental substance and alcohol misuse is usually characterised with features of dependence. The most common drugs implicated in misuse are heroin, benzodiazepines, cocaine and amphetamines. Parental drug and alcohol misuse is associated with child neglect, with a prevalence of around 50% of child abuse cases. Problem drinking is associated with violence, physical abuse and a chaotic lifestyle, all of which pose further risks to the welfare of the child. Low educational attainment, behavioural difficulties and mental health problems are common among involved adults.

Both alcohol and drugs are associated with increased risks of premature delivery and sudden infant death syndrome. Alcohol use in pregnancy can result in foetal alcohol spectrum disorder, with learning and behavioural difficulties seen in affected babies. Intravenous drug misuse can result in the transmission of blood-borne viruses to the unborn child. The baby may also withdraw from the drug (neonatal abstinence syndrome).

Mental health problems

Parental mental health disorders are common and are a significant risk factor that contributes to abuse. Compliance with treatment and access to therapeutic support reduces the risk, as does the presence of a supportive partner. The postnatal period is a period associated with increased risk, as postpartum depression and psychosis can develop in women without a prior psychiatric history.

Learning disability

Learning disability is classified into:

- Mild (IQ 55–70)
- Moderate (IQ 40–55)
- Severe (IQ 25–40)
- Profound (IQ <25)

Learning disability increases the risk of child abuse, especially neglect. Parents may struggle to provide appropriate stimulation for the infant, resulting in developmental delay. There can be poor uptake regarding health surveillance programmes and immunisation, and a failure to attend appointments. These difficulties can escalate with more children. Women with learning difficulties are also more vulnerable themselves, and may struggle to protect their children from abusive partners.

Types of neglect

Neglect is the persistent failure to meet a child's basic needs (Table 2.41). It is the most common form of abuse, and has serious and long-term consequences for a child's developmental outcomes and potentially irreversible impact on emotional development. Neglect is not always deliberate.

Table 2.41: Types of neglect	
Physical neglect	Failure to meet the physical needs of the child. This includes poor hygiene, inadequate clothing or bedding, recurrent infestations or exposure to hazardous substances in the home.
Nutritional neglect	Inadequate provision of food, leading to faltering growth. This can be deliberate or through a lack of understanding of dietary needs.
Medical neglect	Failure to seek (or to comply with) medical advice or administer medications, which compromises a child's health or wellbeing. Failure to attend appointments, poor uptake of immunisation and lack of dental care are included in this category.
Emotional neglect	Persistent lack of emotional availability regarding a child.
Educational neglect	A child's poor attendance at school, and the parents' failure to support learning.
Abandonment	Leaving young children without adult supervision ('home alone').
Failure to provide supervision and guidance	Failure to provide sufficient supervision to ensure that the child is physically safe. There may be multiple attendances with injuries or ingestion of drugs, burns and scalds, or sunburn.

It is unusual for 1 form of neglect to exist in isolation and, generally, children will fall under several subcategories.

Syllabus mapping

General competence

The candidate must:

- Demonstrate good generic communication skills when dealing with children and adolescents.
- Be able to explain, and counsel children and the family on, the conclusions reached.

Safeguarding

Knowledge

The candidate must:

- Be aware of the different categories of non-accidental injury – physical injury, emotional injury, sexual injury, neglect and fabricated illness.
- Know what steps are to be taken when a non-accidental injury is suspected. It is necessary to understand the local referral pathway and the key professionals who can help.

Skills

The candidate must:

- Be able to look at behaviour as a form of communication, and to take this into account when interviewing, examining and assessing children.

Further reading and references

1. British Parliament. Children Act 2004. http://www.legislation.gov.uk/ukpga/2004/31/contents (accessed August 2015).
2. General Medical Council. Protecting Children and Young People: The responsibilities of all doctors. 2012. http://www.gmc-uk.org/guidance/ethical_guidance/13257.asp (accessed August 2015).
3. HM Government. Working together to safeguard children. A guide to inter-agency working to safeguard and promote the welfare of children. 2015. https://www.gov.uk/government/uploads/system/uploads/attachment_data/file/419595/Working_Together_to_Safeguard_Children.pdf (accessed August 2015).
4. Royal College of Paediatrics and Child Health. Child Protection Companion. 2013. http://www.rcpch.ac.uk/child-protection-publications (accessed August 2015).

Chapter 2.5: Case Study 4: 15 Year Old Who Had Unprotected Sex

Dr Lauren Parry

This station assesses your ability to share information with a patient or parent. You will not be assessed on the speed at which you communicate; however, the content and manner in which the consultation is held is important.

Logistics:

Timing: This is a 6-minute station. A knock at 5 minutes will indicate that 1 minute remains before the end of the station. You will have 2 minutes beforehand to read the candidate information provided to prepare yourself.

When the bell rings: On entering the room, the examiner will greet you and take your mark sheet. The examiner will then introduce you to the role player. In this station, you do not have any discussion with the examiner, who will be observing you and scoring your performance.

If you complete your discussion with the role player early, you will be asked to remain in the room until the session has ended.

Candidate role and task:

You are a GP working in a GP practice.

You will be talking to Amy Robertson, a 15 year old girl.

Amy had unprotected intercourse with her 17 year old boyfriend last evening and is now worried about the risk of pregnancy. She is seeking your advice.

Task: Counsel Amy on management options and utilise the opportunity for health promotion.

You are not expected to gather any further medical history during this consultation.

Information given to role player:

You are Amy, a 15 year old girl. You had unprotected intercourse with your 17 year old boyfriend last evening. You are concerned about a possible pregnancy and don't know what to do. Your doctor has agreed to see you at the practice and discuss your concerns.

You are specifically worried that you may get pregnant or catch an infection such as human immunodeficiency virus (HIV). You are looking forward to reassurance and advice on steps to prevent such complications. You are uncomfortable that your parents might find out. You would also like to get some general advice for the future.

A good candidate should leave you feeling reassured and informed.

> **Recommended candidate approach:**
>
> You should be able to put Amy at ease, discuss emergency contraception, and offer counsel on sexual health and safe sex.
>
> You should be able to:
>
> - Explore Amy's concerns with open-ended questions.
> - Be empathic and reassuring.
> - Offer advice on emergency contraception and facilitate Amy's choice of whether to proceed with this.
> - Support Amy in deciding whether to inform her parents and explicitly reassure her that this is her choice.
> - Counsel on sexually transmitted infections (STI) and sexual health/safe sex.
> - Consider whether the 15 year old meets the Fraser guidelines.
> - Discuss the small risk of failure of emergency contraception and offer a follow-up appointment with genitourinary medicine (GUM) clinic.

Top tip!
Understanding the feelings of an adolescent and effective counselling form the mainstay of this scenario. You should be able to elicit Amy's concerns, and discuss the options so as to enable her to take an informed decision. Recognising that she satisfies the Fraser guidelines is vital to establish trust, and carry forward the discussion.

Possible questions from the role player

■ *Please can you help me, doctor, with what I need to do next? I'm really worried about getting pregnant.*

Reassure Amy that she has consulted soon after having unprotected sexual intercourse (UPSI), so emergency contraception has a high chance of being effective and any infection could be picked up promptly. You should explain that there are 3 methods of emergency contraception: 2 'morning-after pills' (MAPs) and a third, the intrauterine copper coil device (IUCD). Amy is likely to guide you into talking about MAPs, as it is the one most favoured by teenagers.

The 2 MAPs available are both taken as stat doses with similar side effects. They differ mainly in their effectiveness based on the length of time after intercourse. Levonorgestrel is licensed up to 72 hours post UPSI and Ulipristal acetate up to 120 hours. You should establish when Amy had sex to guide your choice. The emergency IUD offers ongoing contraception and the Faculty of Sexual and Reproductive Health for doctors (DFSRH) recommends offering it to "all eligible women presenting between 0 and 120 hours of UPSI or within 5 days of expected ovulation, because of the low documented failure rate". You should:

- Establish when Amy's last period was.
- Find out if she has had any other episodes of unprotected sex this cycle (if so, does she need a pregnancy test now? In such a case, an IUD may be unsuitable).
- Check if she is on any other medication (specifically enzyme inducers).
- Explain how to take the medication.

You should offer specific instructions to Amy on the use of hormonal emergency contraception:

- Her next period may be early or late – a barrier method of contraception needs to be used until the next period.
- Seek medical attention promptly if any lower abdominal pain occurs, as this could indicate an ectopic pregnancy.
- Return in 3 to 4 weeks if the subsequent menstrual bleed is abnormally light, heavy or brief, is absent, or if she is otherwise concerned. If there is any doubt as to whether menstruation has occurred, a pregnancy test should be performed at least 3 weeks after UPSI.

Effectiveness of emergency contraception

About 1 to 2 out of a 100 people who take emergency contraception become pregnant. If there is any doubt as to whether Amy's next period is normal, she should be advised to take a pregnancy test in 3 weeks. You may offer Amy a follow-up appointment in 3 to 4 weeks to do a pregnancy test.

Remind Amy that these measures only reduce pregnancy risk for this episode of UPSI. It does not offer any protection against future sexual activity. Therefore, encourage condom use.

The potential side effects of emergency contraception

Generally, Levonorgestrel is tolerated very well. Headaches, nausea and altered bleeding pattern are the most common side effects. The dose must be repeated if vomiting occurs within 2 hours of taking it. Sometimes, it can alter when your next period comes and how heavy it is.

> *Top tip!*
> This is clearly not an easy consultation for a 15 year old to have, and time and effort must be made to congratulate her on attending the appointment, and to make her feel at ease. Structure your time to ensure you cover pregnancy prevention and STI risk, and make plans to help prevent unprotected sex from occurring in the future.

■ *Amy is worried her parents might find out...*

Reassurance is the key here. You should emphasise confidentiality (unless Amy is thought to be in danger). You should encourage her to tell her parents and offer her support in doing this, but reassure her that it is her choice.

Some teenagers find it hard to converse with adults. During examination preparation, think about ways to facilitate the discussion. For example, "some teenagers worry about what their parents will say. Is this bothering you?" or "often parents are reassured that their teenagers have felt able to talk to them and pleased that they are planning safe sex. How do you think your parents might react?"

> *Top tip!*
> You should encourage Amy to tell her parents and offer support for this, but reassure her that this is her choice.

Safeguarding issues

Amy has confided in you that she is having sexual intercourse under the legal age of consent. There is a duty of care to ensure this was complicit sex, without coercion. Underage sexual activity should always be seen as a possible indicator of child sexual exploitation. (Remember: sexual activity with a child under 13 is a criminal offence and should *always* result in a child protection referral.)

You must consider if Amy is competent to make decisions about having sex or having treatment. You should use the Fraser guidelines (see 'Additional Information' below). Therefore, it is imperative to ensure Amy understands the options and potential benefits and side effects of treatment and non-treatment, understands the management plan and is encouraged to speak to her parents.

> *Top tip!*
> You must show you have thought about child protection and Gillick competence/Fraser guidelines.

■ Doctor, what is my risk of getting HIV?

HIV carries very few symptoms. An HIV test is a blood test that can identify the disease, but the test has a window period. Most current tests have a 4-week window period. Abstinence or the condom is the best way to prevent HIV transmission. While it cannot be cured, there are now very effective treatments.

It is important to explain that there are other STIs, and encourage Amy to have a sexual health check-up. A sexual health check-up involves swabs (that Amy can take herself) or a urine test. Amy needs to wait at least 2 weeks after UPSI before having these tests. These can be done at the practice or a GUM clinic.

Other STIs and their symptoms

Chlamydia (the most common treatable STI in Britain, with 5–10% of women under 24 years old potentially infected), and gonorrhoea are the other 2 STIs to be investigated for. Sometimes, these cause vaginal discharge, irregular vaginal bleeding and pelvic pain in women, or urethral discharge and dysuria in men. However, often they have no symptoms. Explain that it is usually not easy to know if a potential partner is infected. There are other infections such as herpes and warts that cause skin rashes. These can be spread just by skin-to-skin contact.

Condoms are the best way to protect against STIs. It is important to use a condom for all sexual activity, not just penetration. Most STIs are treatable but can have long-term consequences if untreated.

> *Top tip!*
> There is plenty of information that can be shared in this communication station. However, you should limit this to what is feasible in the 6 minutes. You may direct Amy to patient information leaflets, the instruction leaflet inside the Emergency Contraception packet, and to teen-friendly websites to support your consultation. Follow-up appointments are another option.

Additional Information

■ *Gillick competence and Fraser guidelines*

These 2 terms relate to whether a child is mature enough to take decisions without discussing it with their parents. These refer to a legal case where Victoria Gillick took her local authority and the Department of Health and Social Security to court in order to try and prevent them from giving contraception to those under 16 without parental consent. The case went to the High Court in 1984 and was dismissed. It then went to The House of Lords in 1985, where the Law Lords, including Lord Fraser, ruled in favour of the original ruling.

The original trial (Gillick vs West Norfolk, 1984) concluded that the child's maturity and understanding and the nature of the consent required should decide the child's capacity. The child must be capable of making a reasonable assessment of the advantages and disadvantages of the treatment proposed, similar to an informed consent. Lord Scarman (Gillick vs West Norfolk, 1985) subsequently added that the child should also have sufficient maturity to understand what is involved.

The Fraser guidelines (Gillick vs West Norfolk, 1985) apply specifically to contraceptive advice. A doctor could proceed to give advice and treatment if he or she is satisfied that:

1. The girl (although under the age of 16 years of age) will understand his advice.
2. He cannot persuade her to inform her parents or to allow him to inform the parents that she is seeking contraceptive advice.
3. She is very likely to continue having sexual intercourse with or without contraceptive treatment.
4. Unless she receives contraceptive advice or treatment, her physical or mental health (or both) are likely to suffer.
5. Her best interests require him to give her contraceptive advice, treatment or both without parental consent.

■ *Different methods of contraception*

Table 2.51 lists the different contraception methods in terms of their benefits and drawbacks.

Table 2.51: Comparison of the different contraception methods			
Method	Examples	Benefits	Drawbacks
Barrier methods	Male condom. Female condom (but this is less user-friendly and less reliable).	The best method to prevent STIs.	May interrupt sexual activity. User-dependent (have a high failure rate if used incorrectly).
Daily or weekly methods	Combined oestrogen and progestogen pills or patches. Progestogen only pills	They are more than 99% effective, but only if the person remembers to take them. May help with heavy or painful periods.	They can cause hormonal side effects, such as spotty skin or mood changes.
Long Acting Reversible Contraceptives	Injectable progestogens (depot) IUCD Mirena coil (IUS) Progestogen implant (Nexplanon)	To be encouraged in teenagers. These are the most effective contraceptives and are not dependent on the user. They can provide contraception for 3 months to 5 years.	Need to be fitted by a trained GP or GUM clinic. May alter period pattern or heaviness. They can cause hormonal side effects, such as spotty skin or mood changes.

Syllabus mapping

General competence

The candidate must:

- Demonstrate good generic communication skills when dealing with children and adolescents.
- Be able to explain, and counsel children and the family on, the conclusions reached.

Adolescent health

Knowledge

The candidate must:

- Understand the different health needs of adolescents and the factors influencing adolescent development.
- Know about contraceptive and sexual health issues, including STIs.

Skills

The candidate must:

- Be able to hold a discussion on all the areas addressed under the 'knowledge' section.

Further reading and references

1. Keegan MB, Diedrich JT, Peipert JF. Chlamydia trachomatis Infection: Screening and Management. *J Clin Outcomes Manag* 2014; 21: 30-8
2. Kong FY, Hocking JS. Treatment challenges for urogenital and anorectal Chlamydia trachomatis. *BMC Infect Dis* 2015; 15: 293. doi: 10.1186/s12879-015-1030-9
3. Larcher V, Hutchinson A. How should paediatricians assess Gillick competence? *Arch Dis Child* 2010; 95: 307-11. doi: 10.1136/adc.2008.148676
4. Post-exposure prophylaxis for HIV. *Drug Ther Bull* 2011; 49: 30-3. doi: 10.1136/dtb.2011.02.0016.
5. Raymond EG, Cleland K. Clinical practice. Emergency contraception. *N Engl J Med* 2015; 372: 1342-8. doi: 10.1056/NEJMcp1406328
6. Webster DP, Donati M, Geretti AM et al. BASHH/EAGA position statement on the HIV window period. *Int J STD AIDS* 2015; 26: 760-1. doi: 10.1177/0956462415579591
7. Wheeler R. Gillick or Fraser? A plea for consistency over competence in children. *BMJ* 2006; 332: 807

Chapter 2.6: Case Study 5: 2 Week Old with Conjunctivitis
Dr Lauren Parry

This station assesses your ability to share information with a patient or parent. You will not be assessed on the speed at which you communicate; however, the content and manner in which the consultation is held is important.

> **Logistics:**
>
> *Timing:* This is a 6-minute station. A knock at 5 minutes will indicate that 1 minute remains before the end of the station. You will have 2 minutes beforehand to read the candidate information provided to prepare yourself.
>
> *When the bell rings:* On entering the room, the examiner will greet you and take your mark sheet. The examiner will then introduce you to the role player. In this station, you do not have any discussion with the examiner, who will be observing you and scoring your performance.
>
> If you complete your discussion with the role player early, you will be asked to remain in the room until the session has ended.

> **Candidate role and task:**
>
> **You are a** GP working in a GP surgery.
>
> You will be talking to Aisha, the 17 year old mother of Adam, a 2 week old baby boy who has conjunctivitis.
>
> You have received the results of Adam's eye swab. Your GP colleague sent the swab to the lab when Aisha brought the 6 day old Adam to the surgery with sticky eyes. The swab is positive for chlamydia.
>
> You have called the mother back to discuss the eye swab results. You prescribe the recommended medication for the baby (oral erythromycin and chloramphenicol eye drops).
>
> You would like to explain to Aisha that she should attend the Genitourinary medicine (GUM) clinic for further investigation and management.
>
> **Task: To explain the need for referral to the GUM or sexual health clinic.**
>
> You are not expected to gather any further medical history during this consultation.

> **Information given to role player:**
>
> You have been called to the surgery to be given the results of Adam's eye swab. The GP has prescribed antibiotics and some eye drops.
>
> You understand that there is an infection in the baby's eyes, but do not understand where it came from.

> The doctor has asked to see you to explain that Adam's eye swab was positive for chlamydia, which is a sexually transmitted disease. The doctor will suggest that you need to attend a sexual health clinic.
>
> You are shocked to discover that the cause of the sticky eyes may be a sexually transmitted disease. You don't understand why you need to go to a different clinic. You are worried that people may find out what the infection is and where it came from.

> **Recommended candidate approach:**
>
> You should communicate your concerns in relation to the chlamydia infection with openness and sensitivity, taking into consideration the mother's embarrassment and lack of knowledge in this area.
>
> You should be able to:
>
> - Sensitively explore Aisha's understanding of sexually transmitted infections (STIs) and STI testing. You should recognise that both the mother and the baby are patients here, but that the task is centred on the mother.
> - The mother should be encouraged to attend a sexual health clinic so that she can be screened for other STIs, to assist with contact tracing, and because follow-up may be necessary. The mother should be reassured about confidentiality, both in the surgery and the GUM clinic.
> - You could reassure the mother that there are many causes of sticky eyes in young children, most commonly due to cold viruses and respiratory tract bacteria. It will not be obvious to people that Adam's infection is due to chlamydia.

Top tip!
Patients are often worried about the stigma of STIs. It is important for you to reassure Aisha that the GP practice and the GUM clinics adhere to strict confidentiality rules.

Possible questions from the role player

■ *Does my partner need to know?*

Chlamydia is a STI. Therefore, it is something that Aisha has contracted during sexual activity. If Aisha has it, it is most likely that her partner does too. Both of them must be treated so that they do not continue to reinfect each other. Both Aisha and her partner should be encouraged to attend the GUM clinic.

You can reassure Aisha that chlamydia is very common, and between 5% and 10% of sexually active women under 24 may be currently infected. However, in most men and women, it doesn't cause symptoms, so most people are unaware they have it. If Aisha is asymptomatic, all her sexual partners in the past 6 months should be contacted and offered treatment.

Top tip!
Be tactful and non-judgemental in your questioning. Aisha may have caught this from her current partner, and she may need time to think about how and when he contracted this infection. However, she herself may have had additional partners. This diagnosis has potential implications for her current relationship.

■ Can I continue to breastfeed?

Chlamydia is not passed on through breast milk. There are drug regimes that are safe to give to lactating mothers, such as erythromycin or amoxicillin. In pregnancy and during lactation, it is advisable to have a test of cure to ensure it has definitely been fully treated.

■ If I do not go to the sexual health clinic, will there be any other problems for me?

Chlamydia is fully treatable and very straightforward to treat. However, if it is not treated, it is likely to persist. An untreated infection can result in abnormal bleeding patterns, abdominal pain, purulent discharge, cervicitis and pain on passing urine. It can then go on to cause pelvic inflammatory disease, which can cause fertility problems and pelvic pain and increases the chances of an ectopic pregnancy.

Top tip!
Explore why Aisha might not want to go to an STI clinic, dispel any myths, and help to look for solutions. Offer supportive patient information leaflets. If you are unable to persuade her to attend the clinic, you may offer some treatment in the surgery and invite her back to explore this again on another occasion.

■ Will I be able to have more children?

Treatment is more than 95% effective. The sooner chlamydia is treated, the less likely it is to cause long-term complications. It is therefore unlikely to prevent Aisha from having more children. You could recommend that Aisha have a sexual health check-up for any future pregnancy to treat any infection and prevent transmission to the baby.

Top tip!
Recommend regular sexual health check-ups, especially when embarking on new relationships. A discussion about condoms may be appropriate.

Additional Information

Rates of ophthalmia neonatorum (conjunctivitis developing in the first 28 days of life) may be as high as 12% in infants born in the Western world, and rates are considerably higher in developing countries. Chlamydia is now the single most common infective cause of neonatal conjunctivitis, and usually presents with watery discharge (rapidly becoming purulent) 5–14 days after birth. Systemic treatment of the infant is important, because if it is present in the eyes, it is almost always present in the respiratory tract. Examination should look for associated rhinitis, otitis media and pneumonia. An infant born to a mother with chlamydia has a 30–40% chance of developing conjunctivitis, and a 10–20% chance of developing pneumonia.

Syllabus mapping

General competence

The candidate must:

- Demonstrate good generic communication skills when dealing with children and adolescents.
- Be able to explain, and counsel children and the family on, the conclusions reached.

Infection, immunity and allergy

Knowledge

The candidate must:

- Be aware of the common infections of the foetus, newborn, and children in Britain, as well as important worldwide infections – e.g. TB, HIV, hepatitis B, malaria, polio.

Ophthalmology

Knowledge

The candidate must:

- Know the common causes and management of red eye.

Skills

The candidate must:

- Be able to hold a discussion on all the areas addressed under the 'knowledge' section.

Further reading and references

1. British Association of Sexual Health and HIV. UK National Guideline for the Management of Genital Tract Infection with Chlamydia trachomatis. 2006. http://www.bashh.org/BASHH/Guidelines/Guidelines/BASHH/Guidelines/Guidelines.aspx (accessed August 2015).
2. Fenton KA, Korovessis C, Johnson AM et al. Sexual behaviour in Britain: Reported sexually transmitted infections and prevalent genital Chlamydia trachomatis infection. *Lancet* 2001; 358: 1851-4
3. LaMontagne DS, Fenton KA, Randall S et al. Establishing the National Chlamydia Screening Programme in England: Results from the first full year of screening. *Sex Transm Infect* 2004; 80: 335-41
4. Rubenstein JB, Tannan A. *Conjunctivitis: Infectious and non-infectious*. In: Yanoff M, Duker JS (ed). Ophthalmology, 4th edition. Elsevier Saunders: China, 2014: 183-91. ISBN 978-1-4557-3984-4

PAGE INTENTIONALLY BLANK

SECTION 3:
THE DATA INTERPRETATION STATION

Chapter 3.1: Introduction
Dr P Venugopalan

Requesting an investigation and interpreting the results obtained in order to decide on the diagnosis and the management of our patients form part of our day-to-day practice. In this station, you will be presented with a short description of a child's clinical history and/or examination findings, along with the results of the investigations. It is important for you to identify the abnormal as well as the relevant normal results, and interpret these in the context of the child's clinical presentation. This station offers you a good opportunity to score high marks.

What to expect

In the data interpretation station, you will be given the scenario (information sheet) while waiting outside the station. This will include both the clinical background of the child and the results of the investigations. You will have at least 2 minutes outside the station to prepare before the start of the test at the station. Examples of data provided could include blood tests, urinalysis, stool charts, audiograms, growth charts, diabetic diaries, peak flow charts, developmental milestones, and laboratory reports. Normal values are also provided on the data sheet. Investigations that are not generally included in this station include radiographs, electrocardiograms (ECGs), electroencephalograms (EEGs), slides and scans.

You enter the station at the ring of a bell, and once inside the station, the examiner will greet you and request the appropriate mark sheet. Please hand over your mark sheet for the station, making sure you have entered your details on it beforehand. The examiner's first question is generally to interpret the data. This is followed by questions based on your interpretation, and usually involves arriving at a diagnosis and formulating a differential diagnosis and management plan. Fluency and confidence in discussing management is essential for a clear pass. A good understanding of the evidence base (for example, NICE guidelines) that underpins good paediatric practice is also essential.

It cannot be emphasised enough that it is important to listen very carefully to the examiner's questions. If uncertain, it is important to clarify this. The examiner would be happy to repeat the question if necessary.

When interpreting the results on your data sheet, it is important to mention not only the abnormal results but also the relevant normal ones that would help you to reach a diagnosis. At times, there are some abnormal results that are only mildly abnormal, and you may feel that these are not important. However, it is necessary to mention these as well, as some of them may later turn out to be helpful in the differential diagnosis.

Managing time in the data interpretation station

Timing: This is a 6-minute station. The entire time in the station is spent conducting a discussion with the examiner on the data provided, the diagnosis, differential diagnoses and management. A knock at 5 minutes will warn you that 1 more minute remains.

It is recommended that you go over the data sheet during the 2 minutes outside the station, and if necessary, make notes on a separate sheet of paper (provided on request) regarding the possible diagnosis, differential diagnoses and management plan.

The data sheet must be returned and left outside the examination room once you have finished the station.

If you finish early, you will be asked to remain in the room until the session has ended.

How consistency is ensured

RCPCH examiners set questions for the station well before the date of the examination, in groups, and agree the standards of performance required from candidates for the various grades awarded. In addition, on the day of the examination, examiners work in pairs to review these standards and adjust them if required. This 'standard setting' process is undertaken before each cycle during the clinical examination to ensure consistency.

'Mark sheets', individualised for each station, help guide examiners in their assessment of candidates. Mark sheets can inform candidates of the different areas examiners consider when awarding marks and, as importantly, areas where marks can be lost. It is worth noting that the final score given to a candidate represents the examiner's overall judgement of the candidate's performance at the station (Appendix 3.11).

The RCPCH has developed 'anchor statements' that examiners refer to when deciding on pass/fail criteria. They use these as further guidance during standard setting and marking. Candidates should review these documents to familiarise themselves with the scoring criteria explained in the anchor statements (Appendix 3.12).

Further reading and references

DCH clinical syllabus: http://www.rcpch.ac.uk/training-examinations-professional-development/assessment-and-examinations/examinations/syllabus (accessed March 2015).

Clinical Cases in Paediatrics: DCH Clinical Examination

Appendix 3.11: Mark Sheet (Front and Back): Data Interpretation Station

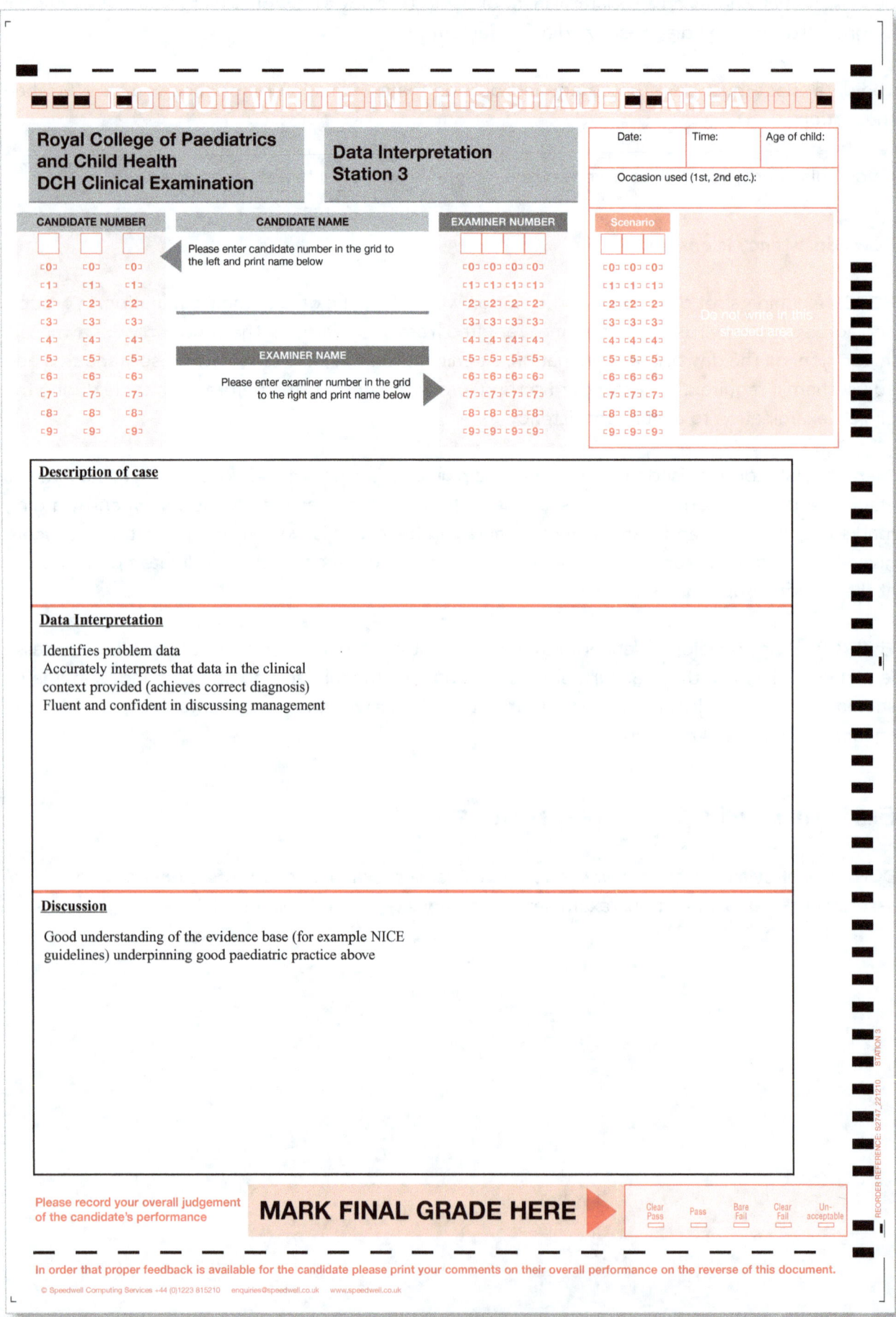

Clinical Cases in Paediatrics: DCH Clinical Examination

☐ Poor approach - Unstructured (please add additional comments)

☐ Failure to deal with the set task (please add additional comments)

☐ Factual inaccuracy (please add additional comments)

Please add any additional comments here:

Appendix 3.12: Anchor Statement: Data Interpretation Station

	Expected Standard/ CLEAR PASS	PASS	BARE FAIL	CLEAR FAIL	UNACCEPTABLE
DATA INTERPRETATION	Identifies problem data Accurately interprets the data in the clinical context provided (achieves correct diagnosis)	Identifies problem data No clinical diagnosis but suggests relevant differential diagnosis	Identifies problem data No clinical diagnosis or limited differential diagnosis	Fails to identify problem data Incorrect clinical diagnosis or inappropriate differential diagnosis	Fails to identify problem data Incorrect and unsafe diagnosis
DISCUSSION	Fluent and confident in discussing management Good understanding of the evidence base (for example NICE guidelines) underpinning good paediatric practice above	Lacks confidence in discussing management Understands evidence base underpinning good paediatric practice	Limited knowledge and understanding of management Limited understanding of evidence-based approach to paediatric practice	Poor knowledge and understanding of management Poor understanding of evidence-based approach to paediatric practice	Unreliable and unsafe response to investigations and management in paediatrics Argumentative and critical of evidence-based approach to paediatric practice

Chapter 3.2: Case Study 1: 15 Year Old with Abdominal Pain
Dr Michael Hii

The station assesses your ability to interpret data in the clinical context provided. You will then undertake a discussion with the examiner, noting the diagnosis and discussing the appropriate management plan.

Logistics:

Timing: This is a 6-minute station. A knock at 5 minutes will denote that 1 minute remains before the end of the station. You will have 2 minutes beforehand to read the candidate information provided to prepare yourself.

When the bell rings: On entering the room, the examiner will greet you, take your mark sheet and proceed with asking questions.

If the discussion with the examiner finishes early, you will be asked to remain in the room until the session has ended.

Candidate role and task:

You are a GP trainee working in a GP practice.

Task: Interpret the data and discuss the management plan with the examiner.

Clinical context

Ben, a 15 year old boy, has come to the clinic to discuss his blood results (Table 3.21). He presented last week with a 2-month history of loss of appetite, weight loss and occasional abdominal pain. He has a normal bowel habit.

Table 3.21: Results of the investigations		
Test	Result	Normal values
WCC	10×10^9/L	$4-11 \times 10^9$/L
Hb	100 g/L	110-130 g/L
MCV	68 fl	74-90 fl
MCHC	28%	31-37%
Platelets	550×10^9/L	$150-400 \times 10^9$/L
Serum sodium	139 mmol/L	135-145 mmol/L
Potassium	5.2 mmol/L	3.5-5.6 mmol/L
Urea	3.3 mmol/L	2.5-5.6 mmol/L
Creatinine	30 micromol/L	20-80 micromol/L
Protein	45 g/L	60-80 g/L
Albumin	25 mg/L	37-50 mg/L
CRP	40 mg/L	<10 mg/L
ESR	35 mm/hr	<10 mm/hr
Urinalysis	Normal	

Examiner questions

- Interpret the data.
- What is the most likely diagnosis?
- What clinical features would you look for in this child?
- What would be your management plan?

Answers

- **_Interpret the data._**
    - Anaemia (hypochromic, microcytic)
    - Raised platelet count
    - Raised inflammatory markers (CRP, ESR)
    - Low serum protein and albumin

- **_What is the most likely diagnosis?_**
    - Inflammatory bowel disease – probably Crohn's disease

If you are stuck, it may be helpful to think of the differential diagnoses.

- Ulcerative colitis
    - Generally presents with rectal bleeding and abdominal pain.
    - May develop anaemia secondary to rectal bleeding.
    - Low serum albumin is less often a feature, due to the absence of small bowel involvement (and consequent protein-losing enteropathy).

- Other causes of abdominal pain
    - Chronic constipation
    - Urinary tract infection
    - Food intolerance
    - Coeliac disease
    - Abdominal migraine
    - Basal pneumonia
    - Non-specific abdominal pain
    - Surgical causes (appendicitis, bowel obstruction, testicular torsion)

> *Top tip!*
> You should correctly identify the low serum protein, raised inflammatory markers and microcytic anaemia, and integrate these with the clinical picture (weight loss and abdominal pain) to diagnose inflammatory bowel disease.

- **_What clinical features would you look for in this child?_**

A detailed history and physical examination should be conducted to look for the symptoms and signs of Crohn's disease (Table 3.22). Presence of significant growth failure, anaemia, and extraintestinal manifestations would point to more extensive bowel involvement.

Table 3.22: Clinical features of Crohn's disease

Symptoms	Signs	Specific to children
Abdominal pain	Anaemia	Growth failure
Diarrhoea	Finger clubbing	Delayed puberty
Weight loss	Mouth ulcers	More extensive disease
Rectal bleeding	Perianal disease (fissure/fistula/abscess)	Rapid progression
Nausea/vomiting	Extraintestinal manifestations (episcleritis, erythema nodosum, arthritis)	
Anorexia		
Joint pain		
Dry/painful eyes		
Lethargy		

Top tip!
You should be able to confidently discuss the clinical features of Crohn's disease in children.

■ What would be your management plan?

Family counselling:
NICE 2012 emphasises the importance of discussing the disease, management options, and prognosis in an age-appropriate manner, while recognising the cognitive and literacy level of the family. Where appropriate, the following also needs to be discussed:
- Possible delay of growth and puberty
- Diet and nutrition
- Fertility and sexual relationships
- Prognosis
- Side effects of the treatment
- Oncological risk
- Surgery
- Transition between paediatric and adult services

Initial treatment options:
- Commence on either an exclusive enteral feed [polymeric (Modulen) or elemental (E028)], or corticosteroids.
- Enteral feed is preferable for children to promote better nutrition and growth.
- Corticosteroids are useful when such enteral therapy is not tolerated.
- 5-aminosalicylate, although less effective in children, can be used with mild forms of the disease.

Second-line medications:
- Long-term immunosuppression, utilising medications such as azathioprine, 6-mercaptopurine or methotrexate, is required for children with frequent relapses who need repeated courses of steroids.
- Biologics such as infliximab and adalimumab are effective in the presence of advanced active disease and in patients who have not responded to conventional therapy.

Surgical intervention is indicated in the presence of:
- Bowel stricture
- Fistula
- Abscess
- Bowel perforation

Patients are encouraged to join patient information websites such as:
- The Crohn's in Childhood Research Association (CICRA: http://www.cicra.org)
- National Association for Colitis and Crohn's Disease (NACC: http://www.crohnsandcolitis.org.uk)

Top tip!
You should have a systematic approach for structuring answers. You should emphasise a child-centred approach and discuss the need to involve other professionals in the management of the patient.

Additional information

Crohn's disease is a chronic, idiopathic inflammatory disease that can affect any part of the gastrointestinal tract from mouth to anus. Currently, there are at least 115,000 Crohn's disease sufferers in the UK. Approximately 25-30% of patients with Crohn's disease are diagnosed before 20 years of age. Children are predisposed to having a more severe version of the disease (small bowel disease) at presentation, and their disease also has a tendency to progress more rapidly compared to their adult counterparts. The disease can be categorised by location (terminal ileal, colonic, ileocolonic, upper gastrointestinal tract) or the nature of the disease (inflammatory, fistulating or stricturing).

Aetiology

The aetiology of Crohn's disease is unknown. Smoking and genetic predisposition are thought to play important roles in the pathogenesis of the disease.

Diagnosis

The diagnosis of Crohn's disease is often delayed compared to ulcerative colitis, mainly due to the decreased prevalence of rectal bleeding. Typical gastrointestinal symptoms of Crohn's disease include abdominal pain and loose stools. Only 25% of patients have the classical triad of abdominal pain, weight loss and diarrhoea, and 22% have rectal bleeding. When the abdominal pain coincides with eating, this may indicate the presence of a small bowel stricture. Positive physical signs include mouth ulcers, finger clubbing, perianal involvement and erythema nodosum. Assessment of growth and pubertal staging is essential in adolescents.

Blood tests often reveal raised inflammatory markers (CRP/ESR), low haemoglobin, low albumin (when there is extensive small bowel involvement), and markedly raised faecal calprotectin level. These laboratory tests may be normal if there is only limited disease, such as in the terminal ileum. It is important that stool samples are tested for infectious causes of diarrhoea, including clostridium difficile.

An endoscopy is necessary to obtain a tissue diagnosis. The presence of epithelioid granuloma (less than 50% of bowel biopsies) and transmural inflammation with skip lesions in the bowel biopsy supports the diagnosis of Crohn's disease. An MRI of the small bowel is useful to detect small bowel involvement. When there is diagnostic difficulty, video capsule endoscopy can be deployed to obtain pictures of the small bowel.

Prognosis

Patients with Crohn's disease often have recurrent relapses with periods of remission or where the disease is less active. However, when there is localised disease (for example, ileocaecal disease), it may remain dormant for many years.

Gastroenterology and hepatology

Knowledge

The candidate must:

- Know the causes of acute and chronic abdominal pain, and recognise when to refer, including the urgency of referral.
- Know the causes of acute and chronic diarrhoea and vomiting, as well as be able to assess and manage these symptoms.
- Know the common causes of upper and lower gastrointestinal bleeding.

Further reading and references

1. Bishop J, Lemberg DA, Day A. Managing inflammatory bowel disease in adolescent patients. *Adolesc Health Med Ther* 2014; 6(5): 1-13
2. National Institute of Clinical Excellence. (CG152) - Crohn's disease: Management in adults, children and young people. 2012. https://www.nice.org.uk/guidance/cg152 (accessed July 2015).
3. Sandhu BK, Fell JM, Beattie RM et al. Guidelines for the management of inflammatory bowel disease in children in the United Kingdom. *J Pediatr Gastroenterol Nutr* 2010; 50 Suppl 1: S1-13

Chapter 3.3: Case Study 2: 13 Year Old with Palpitations

Dr P Venugopalan, Dr Alexandra Da Costa

The station assesses your ability to interpret data in the clinical context provided. You will then undertake a discussion with the examiner, noting the diagnosis and discussing the appropriate management plan.

> **Logistics:**
>
> *Timing:* This is a 6-minute station. A knock at 5 minutes will denote that 1 minute remains before the end of the station. You will have 2 minutes beforehand to read the candidate information provided to prepare yourself.
>
> *When the bell rings:* On entering the room, the examiner will greet you, take your mark sheet and proceed with asking questions.
>
> If the discussion with the examiner finishes early, you will be asked to remain in the room until the session has ended.

> **Candidate role and task:**
>
> **You are a** GP trainee working in a GP practice.
>
> **Task: Interpret the data and discuss the management plan with the examiner.**

Clinical context

Chloe, a 13 year old girl, presents to clinic for a review of her investigations (Table 3.31), which were organised by your colleague. Chloe has had palpitations intermittently over the last year. She is concerned that her heart beats rapidly at times, especially when she is stressed. Her school performance has deteriorated recently, as she has had to miss school on several occasions due to anxiety and poor sleep.

Table 3.31: Results of the investigations		
Test	Result	Normal values
WCC	8.2×10^9/L	$4–11 \times 10^9$/L
Hb	105 g/L	110–130 g/L
MCV	78 fl	74–90 fl
MCHC	32%	31–37%
Platelets	313×10^9/L	$150–400 \times 10^9$/L
Serum sodium	139 mmol/L	135–145 mmol/L
Potassium	5.2 mmol/L	3.5–5.6 mmol/L
Urea	3.3 mmol/L	2.5–5.6 mmol/L
Creatinine	30 micromol/L	20–80 micromol/L
TSH	0.02 mU/L	0.6–4.8 mU/L
Free T4	80 pmol/L	11–22 pmol/L
ECG	Sinus tachycardia	

Examiner questions

- Interpret the data.
- What is the most likely diagnosis?
- What clinical features would support this diagnosis?
- Outline the management principles for this condition.

Answers

- *Interpret the data.*
    - Low thyroid stimulating hormone (TSH)
    - Elevated T4
    - Mild anaemia (normocytic, normochromic)
    - Sinus tachycardia

Figure 3.31 outlines the basic principles that underlie thyroid hormone synthesis. Elevated TSH along with a low T4/T3 point to hypothyroidism, while a low TSH along with elevated T4/T3 would indicate hyperthyroidism. Most laboratories do not measure T3 routinely, but this test should be requested due to the elevated T4 level.

Figure 3.31 Thyroid hormone synthetic pathway (Illustration by Dr P Venugopalan)

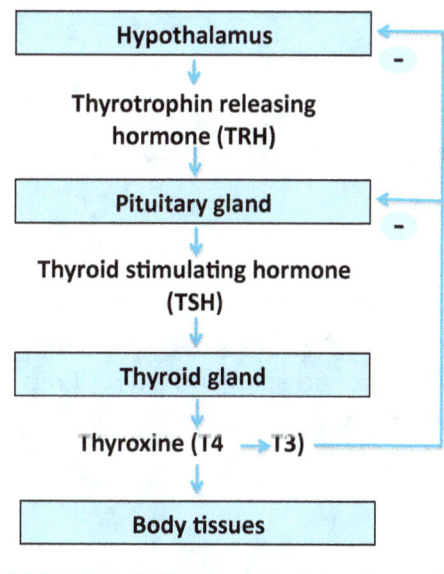

Hypothyroid	Hyperthyroid
TSH ↑	TSH ↓
T4/T3 ↓	T4/T3 ↑

- *What is the most likely diagnosis?*
    - Symptomatic hyperthyroidism (thyrotoxicosis)

Top tip!
You should confidently identify the low TSH and raised T4, and integrate this with the clinical signs (tachycardia) to diagnose thyrotoxicosis.

■ What clinical features would support this diagnosis?

A detailed history and physical examination should be conducted to look for the symptoms and signs of thyrotoxicosis (Table 3.31).

- Recent infections could point to thyroiditis, but most cases in children are autoimmune in origin.
- History of coexisting diabetes or other autoimmune disorders should be elicited.
- Family history of thyroid problems or other endocrine disorders may be forthcoming.
- Possible exogenous exposure to thyroxine should also be clarified.
- It is important to look for any thyroid gland enlargement (goitre) and signs of thyrotoxicosis.

Top tip!
You should be able to demonstrate a good understanding of the clinical features of thyrotoxicosis.

Table 3.31: Clinical features of thyrotoxicosis

Symptoms	Signs	Specific to children
Weight loss	Possible goitre	Tall stature
Sweating	Eye signs – Lid lag, exophthalmos (very rare in children)	Rapid growth
Heat intolerance		Precocious puberty
Agitation	Fine tremor	Advanced bone age
Poor stamina	Tachycardia	Deteriorating school performance
Decreased exercise tolerance	Anxiety	Behavioural disturbances
Menorrhagia	Cardiac compromise/failure	

■ Outline the management principles for this condition.

Investigations

- Serum TSH and thyroid hormones (T4 and T3) help to confirm hyperthyroidism.
- Anti-thyroid antibodies help make the diagnosis of autoimmune thyroid disease.
- Occasionally, a thyroid ultrasound scan and thyroid radioisotope scan will be required to help to locate overactive hot spots.

When do you need to refer?

- Once the diagnosis is confirmed, most children need specialist input.
- In our patient, urgent outpatient referral is indicated, as the patient requires prompt initiation of anti-thyroid medication.

Medications

- Carbimazole (anti-thyroid medication) is first-line treatment.
- Propylthiouracil is not first line, as it carries a risk of idiosyncratic hepatocellular failure.
- Patients and their families must be educated to seek help and get a full blood count when unwell, as carbimazole can cause bone marrow suppression.
- *Beta-blockers or calcium channel blockers* should be considered for immediate relief of symptoms such as tachycardia, as specific therapy takes time to work.

Radioiodine

- This is increasingly the first-line treatment for teenagers.
- It is administered orally to the patient and is taken up by the thyroid gland, leading to destruction of the gland.
- It is inexpensive and a definitive treatment. It can take 3 to 4 months to take effect, and must not be given to pregnant women.
- Therapy requires careful monitoring for side effects, including bone marrow suppression.

Subtotal or near total thyroidectomy

- Surgical removal of a major portion of the gland achieves a 98% cure rate.
- This method of treatment is considered if there is suboptimal response to anti-thyroid medication or radioiodine, especially in patients who are pregnant, have Graves' orbitopathy, or have compression symptoms from their goitre.
- Complications include haemorrhage, hypoparathyroidism and vocal cord paralysis.
- Patients who undergo surgery will need to be followed up over a number of years, as they may develop hypothyroidism.

Top tip!
You should have a systematic approach to structuring your answers, and be confident when discussing your management plan.

Additional information

The thyroid gland is the sole producer of T4, and produces about 20% of T3 (which is about 10 times more biologically active than T4). Apart from a tiny fraction, these circulate bound to thyroxine-binding globulin and other proteins (albumin).

The thyroid hormones have profound effects on growth, neurological development, metabolism and cardiovascular function. These effects can result in tall stature, advanced bone age, weight loss, intolerance of heat, palpitations and tachycardia.

Differential diagnosis

In children and adolescents, 95% of cases with hyperthyroidism are secondary to autoimmune conditions (Graves' disease, Hashimoto's thyroiditis). There is a strong association with other autoimmune conditions, such as diabetes. As in adults, it can rarely be secondary to infection (mostly viral), toxic nodules, or exogenous sources (ingestion of thyroxine, either intentionally or accidentally). In neonates, congenital hyperthyroidism can occur with transplacental transfer of maternal anti-thyroid antibodies, when the mother suffers from Graves' disease or Hashimoto's thyroiditis.

Goitre refers to an enlargement of the thyroid gland, and could be the presenting feature in thyroid disorders (Table 3.32). This may be accompanied by signs and/or symptoms of hypo/hyperthyroidism. Most commonly, this is a diffuse enlargement of the thyroid, with the right lobe being frequently larger than the left lobe. The enlargement of the thyroid is generally mediated by an increase in the pituitary-derived TSH or in antibodies that bind to the TSH receptor, such as the thyroid stimulating immunoglobulins (TSIs) found in Graves' disease. Inflammation or infiltration may cause diffuse and symmetrical enlargement, although the gland is usually asymmetric and nodular.

Table 3.32: Causes of goitre	
Colloid (simple) goitre	
Goitrogen exposure	
Dyshormonogenesis	
Autoimmune thyroid disease	Chronic lymphocytic thyroiditis (Hashimoto's thyroiditis) Graves' disease
Infectious	Subacute (viral) thyroiditis Chronic suppurative thyroiditis
Anatomic abnormalities	Thyroglossal duct cyst Hemiagenesis of the thyroid
Nodular goitre	Solitary nodule (adenoma, carcinoma, cyst) Multinodular goitre secondary to autoimmune thyroid disease

Graves' disease

Graves' disease is the most common cause of hyperthyroidism in children and adolescents. Females are predominantly affected, and a family history of autoimmune thyroid disease is common. Common modes of presentation include declining school performance and behavioural changes. Goitre is almost invariably present and the thyroid has a smooth, rubbery texture. Although lid retraction and lid lag are common findings at diagnosis, exophthalmos occurs in only one third of children, and it is generally mild.

Finding a suppressed TSH level with elevated T4 and/or T3 levels allows one to make the diagnosis of Graves' disease. Antithyroglobulin antibodies and thyroid peroxidase antibody levels may be positive but they are not pathognomonic.

Syllabus mapping

Diabetes and endocrinology

Knowledge

The candidate must:

- Know the causes and management of hypo/hyperthyroidism.

Further reading and references

1. Bahn Chair RS, Burch HB, Cooper DS et al. Hyperthyroidism and other causes of thyrotoxicosis: Management guidelines of the American Thyroid Association and American Association of Clinical Endocrinologists. *Thyroid* 2011; 21(6): 593–646
2. Birrell G, Cheetham T. Juvenile thyrotoxicosis: Can we do better? *Arch Dis Child* 2004; 89(8): 745–50
3. Muirhead S. Diagnostic approach to goitre in children. *Paediatr Child Health* 2001; 6(4): 195–199
4. Williamson S, Greene SA. Incidence of thyrotoxicosis in childhood: A national population-based study in the UK and Ireland. *Clin Endocrinol (Oxf)* 2010; 72(3): 358–63

Chapter 3.4: Case Study 3: 5 Year Old Girl with Dysuria

Dr Anand Kamalanathan, Dr Satyendra Singh

The station assesses your ability to interpret data in the clinical context provided. You will then undertake a discussion with the examiner, noting the diagnosis and discussing the appropriate management plan.

> **Logistics:**
>
> *Timing:* This is a 6-minute station. A knock at 5 minutes will denote that 1 minute remains before the end of the station. You will have 2 minutes beforehand to read the candidate information provided to prepare yourself.
>
> *When the bell rings:* On entering the room, the examiner will greet you, take your mark sheet and proceed with asking questions.
>
> If the discussion with the examiner finishes early, you will be asked to remain in the room until the session has ended.

> **Candidate role and task:**
>
> **You are a** GP trainee working in a GP surgery.
>
> **Task: Interpret the data and discuss the management plan with the examiner.**

Clinical context

Bethany, a 5 year old girl, has presented with painful micturition over the last 3 days. She is afebrile and otherwise well. Examination reveals a slightly red peri-vulvar region and is otherwise unremarkable. Results of a clean-catch urine dipstick are available (Table 3.41).

Table 3.41: Results of the urine dipstick

Leucocytes	+++
Blood	trace
Protein	negative
Nitrite	negative
Urobilinogen	negative

Examiner questions

- Interpret the urine dipstick result.
- What is the significance of the result?
- What is the most likely diagnosis for this child?
- How will you manage this child?

Answers

■ *Interpret the urine dipstick result.*

The urine is:
- Strongly positive for leucocytes
- Weakly positive for blood
- Negative for nitrite and protein

■ *What is the significance of the result?*

Table 3.42: Significance of the urine dipstick results	
Abnormality	Significance
Strongly positive leucocytes	Inflammation; infection site unspecified
Weakly positive for blood	Local inflammation
Negative nitrite	Unlikely that it is urinary tract infection

Leucocytes (pyuria) in the urine are present in children with a urinary tract infection (Table 3.42). However, this can also be a finding with balanitis, vulvovaginitis and in febrile children, even in the absence of a urinary tract infection. Infections of the urinary tract can also occur more rarely without pyuria, seen in children with compromised immune systems and neonates (NICE 2007).

A positive result for blood in the urinalysis may indicate a urinary tract infection. Other causes include nephritis, renal calculi, renal trauma and bleeding disorders.

A positive nitrite result in the urinalysis is likely to indicate a true urinary tract infection. However, a negative nitrite result on a urine dipstick does not rule out urinary infection. Nitrites are the result of bacteria metabolising proteins found in the urine. Therefore, if the urine stays in the bladder for several hours, even normal urine may test positive for nitrites.

If you are stuck, it may be helpful to consider the differential diagnoses (Table 3.43).

Table 3.43: Interpretation based on the urine dipstick result	
Urine dipstick results	Interpretation
Leucocyte and nitrite positive	Treat as a urinary tract infection
Leucocyte negative and nitrite positive	Treat as a urinary tract infection
Leucocyte positive and nitrite negative	Does not necessarily represent a urinary tract infection, but should be correlated with clinical features (fever, vomiting, abdominal/loin pain)
Leucocyte and nitrite negative	Urinary tract infection unlikely
Blood	Haematuria (e.g. nephritis)
Glucose	Diabetes mellitus, renal glycosuria
Protein	Febrile illness, renal causes (nephrotic syndrome)

■ **What is the most likely diagnosis in this child, and what differentials need to be considered?**

- The urinary dipstick result, combined with the clinical picture, suggests vulvovaginitis.
- The results are unlikely to be due to a urinary tract infection.

Top tip!
Consider the data in light of the clinical picture. *A clear pass candidate* will integrate the urine findings with the presence of dysuria in an afebrile child with normal examination, and come to the conclusion of vulvovaginitis as the probable diagnosis.

This child has presented with dysuria, which could be a symptom of a urinary tract infection. However, she is systemically well, without fever, vomiting or abdominal pain, and the urine dipstick only shows leucocytes. Therefore, this is unlikely to be a urinary tract infection.

Another common cause of dysuria is vulval inflammation and irritation. Vulvitis refers to external genital pruritus, a burning sensation, redness or rash. Vaginitis implies inflammation of the vagina, with discharge, malodour and/or bleeding. Common causes of vulvovaginitis include poor hygiene, non-oestrogenised state, infections (bacterial – E. coli, Streptococcus pyogenes, Staphylococcus aureus, Haemophilus influenzae; fungal – Candida) and worm infestation. Other rare causes include foreign bodies and sexual abuse.

Threadworm (pinworm) infection is a common type of worm infestation that presents with symptoms suggestive of vulvovaginitis. The worms reside in the large bowel and come out to the perineum to lay eggs at night. This presents as perianal itching, more common at night. Occasionally, the worms may be seen in stools. Threadworm infection can cause loss of appetite, weight loss, bed-wetting, and vulvovaginitis. The Sellotape test is recommended to document threadworm infestation. This test involves sticking Sellotape to the perineum at night, removing it the next morning, and examining it under a microscope for worms or their eggs.

A detailed history of associated symptoms (such as perineal pain, pruritus, malodorous discharge, and nocturnal pruritus) will help to guide investigation. Information about urinary frequency, fever, abdominal pain, diarrhoea and any previous urinary infections must be sought. Information about hygiene measures and possible chemical irritants (bath soaps, laundry detergents, swimming pools or hot tubs) must be explored.

Physical examination, including examination of the external genitalia, is essential to exclude other causes of dysuria. Signs of inflammation, poor hygiene and any evidence of discharge should be elicited. Any bruising to the genitals should raise the suspicion of sexual abuse.

■ **How will you manage this child?**

Essential investigations when vulvovaginitis is clinically suspected include a urine dipstick and a vaginal swab for culture and sensitivity. The possibility of thrush and threadworms should also be considered. Genital symptoms are occasionally a pointer to child sexual abuse.

Management should focus on the following measures:

1. Provide advice regarding local hygiene.
2. Avoid bubble baths and scented soaps.
3. Use loose-fitting cotton underwear.
4. Salt baths may be useful.
5. Specific treatment of bacterial or fungal infections when identified on low vaginal/perineal swabs.
6. Mebendazole therapy is useful when a threadworm infestation is suspected. Treatment is recommended for the whole family, and repeated a fortnight later. Piperazine is the recommended drug for infants below 6 months.
7. Oestrogen cream applied sparingly to the vulva may relieve the problem in resistant cases by increasing vaginal resistance to infection.
8. Concerns about sexual abuse should prompt a referral to safeguarding agencies or a paediatrician.

Top tip!
Be confident when discussing your management plan. *A clear pass candidate* will have a systematic approach to structuring answers.

Syllabus mapping

Nephro-urology

Knowledge

The candidate must:

- Have the knowledge and an understanding of the manifestations of renal diseases, acute and chronic.
- Demonstrate an understanding of the manifestations and management of urinary tract infections in different age groups.
- Be able to examine the genitalia appropriately and with sensitivity, as well as assess and manage vulvovaginitis (this is unlikely to be tested in an examination).

Further reading and references

1. Anderson B, Thimmesch I, Aardsma N et al. The prevalence of abnormal genital findings, vulvovaginitis, enuresis and encopresis in children who present with allegations of sexual abuse. *J Pediatr Urol* 2014; 10(6): 1216-21
2. National Institute of Clinical Excellence. (CG54) – Urinary tract infection in children. Diagnosis, treatment and long-term management. 2007. https://www.nice.org.uk/guidance/cg54 (accessed July 2015).
3. Rome ES. Vulvovaginitis and other common vulvar disorders in children. *Endocr Dev* 2012; 22: 72-83
4. Van Eyk N, Allen L, Giesbrecht E et al. Pediatric vulvovaginal disorders: A diagnostic approach and review of the literature. *J Obstet Gynaecol Can* 2009; 31(9): 850-62

Chapter 3.5: Case Study 4: 9 Year Old with a Skin Rash

Dr Satyendra Singh, Dr Anand Kamalanathan, Dr Mwape Kabole

The station assesses your ability to interpret data in the clinical context provided. You will then undertake a discussion with the examiner, noting the diagnosis and discussing the appropriate management plan.

Logistics:

Timing: This is a 6-minute station. A knock at 5 minutes will denote that 1 minute remains before the end of the station. You will have 2 minutes beforehand to read the candidate information provided to prepare yourself.

When the bell rings: On entering the room, the examiner will greet you, take your mark sheet and proceed with asking questions.

If the discussion with the examiner finishes early, you will be asked to remain in the room until the session has ended.

Candidate role and task:

You are a GP trainee working in the paediatric outpatient department.

Task: Interpret the data and discuss the management plan with the examiner.

Clinical context

Nine year old Mathew presented to the emergency department with a maculopapular erythematous and itchy rash after eating a chocolate bar. He was treated with oral antihistamines and the rash subsequently subsided. Other than for mild asthma, he is fit and well. He has no previous history of allergies.

Results of blood tests done are available at the outpatient appointment (Table 3.51).

Table 3.51: Results of blood investigations		
Test	Result	Normal values
Total IgE	1250 iu/ml	<120 iu/ml
Specific IgE (hazelnut)	20 kUA/L	Normal: <0.35 kUA/L
Specific IgE (egg)	0.07 kUA/L	Normal: <0.35 kUA/L
Specific IgE (peanut)	98 kUA/L	Normal: <0.35 kUA/L
Specific IgE (milk)	0.35 kUA/L	Normal: <0.35 kUA/L

Examiner questions

- Interpret the result.
- What further information would be helpful in the management of this condition?
- What advice should be given to the family?
- Does this child require an EpiPen prescription?

Answers

- *Interpret the results.*
    - Elevated total IgE
    - Elevated specific IgE to hazelnut
    - Elevated specific IgE to peanut
    - Normal specific IgE to egg and milk

Top tip!
You should be able to correlate the blood results with the clinical presentation, and diagnose an allergy to peanut and hazelnut.

- *What further information would be helpful in the management in this condition?*

It is important to take a detailed history to make a diagnosis and understand the temporal relationship between allergen contact and allergic reaction (Table 3.52). Physical examination should then focus on general nutrition and the signs indicating allergy-related comorbidities (atopic eczema, asthma and allergic rhinitis). Indications for referral to specialist services should also be kept in mind during the assessment.

Table 3.52: History taking for suspected allergy

General history	Allergy-specific history	Pointers to anaphylaxis
Contact with allergen	Tingling of mouth and lips	Wheezing
Time lapse between contact and development of symptoms	Angioedema – Swelling of lips or face	Difficulty breathing
Severity of symptoms	Nausea/vomiting	Sense of swelling around the throat
Duration of reaction	Urticaria (nettle rash or hives)	Dizziness, pallor and drowsiness or hypotension
History of previous reactions and necessary treatment	Abdominal pain	
Personal atopic history	A feeling of tightness around the throat	
Current medication		
Family history of allergy, atopy		

Indications for specialist referral (NICE 2011)

- Faltering growth in combination with gastrointestinal symptoms
- Poor response to a single-allergen elimination diet
- History of 1 or more acute systemic reactions
- History of 1 or more severe delayed reactions
- Confirmed IgE-mediated food allergy and concurrent asthma
- Significant atopic eczema, where multiple or cross-reactive food allergies are suspected by the parent or carer
- Persisting parental suspicion of a food allergy (especially in children or young people with difficult or perplexing symptoms) despite a lack of supporting history
- Strong clinical suspicion of an IgE-mediated food allergy, but allergy test results are negative
- Clinical suspicion of multiple food allergies

■ *What advice should be given to the family?*

As a first step, it is important to clarify with the family what advice was given at the time of presentation, and understand whether the paediatric team saw Mathew when he presented with the reaction. The results of the blood tests should be shared with the family and the risks of future reactions discussed.

The fact that the severity of future reactions cannot be predicted should be emphasised. As such, the need to set in place measures to manage this at the appointment is necessary. The presence of asthma is an important consideration regarding management.

The consultant in charge of the patient should speak to and counsel Mathew and his parents, giving them:

- Information about anaphylaxis, including the signs and symptoms of an anaphylactic reaction. Information leaflets will help reinforce this advice.
- Information about the risk of a biphasic reaction.
- Information on what to do if an anaphylactic reaction occurs and the child has not been previously prescribed an EpiPen:
    - Lie the child flat. If their breathing becomes difficult, allow the child to sit up.
    - Call for an ambulance.
    - If wheezy, give 10 puffs of salbutamol.
    - Stay with the child.
    - There is a role for antihistamines at an early stage of an allergic reaction.
- Advice on how to avoid the suspected trigger (if known).
- Information regarding arrangements for basic life support training.
- Information on the need for referral to a specialist allergy service, and the referral process.
- Information about patient support groups.

Top tip!
You should be confident when discussing your management plan. While waiting outside the station, you could think of a structure to answer similar questions.

Does this child require an EpiPen prescription?

In this case, an EpiPen prescription is not indicated. Possible indications for its requirement in cases of children with suspected nut allergy would include:

- Signs of anaphylaxis in a previous reaction (Mathew did not give a history of respiratory or cardiovascular symptoms).
- Reaction to minute amounts of allergen, like reacting after being touched by someone who had handled nuts (Mathew had ingested the chocolate prior to the symptoms).
- Coexisting asthma requiring inhaled steroids (Mathew gave a history of mild asthma, implying that he is probably only on salbutamol when necessary).
- Living in a remote area with no access to immediate medical facilities or ambulance service (Mathew lives in central London).

It is important that if a pen (injector) is required, training is given to all who would be looking after the child, including teachers. Remember that there are several products in the market, including Jext and Emerade, that all have different injection techniques.

Additional information

In the UK, about 1 in 100 people have an allergy to peanuts and about 1 in 200 people have an allergy to tree nuts. About 1 in 3 people with a nut allergy have an initial reaction to the nut, followed by a second reaction between 1 and 8 hours after the first.

Differentiate between legume and tree nuts:

- Legume – Peanut
- Tree nuts – Walnuts, hazelnuts, almonds, cashews, pecans, brazils, pistachios

Anaphylaxis is a severe, life-threatening, generalised or systemic hypersensitivity reaction. It is characterised by rapidly developing, life-threatening problems involving: the airway (pharyngeal or laryngeal oedema) and/or breathing (bronchospasm with tachypnoea) and/or circulation (hypotension and/or tachycardia).

People who have had a mild or moderate allergic reaction are at risk of, and may subsequently present with, suspected anaphylaxis. Certain groups may be at higher risk, either because of an existing comorbidity (for example, asthma) or because they are more likely to be exposed to the same allergen again (for example, people with venom allergies or reactions to specific food triggers).

After emergency treatment for suspected anaphylaxis, offer a referral to a specialist allergy service (age-appropriate where possible) consisting of healthcare professionals with the skills and competence necessary to accurately investigate, diagnose, monitor and provide ongoing management of, and patient education about, suspected anaphylaxis.

The following can arise as a result of an allergic reaction, and parents/carers/professionals should look out for these whenever an allergic reaction is suspected.

Airway problems:

- Airway swelling, e.g. throat and tongue swelling (pharyngeal/laryngeal oedema)
- Hoarse voice
- Stridor
- Shortness of breath
- Wheezing
- Confusion
- Cyanosis
- Respiratory arrest

Circulation problems:

- Signs of shock – Pale, clammy
- Increased pulse rate
- Low blood pressure – Feeling faint, collapsing
- Decreased conscious level
- Anaphylaxis can cause myocardial ischaemia, and an ECG changes even in individuals with normal coronary arteries.
- Cardiac arrest

Skin/mucosal changes:

- They are often the first feature, and present in over 80% of anaphylactic reactions.
- Skin, mucosal, or both skin and mucosal changes.
- There may be erythema.
- There may be urticaria (also called hives, nettle rash, wheals or welts), which can appear anywhere on the body. The wheals may be pale, pink or red, and may look like nettle stings. They can be of different shapes and sizes, and are often surrounded by a red flare. They are usually itchy.
- Angioedema is similar to urticaria, but involves swelling of deeper tissues, most commonly in the eyelids and lips and sometimes in the mouth and throat.

Life-threatening conditions:

- Sometimes, an anaphylactic reaction can present with symptoms and signs that are very similar to life-threatening asthma – this is most common in children.
- Low blood pressure (or normal blood pressure in children) with a petechial or purpuric rash can be a sign of septic shock.

Non life-threatening conditions (these usually respond to simple measures):

- Faint (vasovagal episode)
- Panic attack
- Breath-holding episode in the child
- Idiopathic (non-allergic) urticaria or angioedema

Syllabus mapping

Infection, immunity and allergy

Knowledge

The candidate must:

- Be able to discuss common food allergies and management of anaphylaxis.

Further reading and references

1. Allergy care pathways for children. Anaphylaxis. RCPCH http://www.rcpch.ac.uk/system/files/protected/page/2011_RCPCH-CarePathway-Anaphylaxis_v1_(18.35).pdf (accessed September 2015).
2. Allergy action plans for children. BSACI. http://www.bsaci.org/about/pag-allergy-action-plans-for-children (accessed September 2015).
3. Muraro A, Roberts G et al. The management of anaphylaxis in childhood: Position paper of the European academy of allergology and clinical immunology. *Allergy* 2007; 62: 857-71
4. National Institute for Health and Care Excellence. (CG116) – Food allergy in children and young people. Diagnosis and assessment of food allergy in children and young people in primary care and community settings. London, 2011. https://www.nice.org.uk/guidance/cg116 (accessed September 2015).

Chapter 3.6: Case Study 5: 2 Month Old with Wheeze

Dr Geetha Fonseka

The station assesses your ability to interpret data in the clinical context provided. You will then undertake a discussion with the examiner, noting the diagnosis and discussing the appropriate management plan.

Logistics:

Timing: This is a 6-minute station. A knock at 5 minutes will denote that 1 minute remains before the end of the station. You will have 2 minutes beforehand to read the candidate information provided to prepare yourself.

When the bell rings: On entering the room, the examiner will greet you, take your mark sheet and proceed with asking questions.

If the discussion with the examiner finishes early, you will be asked to remain in the room until the session has ended.

Candidate role and task:

You are a GP trainee doing your posting in a paediatric assessment unit.

Task: Interpret the data and discuss the management plan with the examiner.

Clinical context

Two month old Adam is referred to the paediatric assessment unit. Adam has had an upper respiratory tract infection for over the last 2 days; this has worsened today into a wet cough and wheeze. He is refusing feeds and has not had a wet nappy in the last 6 hours. He looks pale; his heart rate is 165/min and saturations are 88% in air. The nurse who has triaged him has taken him straight to the resuscitation area and has done a capillary blood gas analysis (Table 3.61).

Table 3.61: Results of the capillary blood gas analysis		
Test	Result	Normal values
pH	7.23	7.35–7.45
pCO_2	7.5 kPa	4.6–6.4 kPa
pO_2	6 kPa	Not reliable
Bicarbonate	22.0 mmol/L	22.0–27.0 mmol/L
Base excess	-2.0 mmol/L	-7.0 to -1.0 mmol/L
Glucose	8.5 mmol/L	4–11 mmol/L
Lactate	1.9 mmol/L	<2 mmol/L

Examiner questions

- Interpret the data.
- What is the most likely diagnosis? Suggest differential diagnoses.
- What clinical features would you look for in this child?
- How would you manage this child?

Answers

- *Interpret the data.*

The data shows an acidaemic blood pH and a high pCO_2 level, with normal bicarbonate and base excess values. This is respiratory acidosis.

Capillary samples reflect reliable pCO_2, bicarbonate (HCO_3^-), and base excess values, consistent with arterial values if the child is well perfused at the time of sampling. However, capillary samples are not reliable for interpretation of pO_2 (Table 3.62).

Table 3.62: Normal capillary and arterial blood gas values		
Result	Capillary blood	Arterial blood
pH	7.35–7.45	7.35–7.45
pCO_2	4.6–6.4 kPa	4.5–6.0 kPa
pO_2	Not reliable	11.0–13.0 kPa
Bicarbonate	22.0–27.0 mmol/L	22.0–28.0 mmol/L
Base excess	-7.0 to -1.0 mmol/L	-2.0 to +2.0 mmol/L

Definitions

The pH changes that happen to the blood should be strictly referred to as 'acidaemia' and 'alkalaemia', and the terms 'acidosis' and 'alkalosis' refer to the processes that lead to the pH changes. However, in the rest of this chapter, we will use the terms 'acidosis' and 'alkalosis' instead, as these are the commonly used terms.

Acidosis refers to a blood pH of less than 7.35. This can result from any situation that causes hydrogen ion to accumulate in the body. It can be induced by a fall in bicarbonate concentration or a rise in pCO_2.

Alkalosis refers to a blood pH of more than 7.45. This results from any disease that causes loss of hydrogen ions from the body. Alkalosis can be induced by a rise in bicarbonate concentration or a fall in pCO_2.

The 4 primary acid-base disorders are respiratory acidosis, metabolic acidosis, respiratory alkalosis and metabolic alkalosis.

Steps to interpreting arterial blood gas results:

Is there acidosis or alkalosis?

- A lower-than-normal pH denotes acidosis and a higher-than-normal pH indicates alkalosis.

Is the primary disturbance respiratory or metabolic?

- *Respiratory* acidosis or alkalosis is indicated by the pCO_2, a high value correlating with respiratory acidosis and a low value correlating with respiratory alkalosis.
- *Metabolic* acidosis or alkalosis is indicated by the bicarbonate value (HCO_3), a high value correlating with metabolic alkalosis and a low value correlating with metabolic acidosis.

Look at the base excess.

- More negative base excess indicates metabolic acidosis, and more positive base excess indicates metabolic alkalosis.

Top tip!
You should be able to diagnose the presence of respiratory acidosis in this baby. You should also suggest normal systemic perfusion in view of the normal bicarbonate and base excess values, but stress the importance of a full clinical examination to confirm this.

■ *What is the most likely diagnosis? Suggest differential diagnoses.*

The most likely diagnosis with this history is acute bronchiolitis.

Differential diagnoses include pneumonia and pulmonary oedema. In babies who present without a history of antecedent upper respiratory tract symptoms, we should also consider other diagnoses such as congenital heart disease with pulmonary oedema, aspiration pneumonia/lobar pneumonias, and congenital anomalies such as a vascular ring.

Bronchiolitis is a viral infection of the lungs, most common among infants younger than a year. Respiratory syncytial virus (RSV) is the most common cause (50% to 75% of hospitalised children). Other agents include parainfluenza viruses (Type 1, 2 and 3), adenoviruses, rhinoviruses, influenza viruses (Type A and B), and enteroviruses.

■ *What clinical features would you look for in this child?*

Symptoms include poor feeding and lethargy, combined with a cough, runny nose and increased work for breathing. Signs include an increase in respiratory rate and heart rate, subcostal and intercostal recession, pallor, mottled skin, hypoxia, audible wheezing, and crepitations and wheeze on auscultation (Table 3.63).

Table 3.63: Assessment of the severity of bronchiolitis			
Mild	Moderate	Severe	Life-threatening
Saturation: >95% in air	Saturation: 92-95% in air	Saturation: <92% in air	
Normal respiratory rate Subtle or no accessory muscle use	Increased respiratory rate (>50/min) Minor accessory muscle use	Markedly increased respiratory rate (>70/min) Nasal flaring, grunting Moderate/marked accessory muscle use	Maximal accessory muscle use Poor respiratory effort Apnoea
Normal heart rate	Increased heart rate	Markedly raised heart rate	
Able to feed	Minimal limitation to feeding, but no signs of dehydration	Dehydrated and unable to feed (<50% normal feed)	
Others	Widespread crackles	Sweaty, tired	Exhausted, cyanosed

Top tip!
You should emphasise the need for a careful assessment of the cardiovascular system for congenital heart diseases when babies present with respiratory distress. However, these babies generally present with a metabolic acidosis or combined respiratory and metabolic acidosis, not a pure respiratory acidosis (as in this case).

■ *How will you manage this child?*

The history and physical examination will help to make a diagnosis and also assess the severity of the illness. Supportive measures form the mainstay of the management.

Criteria for admission

- Apnoea (observed or reported).
- Persistent oxygen saturation of less than 92% when breathing air.
- Inadequate oral fluid intake (50-75% of the usual volume, taking into account risk factors and using clinical judgement).
- Persisting severe respiratory distress (grunting, marked chest recession, or a respiratory rate of over 70/min).

There should be a lower threshold for hospitalisation in the case of children with risk factors for severe disease – for example, patients who are less than 12 weeks old, are premature, have underlying cardiopulmonary disease, or are immunodeficient.

General management

Clear nasal passages – Saline nose drops, especially before feeding. Suction can be used if there are signs of respiratory distress from blocked nasal passages, or if there is a history of apnoea, but should not be used routinely.

- Mild disease with respiratory rates up to 50/min can be managed with oral feeds. Nasogastric tube and frequent smaller feeds should be considered in infants with moderate disease, or those who cannot maintain oral intake due to increased respiratory rates up to 70/min, vomiting or increased work of breathing. In infants with severe disease, with a respiratory rate of >70/min, IV fluids are often required.
- Moderately ill infants often require humidified supplemental oxygen to maintain saturations >92%, often administered preferably by heated humidified high-flow nasal cannula (HHHFNC).
- Non-invasive respiratory support is helpful in moderate to severe cases to reduce the work of breathing and maintain ventilation; this can be in the form of HHHFNC, or continuous positive airway pressure (CPAP). Continued deterioration may warrant invasive ventilation in a minority of cases.
- Hypertonic saline nebulisers (3% saline) provide humidity and loosen the thick secretions, but the recent NICE guidance (2015) no longer recommends they be used.
- Capillary blood gases are only useful in those patients with severe disease and may have a role in those who require respiratory support. Retention of carbon dioxide can be a feature to look for in severe disease due to poor respiratory drive and exhaustion.
- The role of bronchodilators in the care of infants with bronchiolitis remains controversial, and is not recommended on a routine basis.
- Routine testing of nasopharyngeal aspirate for specific viruses is no longer necessary, unless used for isolation/cohorting purposes.
- The results of viral diagnostic tests can be used to limit the inappropriate use of antibacterial therapy and facilitate cohorting of patients and staff to prevent nosocomial transmission of these viruses.
- Routine chest x-ray or laboratory blood tests are unnecessary in the management.

Prevention of bronchiolitis

- At present, we rely upon passive immunisation to prevent serious RSV-related infections in high-risk infants.
- Monthly administration of palivizumab (a monoclonal antibody directed against a key viral surface protein) is associated with a reduction in the rate of hospitalisation for respiratory illnesses among children with a history of prematurity or chronic lung disease.
- RSV prophylaxis should be administered monthly during the RSV season (October to February).

Top tip!
Evidence does not support the use of trial doses of bronchodilators such as salbutamol, as bronchodilators are ineffective in changing the course of bronchiolitis.

Additional information

Causes of respiratory acidosis:
- Depression of respiratory drive – Drugs (opiates), central nervous system (CNS) lesions
- Respiratory muscle weakness – Guillain-Barre syndrome, muscular dystrophy
- Chest wall abnormality or airway obstruction – Kyphoscoliosis, obesity, hypoventilation syndrome
- Disorders affecting gas exchange – Pneumonia, asthma, bronchiolitis, pulmonary oedema

Causes of respiratory alkalosis:
- CNS stimulation – Pain, anxiety, hyperventilation, meningitis
- Tissue hypoxia – Severe anaemia, lack of oxygen
- Lung disease – Pneumonia, asthma, bronchiolitis, asthma, pulmonary oedema
- Drugs – Salicylates

Causes of metabolic acidosis:
- Diabetic ketoacidosis
- Shock leading to tissue hypoxia
- Severe diarrhoeal illness
- Renal failure

Causes of metabolic alkalosis:
- H+ loss – Vomiting, NG suction, loop/thiazide diuretics, Conn's syndrome
- Intracellular shift of H+ ions – Hypokalaemia

Syllabus mapping

Respiratory medicine with ENT

Knowledge

The candidate must:

- Know the causes and management of lower respiratory tract infections.

Metabolic medicine

Knowledge

The candidate must:

- Demonstrate knowledge of electrolyte and acid-base balance, and interpret relevant investigations.

Further reading and references

1. Acid-base balance (Appendix A). In: *Advanced paediatric life support. The practical approach* 4th ed. Advanced life support group. Blackwell publishing, Manchester, 2005: 279-84. ISBN 0-7279-1847-8
2. Baraldi E, Lanari M, Manzoni P et al. Inter-society consensus document on treatment and prevention of bronchiolitis in newborns and infants. *Ital J Pediatr* 2014; 24: 65
3. Blood gas analysis and pulse oximetry. In: *Advanced Life Support*, 6th edition. Resuscitation Council (UK), London, 2011: 157-65. ISBN 978-1-903812-22-8
4. National Institute for Health and Care Excellence. (NG9) - Bronchiolitis in Children. London, 2015. https://www.nice.org.uk/guidance/ng9/resources/bronchiolitis-in-children-51048523717 (accessed September 2015).
5. Capillary blood gas results. http://www.childrensmn.org/manuals/lab/Chemistry/042514.pdf (accessed September 2015).
6. Driscoll P, Brown T, Gwinnutt C, Wardle T. *Simple guide to blood gas analysis*. John Wiley & Sons, 1997.
7. Friedman JN, Rieder MJ, Walton JM. Bronchiolitis: Recommendations for diagnosis, monitoring and management of children one to 24 months of age. *Paediatr Child Health* 2014; 19: 485-91
8. Zavorsky GS, Cao J, Mayo NE et al. Arterial versus capillary blood gases: a meta-analysis. *Respir Physiol Neurobiol* 2007; 155: 268-79

SECTION 4:
THE STRUCTURED ORAL STATION

Chapter 4.1: Introduction
Dr Olive Hayes

The ability to problem-solve, consider various diagnostic possibilities and then undertake targeted investigations is an essential part of medical practice. The structured oral station tests your knowledge and understanding of common problems in child health. The topics discussed in this station are generally those that are not covered in other stations. The examiner is looking for a clear thought process based on the knowledge of common health problems and the application of this in practice. Ethical issues may also be included in this station. This station may, in the future, also include pictures, radiographs or video clips, which would serve as the basis from which further discussion is held.

What to expect

This structured oral station is part of the 'talking cycle' of the examination. You will be given a scenario and asked a preset number of questions by the examiner. The main aim of this station is to test your knowledge of common clinical problems and the application of that knowledge. You should have knowledge of the common guidelines used in paediatric practice. In addition, examiners are looking for a structured approach, sound (or, at the minimum, safe) clinical judgement, and consideration of any ethical issues that may apply to the specific scenario.

In the structured oral station, you will be given the clinical scenario on an information sheet while waiting outside the station. You will have at least 2 minutes outside the station to prepare before the start of the station.

It is important that you refer to the DCH syllabus published by the RCPCH when preparing for the examination, as the question from the structured oral may come from any section. This station does lend itself to scenarios that are more difficult to test in a clinical station – for example, ethical dilemmas, safeguarding situations or scenarios with a number of diagnostic possibilities that require consideration. This station can also include the acute management of common medical emergencies that would be difficult to test in other clinical stations.

When you enter the station, the examiner will greet you and request your mark sheet, making sure you have entered your details (name and candidate number) on it. The examiner will then ask a few questions, usually 3 to 4, based on this scenario. Where videos or pictures form the basis for the station, the examiner will show these at the start of the station and then proceed to ask questions. A fluent and confident approach in discussing management is essential for a clear pass. A good understanding of the evidence base (for example, NICE guidelines) underpinning good paediatric practice is also essential.

Managing time in the structured oral station

Timing: This is a 6-minute station. The entire time of 6 minutes is spent conducting a discussion with the examiner on the information provided, the diagnosis, differential diagnoses and management. A knock on the door at 5 minutes will warn you that 1 more minute is remaining.

It is recommended that you go over the information sheet during the 2 minutes you are waiting outside the station. This information should be read carefully. It is useful to pick out the salient points from the scenario, such as the age of the child, important symptoms and relevant family information, as this may point towards specific diagnostic possibilities. It is not uncommon for important clues to the diagnosis to be missed on the initial reading. The scenarios are not long, and there is ample time to prepare.

If necessary, make notes on a separate sheet of paper (provided on request) on the possible diagnosis, differential diagnoses and management plan.

The information sheet must be returned and left outside the examination room once you have finished the station.

If you finish early, you will be asked to remain in the room until the session has ended.

How consistency is ensured

RCPCH examiners set questions for the station well before the date of the examination, in groups, and agree the standards of performance required from you for the various grades awarded. In addition, on the day of the examination, examiners work in pairs to review these standards and adjust them if required. This 'standard setting' process is undertaken before each cycle during the clinical examination to ensure consistency.

Mark sheets, individualised for each station, help to guide examiners in their assessment. Mark sheets can inform you of the different areas examiners consider when awarding marks and, as importantly, areas where marks will be deducted (Appendix 4.11).

The RCPCH has developed 'anchor statements' that examiners refer to when deciding on pass/fail criteria. They use these as further guidance during standard setting and marking. You should review these documents to familiarise yourself with the scoring criteria explained in the anchor statements (Appendix 4.12).

Further reading and references

DCH clinical syllabus: http://www.rcpch.ac.uk/training-examinations-professional-development/assessment-and-examinations/examinations/dch-clinical#syllabus

Appendix 4.11: Mark Sheet (Front and Back): Structured Oral Station

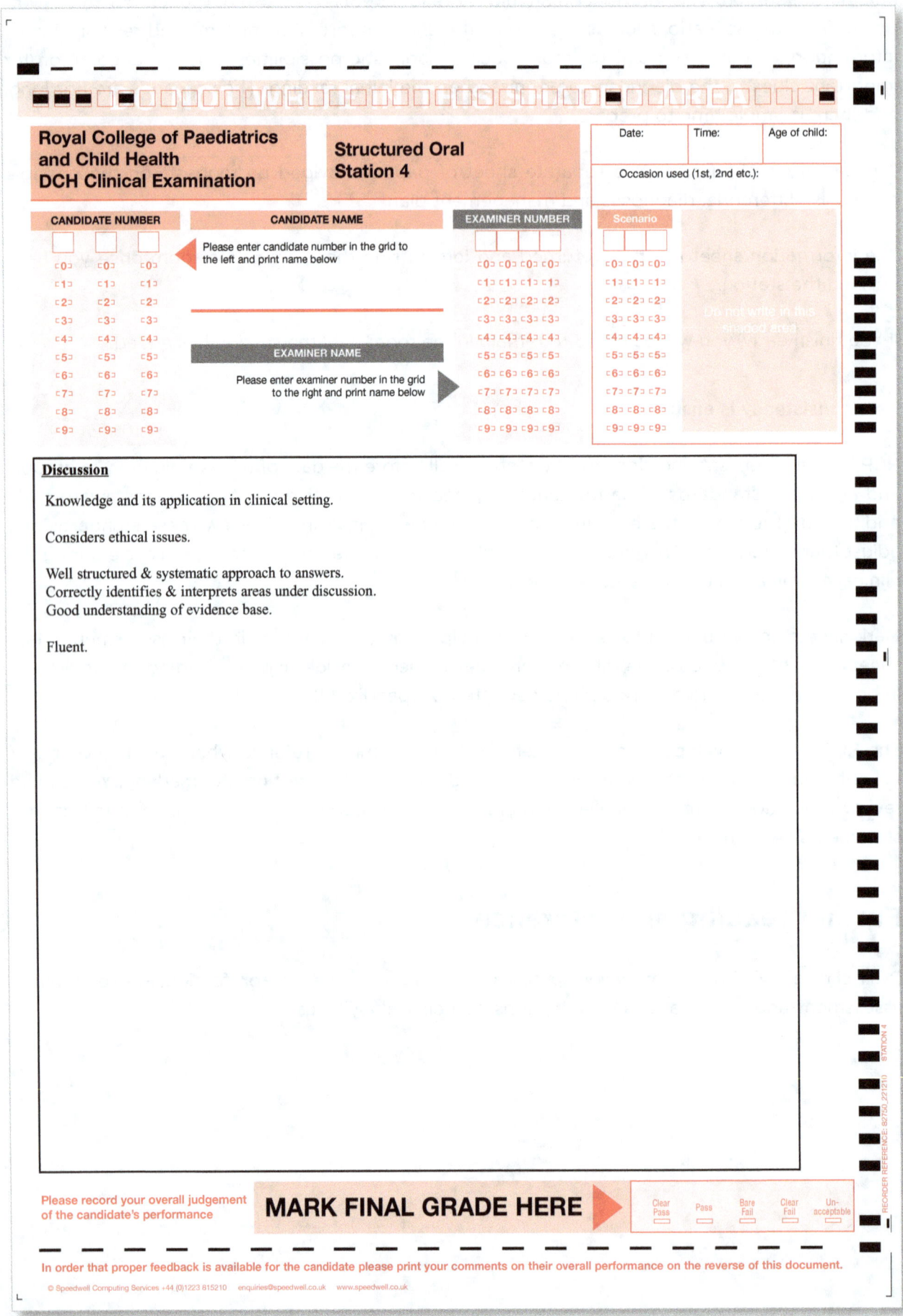

Clinical Cases in Paediatrics: DCH Clinical Examination

☐ Poor approach - Unstructured (please add additional comments)

☐ Failure to deal with the set task (please add additional comments)

☐ Factual inaccuracy (please add additional comments)

Please add any additional comments here:

Appendix 4.12: Anchor Statement: Structured Oral Station

	Expected Standard/ CLEAR PASS	PASS	BARE FAIL	CLEAR FAIL	UNACCEPTABLE
DISCUSSION	Knowledge and its application in clinical setting. Considers ethical issues. Clear, appropriate and professional.	Able to solve problems. Reasonable clinical thinking.	Some ability in problem solving. Muddled clinical thinking.	Little ability in problem solving. Muddled clinical thinking. Examiner has to work hard to give assistance.	Poor grasp of clinical concepts. Argumentative or dogmatic in approach.

Chapter 4.2: Case Study 1: 7 Month Old with an Abnormal Head Shape
Dr Ingran Lingam, Dr Saher Zakai

This station assesses your ability to undertake a discussion with the examiner around a commonly presenting paediatric problem.

> **Logistics:**
>
> *Timing:* This is a 6-minute station. A knock at 5 minutes will denote that 1 minute remains before the end of the station. You will have 2 minutes beforehand to read the candidate information provided to prepare yourself.
>
> *When the bell rings:* On entering the room, the examiner will greet you, take your mark sheet and proceed with asking questions.
>
> If the discussion with the examiner finishes early, you will be asked to remain in the room until the session has ended.

> **Candidate role and task:**
>
> **You are an** ST3 GP trainee.
>
> **Task: A mother brings her 7 month old baby with concerns about a funny head shape. Undertake a discussion with the examiner on the differential diagnosis and management.**

Examiner questions

- What is your differential diagnosis?
- How will you assess this child?
- Discuss the management options.

Answers

- *What is your differential diagnosis?*

The most common cause of an abnormal skull shape is positional plagiocephaly or brachycephaly, with a prevalence as high as 48% among healthy newborns. When evaluating a child with an abnormal head shape, the possibility of craniosynostosis must be considered.

The term 'plagiocephaly' is a Greek derivative that means 'oblique head'. Positional plagiocephaly refers to a distorted head shape with flattening on 1 side, giving the appearance of a parallelogram if viewed from above. Brachycephalic head shapes are flattened at the back, resulting in a wider and flattened skull shape. These shapes are the result of the moulding of the skull bones that are not yet fused, such as in a newborn. The supine position of the baby and the 'back to sleep' initiative to reduce 'cot deaths' has led to increased risks of prolonged pressure on 1 side of the head. Many babies in the first 3 to 6 months of their life develop a preferred head position in sleep that contributes to the development of plagiocephaly.

Craniosynostosis, on the other hand, is a rare condition resulting in the premature fusion of the skull plates. The premature closure of cranial sutures restricts cranial expansion on the affected side, resulting in an abnormal skull shape. The resulting shape of the skull is dependent on the sutures involved. Unrecognised, craniosynostosis can result in symptoms of raised intracranial pressure (headaches, visual disturbances), and can lead to significant developmental delay and learning difficulties (Table 4.21).

Table 4.21: Differentiating positional plagiocephaly from craniosynostosis

	Positional plagiocephaly	Craniosynostosis
Age at presentation	Typically 3–6 months of age	Usually at birth or shortly afterwards
Head shape	Primarily occipitoparietal flattening with contralateral frontal flattening	Sagittal suture fusion: long, narrow skull Unilateral coronal suture fusion: ipsilateral flattened forehead Bilateral coronal suture fusion: flat, prominent forehead and brow Metopic suture fusion: triangular, pointed scalp Lambdoid suture fusion: occipital flattening
Symptomatology	Clinically well and asymptomatic	May have features of raised intracranial pressure in advanced cases (vomiting, irritability, decreasing consciousness)
Associated anomalies	Not dysmorphic	May be associated with syndromes (e.g. Apert, Crouzon)

Top tip!
Although associated with some risk of positional skull deformity, healthy young infants should be placed down to sleep on their backs. The practice of putting infants to sleep on their backs has been associated with a marked reduction in the incidence of sudden infant death syndrome. Positional plagiocephaly is generally benign and self-resolving.

■ **How will you assess this child?**

Infants with plagiocephaly are primarily well with no symptoms. Parents or carers often identify the asymmetrical head shape. The child does not have any intracranial or neurodevelopmental sequelae. Although it is primarily a cosmetic issue, it is often a source of parental anxiety. This is made worse by the presence of adverts in the market on therapies such as the 'helmet' and the 'pillow', which, in fact, offer no significant or confirmed benefit.

History: Key features in the history that point towards a diagnosis of positional plagiocephaly include favoured positions during sleep, prematurity and a background of restricted movement in utero (Table 4.22). Risk factors associated with the development of positional plagiocephaly include oligohydramnios, twin pregnancies, prematurity, motor delay and a preferred sleep position. It is important to consider additional factors that may result in prolonged periods in fixed positions, such as congenital torticollis, visual abnormalities (e.g. amblyopia), scoliosis or any underlying disorders limiting the initiation or coordination of movement.

Examination: Examination should focus on documenting a description of the head shape, presence of facial asymmetry, torticollis, visual disturbances, and neurodevelopment. This should include a clinical assessment of the suture lines and fontanelles. It is also important to determine if there are any predisposing factors that restrict head movements – e.g. sternomastoid tumours.

The primary differential diagnosis of positional plagiocephaly is craniosynostosis, which is the presence of the premature fusion of sutures that result in an abnormal head shape. When premature suture fusion occurs, skull growth is usually restricted in a direction perpendicular to the fused suture and enhanced in a plane parallel to it, trying to provide space for the growing brain. The subsequent head shape, as mentioned above, is thus dependent on which sutures have fused prematurely.

Table 4.22: Key points to note in an assessment

History	Examination	Investigations
Neonatal history or prematurity	Assess the head shape	Consider investigations with skull x-ray if:
Neurodevelopment	Measure the head circumference and plot on the chart	• Significant facial asymmetry
Sleep position		
Symptoms of raised intracranial pressure	Examine fontanelles and sutures	• Suspected abnormal fusion of sutures
	Assess neurology	
Family history of abnormal head shapes and bone/brain diseases		Confirmation of craniosynostosis requires a CT scan of the head with bone windows

Top tip!
Assessment of an infant with an abnormal head shape focuses on differentiating benign positional plagiocephaly or brachycephaly from more sinister causes, such as craniosynostosis or genetic syndromes. Because the diagnosis of positional skull deformity is made on the basis of history, findings from physical examination, and resolution over time with positional intervention, imaging studies are unnecessary in most babies.

■ Discuss the management options.

Positional plagiocephaly is a benign disorder, and parents should be reassured that if simple measures are undertaken, the skull shape returns spontaneously to normal without any other intervention in the vast majority of children. Parental compliance with the management plan is pivotal to lessening the likelihood and severity of positional skull deformity.

Infants should be positioned so that the rounded side of the head, and not the flat side, is placed dependent against the mattress. The position of the crib in the room may also be adjusted to encourage the infant to look away from the flattened side when focusing on parents. Supervised tummy time on a firm surface when the infant is awake and being observed will help reduce the pressure to the back of the head. If torticollis is present, neck-motion exercises should be taught to the parents as part of the management plan. Rolled towels or ring-shaped cushions can be used to prevent infants from trying to adopt the frequently favoured position. Furthermore, parents can ensure the child does not spend prolonged periods of time in car seats or pushchairs. It is important to monitor head shape closely until there is discernible improvement. Monitoring should continue until the infant is old enough to sit, crawl, and spend less time on his or her back, and until any associated torticollis is completely corrected.

There is no clear evidence to support the use of helmets in positional plagiocephaly. When used, helmets must be worn for at least 23 hours a day and have been associated with contact dermatitis, pressure sores and skin irritation. Furthermore, infants wearing helmets may also suffer significant social and psychological distress. This intervention is not routinely funded by the National Health Service in the UK.

Preventive counselling has an important role in reducing the prevalence and severity of positional plagiocephaly. The newborn's skull is maximally deformable in the first 2 to 4 weeks of life. Parents should be instructed to lay the infant down to sleep in the supine position while alternating head positions (i.e. left and right occiputs). When awake and being observed, the infant should spend time in the prone position for at least 30 to 60 minutes per day. Infants should spend minimal time in car seats (when not a passenger in a vehicle) or other seating that maintains the supine position. Routine tummy time, besides reducing positional skull deformity, has been shown to enhance infant motor developmental scores during the first 15 months of life.

Infants with suspected craniosynostosis, abnormal neurology or neurodevelopmental concerns should be urgently referred to a paediatrician. Referral is also required if there is progression or lack of improvement in the skull deformity by the age of 6 months, despite positional adjustments. Careful clinical evaluation and plain skull x-rays may offer a clue to the diagnosis of craniosynostosis. However, a CT scan of the head with bone windows is required in case there is doubt in order to make the diagnosis.

Infants with craniosynostosis require surgical correction and skull reconstruction. Early surgical intervention results in less invasive procedures, as an infant's normal brain growth assists in remodelling the skull postoperatively. Minimally invasive surgery is now available to some infants identified with craniosynostosis in the first months of life.

> *Top tip!*
> Imaging studies should be reserved for infants born with deformities or those who do not improve over the first several weeks with repositioning. Significant concerns warranting further radiological investigations also would indicate a need for referral to secondary/tertiary care.

Syllabus mapping

Paediatric surgery

Knowledge

The candidate must:

- Be aware of the causes and approach to a dysmorphic baby.
- Be aware of the common disorders in the newborn and the management of these disorders.

Further reading and references

1. Hutchison BL, Stewart AW, Mitchell EA. Deformational plagiocephaly: A follow-up of head shape, parental concern, and neurodevelopment at ages 3 and 4 years. *Arch Dis Child* 2011; 96: 85-90
2. Laughlin J, Luerssen TG, Dias MS. Prevention and Management of Positional Skull Deformities in Infants. *Pediatrics* 2011; 128: 1236-41. doi: 10.1542/peds.2011-2220
3. Pogliani L, Mameli C, Fabiano V et al. Positional plagiocephaly: what the pediatrician needs to know: A review. *Child's Nerv Sys* 2011; 27: 1867-76. doi: 10.1007/s00381-011-1493-y
4. Saeed NR, Wall SA, Dhariwal DK. Management of positional plagiocephaly. *Arch Dis Child* 2008; 93: 82-4. doi: 10.1136/adc.2006.093740

Chapter 4.3: Case Study 2: 8 Year Old with Bed-Wetting

Dr Salah Mansy, Dr Soluchi Amobi

This station assesses your ability to undertake a discussion with the examiner around a commonly presenting paediatric problem.

> **Logistics:**
>
> *Timing:* This is a 6-minute station. A knock at 5 minutes will denote that 1 minute remains before the end of the station. You will have 2 minutes beforehand to read the candidate information provided to prepare yourself.
>
> *When the bell rings:* On entering the room, the examiner will greet you, take your mark sheet and proceed with asking questions.
>
> If the discussion with the examiner finishes early, you will be asked to remain in the room until the session has ended.

> **Candidate role and task:**
>
> **You are an** ST3 GP trainee.
>
> Eric is an 8 year old boy with bed-wetting. Eric's mother is very concerned by his bed-wetting and has brought him to the outpatient clinic. Eric has never been totally dry, but the frequency of bed-wetting has increased over the last 4 months, when they moved home.
>
> **Task: Undertake a discussion with the examiner.**

Examiner questions

- What is the likely cause of this child's nocturnal enuresis?
- How do his clinical features help to differentiate from other causes?
- How do you investigate these children?
- What treatment options are available for nocturnal enuresis?
- When should you refer for further assessment/investigation?

Answers

- ***What is the likely cause of this child's nocturnal enuresis?***

This child has primary nocturnal enuresis, made worse by the recent change of home and possibly school.

Enuresis refers to involuntary wetting during sleep without any inherent suggestion of the frequency of bed-wetting or pathophysiology (NICE 2010). The diagnosis of enuresis is made when urine is voided twice a week for at least 3 consecutive months, or when clinically significant distress occurs in areas of the child's life as a result of the wetting. Enuresis generally happens at night (nocturnal enuresis), but can also occur during daytime (diurnal enuresis). Enuresis can be primary or secondary.

In primary enuresis, the child has not been dry at night without assistance for 6 months or more at any time since birth. This gets better, with support, as the child grows older. The prevalence of bed-wetting decreases with age. Bed-wetting less than 2 nights a week has a prevalence of 21% at 4 years and 8% at 9 years. More frequent bed-wetting is less common, and has a prevalence of 8% at 4 years and 1.5% at 9 years. The cause of primary enuresis is not established as yet. Several suggestions – including disturbed physiology/maturational delay (e.g. sleep arousal difficulties, polyuria and bladder dysfunction) – may predispose one to primary nocturnal enuresis. Bed-wetting often runs in families, implying a genetic predisposition.

In secondary enuresis, the child wets at night after being dry for 6 months or more without assistance. The history is very important in order to find the cause or trigger for secondary enuresis. Common causes/triggers include urinary tract infection, constipation or soiling, diabetes mellitus or diabetes insipidus, physical or neurological problems, developmental delay or behavioural problems, family or emotional problems, or maltreatment.

Daytime enuresis can coexist with nocturnal enuresis, and children and young people with bed-wetting may also have symptoms related to the urinary tract during the day. These symptoms may include daytime frequency (i.e. passing urine more than 7 times a day), daytime urgency, daytime wetting, passing urine infrequently (fewer than 4 times a day), abdominal straining or poor urinary stream, and pain on passing urine. A history of daytime urinary symptoms may be important in determining the approach to the management of bed-wetting.

> *Top tip!*
> A thorough history is crucial to establish the cause of enuresis. It is important to know whether the child has primary or secondary enuresis, as secondary enuresis often has a trigger factor. Presence of daytime symptoms will also influence management strategies.

■ *How do his clinical features help to differentiate from other causes?*

History: A careful review of the history of bladder control would help to establish if this is primary or secondary enuresis. The frequency of bed-wetting, time of bed-wetting, fluid intake, volume of urine passed, snoring at night, daytime symptoms, and toilet patterns should be sought. In the majority of children with primary enuresis, an identifiable cause is not revealed, although the family history may reveal similar problems in other members.

With secondary or complicated enuresis, an identifiable and treatable cause is more likely. Frequency of urination, dysuria, or systemic symptoms such as fever could point to an underlying urinary tract infection. Polyuria, polydipsia and weight loss point to diabetes mellitus, or diabetes insipidus. Psychogenic polydipsia can also present with urinary symptoms. Pain in the absence of a urinary infection may be associated with detrusor muscle instability. A thorough history of bowel habits would help to elicit the presence of constipation, which is sometimes not given the importance that it deserves. A history of bullying at school, anxiety or sexual abuse should also be sought.

Examination: Observation of the child's behaviour in the clinic and interaction with the parents might point to a behavioural problem, maltreatment or disturbed family dynamics.

A thorough physical examination that notes the general physique and plots the weight, height and head circumference on the growth chart might indicate underlying medical problems. The presence of dysmorphic features helps in the diagnosis of genetic disorders and syndromes. Signs of self-harm highlight underlying emotional disturbance. A full developmental assessment is warranted in all children with enuresis.

There should be an abdominal examination for a distended bladder, faecal masses or other masses, which point to bladder or bowel problems. Examination of the back for sacral dimples, hairy patches or lipoma draws attention to underlying spinal anomalies. A thorough neurological examination is important to look for subtle neurological signs that suggest cerebral palsy, hemiplegia/quadriplegia or underlying neuromuscular disease. An inspection of the back, external genitalia and the anal orifice (in the presence of a chaperone and after taking a verbal consent from the parents) might show signs of vertebral anomalies, congenital anomalies of external genitalia or the absence of anal tone.

> *Top tip!*
> A comprehensive history and physical examination are essential to identifying underlying causes of enuresis.

■ How do you investigate this child?

Diagnosis is mostly clinical, and investigations play a minor role in the diagnosis of primary monosymptomatic enuresis. A urine dipstick and, if abnormal, a urine microscopy and culture are often helpful.

In secondary or complicated enuresis, investigations are guided by clinical suspicion. Selected children may require further investigations such as tests for renal functions including serum and urine osmolality. Urodynamic studies lead to a diagnosis of an unstable bladder in a minority of children.

■ What are the treatment options for nocturnal enuresis?

All ages: The treatment of nocturnal enuresis should not only focus on the child but also include the family and the environment. Engaging the child and the family while offering a clear explanation of all available treatment options form the basis of a successful outcome. Inform children and young people with bed-wetting and their parents or carers that bed-wetting is not the child or young person's fault and that punitive measures should not be used in the management of bed-wetting. Offer advice on reducing the impact of bed-wetting (e.g. bed protection, washable and disposable products). Providing written information tailored to the patient's needs would enhance compliance.

The importance of general advice on fluid intake, diet, sleep, hygiene, toileting behaviour and reward systems for agreed behaviour (rather than dry nights) cannot be overemphasised. Advise parents or carers to encourage the child to use the toilet to pass urine at regular intervals during the day and before sleep (typically between 4 to 7 times in a day). Attention to any underlying health problems or triggers, such as urinary infections, constipation, diabetes or bullying, may give immediate results.

Over 7 years old: NICE (2010) recommend the use of the alarm if there is no response to general advice (advice on fluids, toileting or an appropriate reward system), and the child and family accept the alarm as a treatment option. It should be considered only in children over the age of 7 years. It has a high success rate, and can also be used to manage any relapses. However, alarms are not appropriate if bed-wetting is very infrequent (i.e. less than 1 to 2 bed-wetting incidents per week), or where parents or carers are having emotional difficulty coping with the burden of bed-wetting, or are expressing anger, negativity or blame towards the child or young person.

Desmopressin is the next treatment option. Offer Desmopressin to children and young people over 7 years, if the priority is for a rapid-onset and/or short-term improvement in bed-wetting or where an alarm is considered inappropriate. Recommended initial doses are 200 micrograms for Desmotabs and 120 micrograms for DesmoMelt. The medicine should be taken at bedtime and it is important to restrict fluids from 1 hour before to 8 hours after taking desmopressin, in order to prevent dilutional hyponatremia. The response to desmopressin should be assessed at 2 and 4 weeks. If there is a good response, the medication can be continued for 3 months and then stopped to reassess. Consider increasing the dose if there is no response. Desmopressin can be used for short periods such as during travel, sleepovers, etc. It can also be combined with the use of alarms and other medications such as anticholinergics.

Under 5's: For children below 5 years, it is common practice not to offer active management. Instead, a detailed history and general physical examination, followed by reassurance and general advice, are recommended.

5 to 7 year olds: Treatment for children between 5 and 7 years of age should be individualised, and they should be offered what is considered appropriate for each child.

Anticholinergics and tricyclic antidepressants could be used in consultation with a specialist in bed-wetting if the other treatment options are unsuccessful. These are not recommended as first-line treatment.

> *Top tip!*
> Engage the child and the family in the management plan from the outset to ensure compliance and better outcomes.

■ When should you refer for further assessment/investigation?

Health visitors and GPs have an important role to play in the initial assessment and management of enuresis. Community paediatricians with a special interest in enuresis help in the management of primary enuresis, while hospital paediatricians have an important role to play in the identification and management of any underlying pathology that can coexist or cause symptoms.

Referral criteria:

- Children with a poor response to general advice, alarm and/or desmopressin treatment – To assess for factors associated with a poor response such as overactive bladder, an underlying disease, or social and emotional factors.
- Children with persistent primary daytime enuresis and voiding problems or recurrent urine infections – To look for urinary tract abnormalities.

- Children with a neurological disorder or a history suggestive of detrusor instability – To consider the need for urodynamic studies.
- Children with deliberate bed-wetting, where parents or carers are punishing the child in spite of professional advice to the contrary, or secondary enuresis that is otherwise unexplained and resistant to therapy – Suspect safeguarding issues (NICE 2010).

Top tip!
Management of enuresis may take several months before a satisfactory outcome. Have a low threshold for referring non-responders to a paediatric specialist for further multidisciplinary input.

Syllabus mapping

Behavioural problems

Knowledge

The candidate must:

- Understand the principles of managing common behaviour problems such as temper tantrums, breath-holding attacks, sleep problems, the crying baby, oppositional behaviour, enuresis and encopresis, school refusal and bullying.

Skills

The candidate must:

- Be able to look at behaviour as a form of communication and to take this into account when interviewing, examining and assessing children.
- Have begun to develop an approach to the assessment of behaviour problems that uses observation as well as history taking.

Nephro-urology

Knowledge

The candidate must:

- Have a knowledge and understanding of the manifestations of renal diseases, both acute and chronic.
- Demonstrate an understanding of manifestations and management of urinary tract infections in different age groups.
- Understand the principles of managing enuresis.

Further reading and references

1. Butler RJ, Heron J. The prevalence of infrequent bedwetting and nocturnal enuresis in childhood: A large British cohort. *Scandinavian Journal of Urology and Nephrology* 2008; 42: 257–64
2. National Institute Health and Care Excellence. (CG111) – Nocturnal enuresis. The management of bedwetting in children and young people. London, 2010. http://www.nice.org.uk/guidance/cg111/resources/guidance-nocturnal-enuresis-pdffor

Clinical Cases in Paediatrics: DCH Clinical Examination

Chapter 4.4: Case Study 3: 8 Month Old with an Inguinal Swelling
Dr Caroline Pardy, Mr Varadarajan Kalidasan

This station assesses your ability to undertake a discussion with the examiner around a commonly presenting paediatric problem.

> **Logistics:**
>
> *Timing:* This is a 6-minute station. A knock at 5 minutes will denote that 1 minute remains before the end of the station. You will have 2 minutes beforehand to read the candidate information provided to prepare yourself.
>
> *When the bell rings:* On entering the room, the examiner will greet you, take your mark sheet and proceed with asking questions.
>
> If the discussion with the examiner finishes early, you will be asked to remain in the room until the session has ended.

> **Candidate role and task:**
>
> **You are an** ST3 GP trainee.
>
> **Clinical context:** Joseph is an 8 month old boy whom you are seeing in your GP surgery. His mother is concerned about a swelling in his groin. This swelling is noticed occasionally on the right side of his groin, and is prominent when he cries. At the neonatal check, the doctors had noted that his right testicle was not palpable in the scrotum, and had promised a review appointment, but this has not yet materialised.
>
> **Task: Undertake a discussion with the examiner on the differential diagnosis and management.**

Examiner questions

- What is the likely cause of this child's inguinal swelling?
- How do the clinical signs help to differentiate from the other main causes?
- Does he require any investigations? When should you refer for further assessment/investigation?
- What are the management options?

Answers

- ***What is the likely cause of this child's inguinal swelling?***

The fact that the right testis was not palpated in the scrotum at the 6-week check suggests a diagnosis of a right, undescended testis. However, the history suggests a swelling that is prominent when the child cries. Thus, you need to check for an inguinal hernia as well in this child, as it is not uncommon for these 2 to coexist. In addition, you need to distinguish a retractile testis from an undescended testis.

Top tip!
A good candidate will recognise that an undescended testis can coexist with an inguinal hernia, and should emphasise that these diagnoses are not mutually exclusive.

An undescended testis (cryptorchidism) is a relatively common congenital anomaly, reported among 1–5% in-term newborn males. However, there is considerable spontaneous descent in the first year of life and, by the age of 1 year, only about 1–2% remain undescended. Unilateral incomplete descent is 4 times more common than bilateral. Recognised risk factors include prematurity, low birth weight, a first-degree relative with a history of undescended testes, and the presence of another genital abnormality (e.g. hypospadias) (NICE 2014). During pregnancy, the testicles form inside the baby's abdomen, and then slowly move down into the scrotum from about 2 months before birth. Undescended testicles occur when the testicles do not move into the scrotum by the time the baby is born. The descent may be arrested anywhere along the path of descent from the abdominal cavity to high up in the scrotum or to an ectopic position outside the scrotum (e.g. perineum or inner thigh). Diagnosis and appropriate management are important, as an undescended testis carries an increased risk of torsion due to abnormal fixation, a 4–8 times increased risk of malignancy if the testis is intra-abdominal at birth, and reduced fertility if the testis remains undescended.

Inguinal hernia is again common in the newborn, and results from persistent patency of the processus vaginalis, which normally closes by birth (Figure 4.41). The swelling generally reduces in size or disappears when the baby is relaxed and lying down. Complications include incarceration (when the hernia contents become entrapped in the sac and are difficult or impossible to reduce), strangulation (when the circulation to the contents is compromised), and intestinal obstruction. As a result, an inguinal hernia needs referral to a paediatric surgeon as soon as it is diagnosed or suspected.

A hydrocele is a scrotal swelling that results from a collection of peritoneal fluid around the testicles in the tunica vaginalis (Figure 4.41). In children, this almost always represents the presence of a patent processus vaginalis communicating with the peritoneal cavity. They may fluctuate in size when there is a large communication with the peritoneal cavity. Most hydoceles resolve by the age of 2, but, occasionally, they are large or persist and may require surgical intervention. A hydrocele can coexist with an inguinal hernia; thus, all cases require careful clinical assessment.

■ How do the clinical signs help to differentiate from the other main causes?

A careful history and examination will help to arrive at the correct diagnosis. The most common causes of inguinal swellings are inguinal hernia, hydrocele, undescended testis and inguinal lymph nodes. An undescended testis and a hernia may coexist, and form the main differential in this child. Hydroceles, particularly in ambulant older children, often enlarge gradually during day while active and shrink at night while resting, and can also increase in association with other problems that raise intra-abdominal pressure (e.g. coughing with upper respiratory infections). An inguinal lymph node does not usually significantly vary in size on a day-to-day basis. In older children, varicoceles also need to be considered in the differential diagnosis.

Undescended testis

Once it is determined that the groin swelling in this child is a testis, the next step is to distinguish whether it is an undescended testis or a retractile testis (Table 4.41).

Table 4.41: Features to distinguish an undescended from a retractile testis		
	Undescended testis	**Retractile testis**
Is the testis visible in the scrotum occasionally?	No	Yes
Is the testis palpable?	Not always. Testis may be intra-abdominal, and not palpable	Always palpable
Are the testes equal in size?	May be smaller than the normally descended testis	Generally equal in size
Is the scrotum well developed?	May be smaller on the side of the undescended testis	Scrotum normal in size
Can the testis be brought into the scrotum?	May reach the root of the scrotum, but does not stay in the scrotum	Can be brought comfortably into the scrotum and stays there for at least a few seconds after being drawn down

Inguinal hernia and hydrocele

Table 4.42 lists the important differences between an inguinal hernia and a hydrocele. An undescended testis may be associated with an inguinal hernia, and the latter needs to be considered when there is a history of change in the size of the swelling when the child cries. Occasionally, a hydrocele behaves like a hernia in that it can be reduced (slowly) and this is probably because the communication with the peritoneal cavity is large enough for fluid to move through it more freely. Both a hernia and a hydrocele are caused by a patency of the processus vaginalis (Figure 4.41). If the communication with the peritoneal cavity is large enough to enable a protrusion of abdominal contents, a hernia results; a smaller communication results in a hydrocele (Figure 4.41).

Figure 4.41: Diagrams showing the different inguino-scrotal swellings, along with the normal anatomy. 1 Peritoneal cavity; 2 Spermatic cord structures; 3 Obliterated processus vaginalis; 4 Epididymis; 5 Testis; 6 Tunica vaginalis; 7 Scrotum; 8 Encysted hydrocele of the cord; 9 Patent processus vaginalis; 10 Hydrocele; 11 Contents of hernial sac, usually the bowel (Illustration by Dr P Venugopalan)

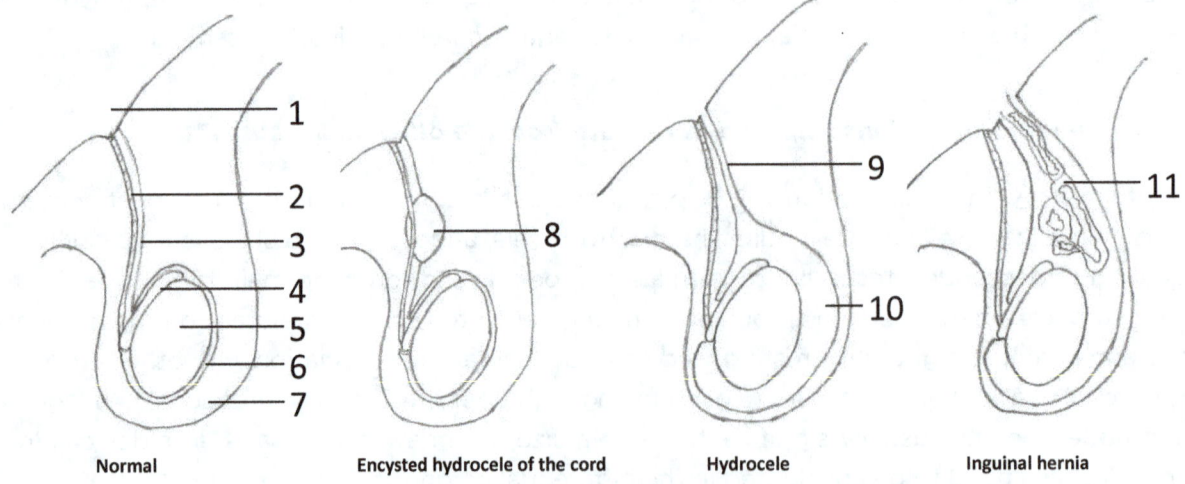

Top tip!
A hernia varies in size and, sometimes, it is not possible to demonstrate it when you examine the child in the clinic. One may have to rely on a good history from the parents. (Many parents now come with a photograph on their phones!)

Table 4.42: Features to distinguish an inguinal hernia from a hydrocele		
	Inguinal hernia	Hydrocele
Reducible	Yes. Unless obstructed or incarcerated	No (Except with a widely communicating hydrocele, which may behave like a hernia)
Transillumination	Negative	Positive
Cord palpable proximal to the swelling	No	Yes
Fluctuation	No. Attempts to elicit fluctuation may result in the hernia getting reduced	Yes, but can be very tense

Groin lymph nodes

Groin lymph nodes are more commonly enlarged in toddlers and older children, due to the frequency of injuries and infections in the lower limbs. The history is shorter, and the swellings are often multiple and of varying size. It may be possible to elicit signs of inflammation such as tenderness and redness in acute presentations. You need to examine the lower limbs and genitals in search of a focus of infection. There is no history of frequent change in size and these are not reducible.

■ *Does he require any investigations? When should you refer for further assessment/investigation?*

The history and clinical examination are usually sufficient to arrive at a diagnosis. In this case, no investigation is required, and Joseph should be referred to a paediatric surgeon for further management. Imaging for undescended testis (e.g. ultrasound or MRI) is not recommended, as it does not alter the clinical management of the child even if the testis is not palpable.

An undescended testis needs to be brought down into the scrotum and fixed to the scrotum by an operation (orchidopexy). Current guidelines recommend that this procedure should be performed between the ages of 6 months to 1 year. In most centres, the operation is scheduled around the age of 1 year. Joseph is now 8 months old and, therefore, needs referral to the paediatric surgical outpatient services.

If a competent doctor (GP, paediatrician or paediatric surgeon) is confident of the diagnosis of a retractile testis, then the majority do not require follow-up or treatment. Most centres do not comply with the European Association of Urology's recommendation to follow all these children until puberty. A small number of children present with a testis that seems to 'ascend' and may need orchidopexy at a later date. Parents should be advised of this and if there is any suggestion, as the child gets older, that the position of the testis has not improved, they must seek further advice.

■ *What are the management options?*

The palpable undescended testis will need orchidopexy. This is done under general anaesthesia as a day-case procedure, and has a high success rate of 98%. The potential complications are damage to the vas deferens and the testicular vessels. The latter may lead to testicular atrophy.

If the testis is **impalpable**, then the child is re-examined under anaesthesia. If still impalpable, a laparoscopy is performed to determine the presence and position of the testis. In approximately one third of cases, the testis may be absent. If the testis is present intra-abdominally, the surgeon will make a decision on the feasibility of performing a single stage orchidopexy or if a staged procedure (Fowler-Stephens) will be required. It is to be noted that intra-abdominal testes have a higher rate of testicular atrophy after orchidopexy, especially if a staged procedure is required; however, leaving it in carries the risk of testicular malignancy.

An **inguinal hernia** is treated by surgical repair (herniotomy), which is done as a day procedure under general anaesthetic.

A **hydrocele** in a young child may be observed till the child is 2 to 3 years old, as many of these resolve spontaneously. The exceptions to this may be massive, symptomatic or complicated secondary hydroceles.

Inguinal lymphadenopathy, if secondary to an infection, needs treatment with appropriate antibiotics. Occasionally, the node may suppurate and may need incision and drainage of the abscess.

Testicular torsion refers to the testis rotating on the spermatic cord, and is a recognised complication of undescended testis. When torsion of an undescended testis occurs, the swelling and pain is in the groin and should be distinguished from an incarcerated or obstructed hernia. Testicular torsion may also occur in descended testis in the scrotum. Acute onset of pain and increased swelling of the scrotum should alert the parents and the physician. The scrotum looks swollen and feels tender, and the child resists further examination. Diagnosis is clinical and urgent surgical intervention, preferably within 4 hours of onset of symptoms, as this can save the testis from atrophy. The surgery involves untwisting the spermatic cord and fixing the testis to the bottom of the scrotum to prevent recurrence.

Top tip!
Testicular torsion is an emergency, and candidates should be prepared to discuss the different aspects of the management. Most importantly, the need to visit a specialist centre as soon as the diagnosis is suspected should be appreciated.

Syllabus mapping

Paediatric surgery

Knowledge

The candidate must:

- Be able to recognise and manage common surgical disorders of the abdomen and urogenital tract.

Further reading and references

1. Nah SA, Yeo CS, How GY et al. Undescended testis: 513 patients' characteristics, age at orchidopexy and patterns of referral. *Arch Dis Child* 2014; 99: 401–6. doi: 10.1136/archdischild-2013-305225
2. National Institute of Health and Care Excellence. (CG37) – Postnatal care. London, 2014. http://www.nice.org.uk/guidance/cg37/resources/guidance-postnatal-care-pdf (accessed August 2015).
3. National Institute of Health and Care Excellence. Clinical Knowledge Summaries – Undescended testes. London, 2014. http://cks.nice.org.uk/undescended-testes (accessed August 2015).
4. Steinbrecher H. The undescended testis: working towards a unified care pathway for 2014. *Arch Dis Child* 2014; 99: 397–8. doi: 10.1136/archdischild-2013-305459
5. Virtanen HE, Bjerknes R, Cortes D et al. Cryptorchidism: Classification, prevalence and long-term consequences. *Acta Paediatr* 2007; 96: 611–6
6. Zamakhshary M, To T, Guean J et al. Risk of incarceration of inguinal hernia among infants and young children awaiting elective surgery. *CMAJ* 2008; 179: 1001–5

Chapter 4.5: Case Study 4: 4 Year Old with a Limp

Dr Saher Zakai, Dr Ingran Lingam

This station assesses your ability to undertake a discussion with the examiner around a commonly presenting paediatric problem.

Logistics:

Timing: This is a 6-minute station. A knock at 5 minutes will denote that 1 minute remains before the end of the station. You will have 2 minutes beforehand to read the candidate information provided to prepare yourself.

When the bell rings: On entering the room, the examiner will greet you, take your mark sheet and proceed with asking questions.

If the discussion with the examiner finishes early, you will be asked to remain in the room until the session has ended.

Candidate role and task:

You are an ST3 GP trainee.

Tom is a 4 year old boy who presents to your surgery for the second time in a week. A colleague reviewed him 3 days previously because he was limping. Analgesia was prescribed. Tom is still reluctant to walk. He remains afebrile and is otherwise well. His mother is concerned he could be suffering from Perthes disease.

Task: Undertake a discussion with the examiner.

Examiner questions

- What is the most likely diagnosis? Discuss the common differentials.
- What investigations would you consider?
- In our 4 year old child, the initial investigations reveal a normal full blood count and a normal C-reactive protein of <5 microgram per litre. Inform the candidate of these results and ask the candidate to consider their next course of action.

Answers

- ***What is the most likely diagnosis? Discuss the common differentials.***

The most likely diagnosis in this child is transient synovitis; however, it is also important to consider trauma, foreign bodies, septic arthritis (unlikely), as well as more rare causes including acute lymphoblastic leukaemia, juvenile arthritis, and Perthes disease (Table 4.51).

The most common cause of an acute limp is trauma; however, careful clinical assessment is required to exclude uncommon, but serious differential diagnoses. Key features in the history include characteristics of the pain (site, triggers, weight-bearing), associated systemic features, travel history and recent medications (e.g. recent antibiotics partially treating septic arthritis). Identifying the precise location of the pain may be difficult in young children, and thus it is important to assess the joints above and below the suspected area of pathology. It is especially important to examine the abdomen, pelvis, testes and spine as part of the hip examination.

Top tip!
A limp is a symptom, not a diagnosis. A detailed clinical evaluation is required to determine the underlying cause. Pain localised to a joint may be referred from pathology elsewhere. Evaluating hip pain includes assessing the spine, abdomen, pelvis and knee.

Table 4.51: Differential diagnosis stratified by age of presentation

	Differential diagnosis	Clinical features
0–3 years	Toddler's fracture	Undisplaced spiral fracture, usually in the distal two thirds of the tibia. Caused by a sudden twist after an often unwitnessed fall in preschool infants. May have localised tenderness over the tibial shaft.
	Developmental hip dysplasia	Painless limp since starting to walk. May have a Trendelenburg gait (unilateral) or a waddling gait (bilateral). Examination findings include limited abduction, leg-length discrepancy and asymmetrical skin creases.
	Neuroblastoma	Neuroblastoma is the most common extra-cranial tumour in children. It usually presents as an abdominal mass, although it can rarely present as a limp or limb paralysis. Red flags suggesting malignancies are listed in Table 4.52.
4–10 years	Transient synovitis	More common in boys. Usually in patients who have a history of recent upper respiratory or gastrointestinal infection. Patients are systemically well and present with an acute limp, reluctance to weight-bear and restricted passive hip movements. Inflammatory markers are usually normal.
	Perthes disease	Typically affects boys (4–8 years) and results in avascular necrosis of the femoral head. Presents with an insidious onset limp that worsens over weeks, or may present with hip or leg pains (referred) that is worse with activity. Inflammatory markers are normal and radiographic changes may not be apparent in early disease.
	Acute lymphoblastic leukaemia	Signs and symptoms often reflect bone marrow infiltration, including signs of anaemia, thrombocytopenia and lymphopenia, as well as bone pain/limping. A small proportion of infants present with limb pain alone, which may delay diagnosis.
11–16 years	Slipped upper/capital femoral epiphysis	More common in boys. Other risk factors include obesity, hypothyroidism and hypopituitarism. Usually unilateral, though bilateral in 25–40% of cases. May present acutely with sudden severe hip or (referred) knee pain, limp and limited internal rotation and abduction. May also present with milder chronic symptoms.
	Bone tumours	Benign bone tumours (e.g. osteoid osteomas) present with localised pain, which is often worse at night and relieved by non-steroidal anti-inflammatory medication. Malignant bone tumours (e.g. osteosarcomas) present as relatively painless tumours, with local tissue destruction and early metastasis to the lung.
	Osgood-Schlatter disease	Primarily affects young teenagers who play sports. Presents with pain just below the patella, worse on activity and may last up to 2 years. The knee itself is unaffected.
	Sinding-Larsen disease	Presents with anterior knee pain and tenderness in the inferior aspect of the patella. Symptoms are worse with activity. Repeated traction between the patella and patellar ligament results in abnormal ossification, usually in the inferior pole of the patella.

Table 4.51 continued...

Table 4.51: continued

	Differential diagnosis	Clinical features
All age groups	Septic arthritis	Fever, complete non-weight-bearing, and raised inflammatory markers (refer to Table 4.52 and the 'additional information' section for more details).
	Non-accidental injury	Delayed presentation, inconsistencies in history, and unusual location/pattern of injury for the child's development (refer to Table 4.52 and the 'additional information' section for more details).
	Juvenile idiopathic arthritis	Often an intermittent limp that is worse in the morning or after periods of inactivity. May present with regression of motor milestones. Joint swelling may be subtle, involving single joints (oligoarticular) and multiple joints (polyarticular). May develop systemic symptoms.
	Haematological causes (e.g. sickle cell disease)	Vaso-occlusive episodes that commonly affect the long bones of the arm and leg. The pain may be severe and last for minutes to days.
	Acute abdominal pain	Limping may be a presenting feature of abdominal pathology – e.g. appendicitis, testicular torsion, urinary infections, inguinal hernias, etc.

■ *What investigations would you consider?*

Initial investigations in a systemically unwell child may include a full blood count, blood film, c-reactive protein and erythrocyte sedimentation rate. Regarding systemically well children with a limp who are able to weight-bear, there is no clear clinical consensus or national guidance on the need for immediate investigation. Clinical management varies from 'watchful waiting' to baseline blood tests.

Top tip!
Urgent investigations should be performed in those with 'red flag' features, including a young age (less than 3 years), being febrile or unwell, non-weight-bearing and restricted hip movements on examination (Table 4.52).

Table 4.52: Condition-specific 'red flags'

Septic arthritis	Predictive score for septic arthritis (Kotcher et al.): • Fever >38°C • Unable to weight-bear • ESR >40 mm/h • Serum WCC >12 x 10^6/L Probability of septic arthritis with 2 features is 40%, 3 features 93% and all features >99%. Other features include severe pain with distress at passive movements, night pain and waking pain, and adopting a passive limb position that accommodates joint effusion.
Malignancy	Localised bone pains Pallor, easy bruising, hepatosplenomegaly Lethargy, weight loss, night sweats, fever Back pain in an unwell child
Non-accidental injury	Delay in presentation Unwitnessed injury Injury inconsistent with history or the child's development Repeated presentations to health services Unkempt appearance/poor hygiene

■ **In our child, the full blood count and CRP were normal. What is the next course of action?**

The results of the investigations are reassuring and indicate transient synovitis is the most likely diagnosis. Treatment involves regular analgesia and encouraging mobilisation when the pain settles. Symptoms should resolve within 2 weeks but if persistent, further review is warranted.

Persistent limping beyond 3 weeks increases the likelihood of juvenile idiopathic arthritis. Further investigations include an ultrasound of joints to detect effusions, plain radiographs and referral to a paediatrician.

Top tip!
Safety netting and appropriate follow-up is essential. Worsening or persistent symptoms warrant referral to specialist services.

Additional Information

Transient synovitis

Transient synovitis of the hip (also called irritable hip) is the most common cause of sudden hip pain in children, and is often reactive to a viral infection (in the respiratory or digestive tract). It commonly affects children aged 3 to 10 years, and affects boys twice as often as girls. A history of trauma may be elicited.

Diagnosis is clinical. When in doubt, blood tests (particularly FBC, ESR and CRP) and a hip ultrasound help to differentiate transient synovitis from septic arthritis.

Transient synovitis often resolves within 5 to 7 days without any specific treatment. Anti-inflammatory medications such as ibuprofen may help to decrease pain and shorten the duration of symptoms. Treatment often includes limiting activity to make the child more comfortable.

Developmental dysplasia of the hip

Developmental dysplasia of the hip is a condition where there is underdevelopment of the hip joint with or without dislocation. Types of developmental dysplasia of the hip include subluxation, dysplasia, and dislocation, and result from either laxity of the supporting capsule or an abnormal acetabulum. Developmental dysplasia of the hip occurs in about 1 in 1,000 babies.

The aetiology is not clear. The contributing factors include a positive family history, prematurity, female babies, oligohydramnios, breech presentation, and a first-born baby. Neuromuscular disorders involving the spine and lower limbs increase the risk.

It is important to assess the hips of all newborn babies with a view to early diagnosis. Later on in life, asymmetrical gluteal folds and delayed walking may be the presenting feature. Any suspicious hips will need an ultrasound and referral to the specialists, as per local protocol.

The goal of treatment is to relocate the head of the femur into the acetabulum. This then allows the structures of the rapidly developing hip joint (femur, acetabulum, supporting ligaments, etc.) to become established normally. The Pavlik harness is often the first treatment for children under the age of 6 months. For children over 6 months of age, or if the Pavlik harness is not effective, closed reduction followed by a hip spica case for about 12 weeks may be necessary. If this fails, open reduction may be required.

Perthes disease

Perthes disease results from reduced blood supply (avascular necrosis) to the femoral epiphysis, leading to the softening of the femoral head. With subsequent healing, the femoral head gets deformed, leading to disability. The disease affects about 1 in 1,200 children in the UK, commonly between 4 and 8 years of age. Boys are more affected than girls.

Initial presenting features are hip or groin pain or a limp. Occasionally, referred pain to the knee may be the first symptom. Later, features include wasting of the muscles of the upper thigh, shortening of the leg and stiffness of the hip causing pain. Hip radiography shows a femoral head that is broken or damaged; the typical appearance is a 'flattened' femoral head when it should normally look rounded in the hip socket. However, the x-ray can be normal in the early stages of the disease, before the 'softened' bone breaks. An x-ray every few months can show the progress of the breakdown, and then the healing as new fresh bone is made and gradually 'remodelled'. A bone scan and an MRI are generally performed in these children to confirm the diagnosis.

Management aims to promote the healing process and to ensure that the femoral head remains well seated in the acetabulum as it heals and regrows. Conservative management involves restricting activities to low-impact activities, such as swimming and home exercises. Over 50% of children, particularly those under 5 years, do well this way. The aim of treatment is to encourage the use of the hip in a full range of motion and to ensure that the femoral head remains within the acetabulum as it heals and remodels. Bed rest and/or crutches may be needed for a short period of time if the initial symptoms are severe. Plaster casts or a special brace may also be considered in more severe cases or in older children. Surgery may be considered in some cases, particularly older children or those more severely affected.

Syllabus mapping

Musculoskeletal medicine

Knowledge

The candidate must:

- Know the differential diagnosis of a limp.
- Be able to discuss causes of acute and chronic arthritis.

Further reading and references

1. Herman MJ, Martinek M. The limping child. *Pediatr Rev* 2015; 36: 184–97. doi: 10.1542/pir.36-5-184
2. Huntley JS. Diagnosing and managing hip problems in childhood. *Practitioner* 2013; 257:19, 22-5, 2-3
3. Kocher MS, Zurakowski D, Kasser JR. Differentiating between septic arthritis and transient synovitis of the hip in children: An evidence-based clinical prediction algorithm. *J Bone Joint Surg Am* 1999; 81: 1662–70
4. Sawyer JR, Kapoor M. The limping child: A systemic approach to diagnosis. *Am Fam Physician* 2009; 79: 215–24
5. Sidwell R, Thomson M. *Concise Paediatrics*. Cambridge University Press: New York, 2006. ISBN 0521697247
6. Smith E, Anderson M, Foster H. The child with a limp: A symptom and not a diagnosis. *Arch Dis Child Educ Pract* 2012; 97: 185–93. doi: 10.1136/archdischild-2011-301245

Chapter 4.6: Case Study 5: 3 Month Old with an Immunisation Reaction

Dr Delair Khider, Dr P Venugopalan

This station assesses your ability to undertake a discussion with the examiner around childhood immunisations.

> **Logistics:**
>
> *Timing:* This is a 6-minute station. A knock at 5 minutes will denote that 1 minute remains before the end of the station. You will have 2 minutes beforehand to read the candidate information provided to prepare yourself.
>
> *When the bell rings:* On entering the room, the examiner will greet you, take your mark sheet and proceed with asking questions.
>
> If the discussion with the examiner finishes early, you will be asked to remain in the room until the session has ended.

> **Candidate role and task:**
>
> **You are an** ST3 GP trainee.
>
> A 3 month old baby had his second routine immunisation at the GP surgery. He developed pain, swelling and redness at the site of the injection of the combined vaccine. This lasted for a few hours and, by the end of that day, these signs had resolved.
>
> **Task: Undertake a discussion with the examiner.**

Examiner questions

- What is your advice regarding the next immunisation?
- What are immunisation reactions?
- What is the schedule for routine immunisation in preschool children?
- What are the contraindications to immunisation?

Answers

- ***What is your advice regarding the next immunisation?***

Give subsequent immunisations according to the immunisation schedule (see below). Pain, swelling or redness at the site of the injection occurs commonly after immunisation, and is not a contraindication for further doses.

Patients, parents or carers should be given advice about possible adverse events following immunisations (AEFIs) and how such events should be managed. The leaflets on vaccinations provided by the Department of Health give information about AEFIs and include advice on their management.

Fevers over 37.5°C are common in children and are usually mild. Advice on the use and appropriate dose of paracetamol or ibuprofen liquid to treat a fever should be given at the time of immunisation. Local reactions are usually self-limiting and do not require treatment. If they appear to cause discomfort, then paracetamol or ibuprofen should be given. Do not use aspirin in children for such reactions.

> *Top tip!*
> There is no indication for prophylactic antipyretic use, anticipating local or systemic reactions.

■ What are immunisation reactions?

- Common reactions include pain, swelling or redness at the site of the injection, and these should be anticipated.
- Local adverse reactions generally start within a few hours of the injection and are usually mild and self-limiting. Although these are often referred to as 'hypersensitivity reactions', they are not allergic in origin, but may be either due to high titres of antibody or a direct effect of the vaccine product – e.g. endotoxin in whole-cell bacterial vaccines. The occurrence or severity of such local reactions does not contraindicate further doses of immunisation with the same vaccine or vaccines containing the same antigens.
- Systemic adverse reactions include fever, malaise, myalgia, irritability, headaches and loss of appetite. The timing of systemic reactions will vary according to the characteristics of the vaccine received, the age of the recipient and the biological response to that vaccine. For example, a fever may start within a few hours of tetanus-containing vaccines, but occurs 7 to 10 days after the measles-containing vaccine. The occurrence of such systemic reactions does not contraindicate further doses of the same vaccine or vaccines containing the same antigens.
- The 'Green Book' has the latest information on vaccines and vaccination procedures for vaccine preventable infectious diseases in the UK.

Time frames for vaccine-related reactions

Reactions to vaccines generally occur within specified time frames. Adverse reactions to inactivated vaccines generally occur within 48 hours following vaccination.

Many of the reactions that occur after the receipt of live viral vaccines are due to effective replication of the vaccine viruses. This is the case for all live vaccines. For example, in the case of the MMR vaccine:

- Reactions to the measles component (malaise, fever, rash) occur 6 to 11 days after vaccination because this is the amount of time it takes for the measles virus to replicate.
- Reactions to the rubella component (pain, stiffness or swelling of joints) usually occur 2 to 3 weeks after vaccination, but may occur up to 6 weeks after vaccination.
- Reactions to the mumps component (parotid swelling) usually occur 2 to 3 weeks after vaccination, but may occur up to 6 weeks after vaccination.

Live vaccines:

- With the exception of BCG, the frequency of adverse events falls with the number of doses of live vaccines. An example is the MMR vaccine: if an antibody is made in response to the vaccine following an initial dose, it neutralises the vaccine virus in subsequent doses.

Inactivated vaccines:

- The frequency and severity of adverse events may increase with the number of doses of inactivated vaccines. Examples include reactions to the tetanus and pertussis vaccines. If antibody levels are high following a previous vaccination of tetanus or pertussis, this antibody binds to the vaccine antigen in a subsequent dose of the vaccine. This causes an inflammatory response (such as a sore arm).

Top tip!
Most of the local and systemic adverse reactions to vaccination do not warrant or justify any change to subsequent immunisations.

■ What is the schedule for routine immunisation in preschool children?

The recommendations can vary from time to time and in different countries. Table 4.61 outlines the current recommendations for children in the UK.

Table 4.61 Routine immunisation schedule for preschool children in the UK		
When to immunise	What is given	How it is given
Age – 2 months	Diphtheria, tetanus, pertussis, polio, Haemophilus influenzae type b (DTaP/IPV/HiB)	One injection Pediacel
	Pneumococcal (PCV)	One injection Prevenar
	Rotavirus	One oral application
Age – 3 months	Diphtheria, tetanus, pertussis, polio, Haemophilus influenzae type b (DTaP/IPV/HiB)	One injection Pediacel
	Meningitis C (MenC)	One injection NeisVac-C or MeningiteC
	Rotavirus	One oral application
Age – 4 months	Diphtheria, tetanus, pertussis, polio, Haemophilus influenzae type b (DTaP/IPV/HiB)	One injection Pediacel
	Pneumococcal (PCV)	One injection Prevenar
	Meningitis C (MenC)	One injection NeisVac-C or MeningiteC
Age – 12 months	Haemophilus influenzae type b, meningitis C (HiB/MenC)	One injection Menitorix
Age – 13 months	Measles, mumps, rubella (MMR)	One injection Priorix or MMR II
	Pneumococcal (PCV)	One injection Prevenar
Age – 3 years and 4 to 5 years	Diphtheria, tetanus, pertussis, polio (dTaP/IPV or DTaP/IPV)	One injection Repevax or Infanrix-IPV
	Measles, mumps, rubella (MMR)	One injection Priorix or MMR II

Top tip!
Immunisation schedules are updated regularly, and it is important to keep update with the latest recommendations.

■ ***What are the contraindications to immunisation?***

Almost all children can safely receive all vaccines. It is emphasised that minor illnesses, without fever or systemic upsets, should not lead to a postponement of the immunisation. If acutely unwell, immunisation may be postponed until fully recovered. This is to avoid wrongly attributing any new symptom or the progression of existing symptoms to the vaccine. In individuals with an evolving neurological condition, certain immunisations should be deferred until the neurological condition has been resolved or stabilised.

However, all vaccines are contraindicated in those who have had:

- A confirmed anaphylactic reaction to a previous dose of a vaccine containing the same antigens.
- A confirmed anaphylactic reaction to another component contained in the relevant vaccine – e.g. neomycin, streptomycin or polymyxin B (which may be present in trace amounts in some vaccines).

Live vaccines should not be given to:

- Patients actively being treated for malignancy (chemotherapy, or generalised radiotherapy).
- Patients within 6 months of such treatment.
- Transplant patients on immunosuppressive drugs.
- Patients within 12 months of completing all immunosuppressive treatment and following bone marrow transplant.
- Within 3 months of adults receiving 40 milligram (mg) per day of prednisolone for more than a week.
- Within 3 months of children receiving certain doses of prednisolone (2 milligram (mg) per kilogram per day for 1 week or 1 milligram (mg) per kilogram per day for 1 month).
- When steroids and immunosuppressive drugs are being given together (the specialist in charge should be consulted).
- Patients with impaired cell-mediated immunity or immunodeficiency syndromes such as Wiskott-Aldrich syndrome, and severe combined immunodeficiency syndromes.
- Patients with immunosuppression due to HIV.

If immunoglobulin has been administered within the preceding 3 months, it may interfere with the immune response to live viral vaccines, as it may contain antibodies to measles, varicella and other viruses. Live viral vaccines should therefore not be given until 3 months after the administration of immunoglobulin. In addition, live viral vaccines should be administered at least 3 weeks before an injection of immunoglobulin. This does not apply to yellow fever, as immunoglobulin used in the UK is unlikely to contain high levels of antibody to this virus.

Egg allergy

Individuals with a confirmed anaphylactic reaction to egg should not receive the yellow fever vaccine. Individuals who have an egg allergy may be at increased risk of a reaction to some influenza vaccines.

All children with an egg allergy should receive the MMR vaccination as a routine procedure in primary care. Recent data suggest that anaphylactic reactions to the MMR vaccine are not associated with hypersensitivity to egg antigens but to other components of the vaccine (such as gelatin). Children who have had documented anaphylaxis to the vaccine should be assessed by a specialist in allergies.

Top tip!
Where there is doubt, rather than withholding the vaccine, advice should be sought from an appropriate consultant paediatrician or physician, the immunisation coordinator, or a consultant in health protection.

Additional information

Immunisation, which refers to protection from infection, can be achieved by natural disease or vaccination. Infection and vaccination provide **active immunity**, which is usually long-lasting. **Passive immunity** is passed from mother to infant through the placenta, or when receiving blood or blood products such as immunoglobulin. Passive immunity usually gives immediate protection, but the benefit lasts only for a short period of time. There is no evidence to suggest that vaccines can overload the immune system.

Inactive vaccines are made of killed or part of a killed organism, are weakly immunogenic and are less effective than an active vaccine in giving lifelong immunity. Thus, they are often combined with an adjuvant to improve their efficacy (Table 4.62).

Table 4.62: Inactivated vaccines	
Advantages	Disadvantages
They are relatively stable.	They usually require more than 1 dose.
Their constituents are more clearly defined.	Local reactions are more common than with live attenuated vaccines.
They are unable to cause the infection.	An adjuvant may be needed to stimulate or enhance the immune response.

Live vaccines are made of live organisms that are weakened or attenuated, and so do not cause the disease or only cause a mild form of it. They usually promote a full and lasting antibody response after 1 or 2 doses. Examples include MMR, yellow fever, varicella, oral typhoid, oral polio, and BCG, and they have several advantages (Table 4.63).

Table 4.63: Live attenuated vaccines	
Advantages	Disadvantages
They are highly immunogenic, usually promoting a full, long-lasting antibody response after 1 or 2 doses.	With some live vaccines, a mild form of the disease may rarely occur (e.g. a rash following the measles-containing vaccine).
	They can, in some situations, cause severe or fatal infections in immunocompromised individuals due to extensive replication of the vaccine virus strain.
	There is the potential for live attenuated vaccines to revert to their pathogenic form and cause serious illness. It is for this reason that the live polio vaccine (Sabin) has been replaced in many countries by the inactivated vaccine (Salk).

Combination vaccines make it easier to give several vaccines at 1 time – for example, DTaP/IPV/Hib, MMR and combined hepatitis A and hepatitis B. Combination vaccines reduce the number of injections and clinic visits needed.

Syllabus mapping

Infection, immunity and allergy

Knowledge

The candidate must:

- Understand the principles and the rationale behind the national immunisation programme for children in Britain.
- Know the indications, contraindications and complications of routine childhood immunisations, and be able to advise parents about immunisations.

Further reading and references

1. Bonhoeffer J, Siegrist CA, Heath PT. Immunisation of premature infants. *Arch Dis Child* 2006; 91: 929-935
2. Casiday RE, Cox AR. Restoring confidence in vaccines by explaining vaccine safety monitoring: is a targeted approach needed? *Drug Saf* 2006; 29: 1105-9
3. Gov.uk. Immunisation against infectious disease: The green book. 2013. https://www.gov.uk/government/publications/contraindications-and-special-considerations-the-green-book-chapter-6 (accessed August 2015).
4. Gov.uk. UK immunisation schedule: The green book. 2013. https://www.gov.uk/government/publications/immunisation-schedule-the-green-book-chapter-11 (accessed August 2015).

SECTION 5:
THE CLINICAL ASSESSMENT STATION

Chapter 5.1: Introduction
Dr Anna Mathew, Dr Rachel Varughese

A focused but thorough clinical examination is the foundation of good clinical practice. In this station, you will be presented with a child with a problem in any system of their body, so it is important to be confident in the examination of all systems.

In the DCH clinical examination, there is only 1 clinical assessment station, so candidates should be prepared to undertake examination of any system of the body. Adequate preparation is also required to undertake the necessary discussion that would follow the demonstration and the interpretation of the child's clinical findings.

What to expect

In the clinical assessment station, you will be given a task. You will be asked to:

- Examine a whole system (e.g. "please examine this child's respiratory system").
- Examine a part of a system (e.g. "please examine this child's legs").
- Just observe and report what you see (e.g. "please describe this child's facial features").

Where simple observation has been requested, the child should have features that the examiners are expecting you to notice. In such instances, if it is not possible to suggest a diagnosis, simply describing what is observed will be useful and could be all that the examiner is looking for. Some children with dysmorphism may not have a specific diagnosis; however, you should be familiar with the facial features of the most common chromosomal abnormalities.

It cannot be emphasised enough that it is important to **listen very carefully** to the examiners instructions and undertake only what has been asked. If uncertain, it is important to clarify this, as the examiner would be happy to repeat the 'opening statement' given.

Once instructions have been given, the examiner will observe the candidate's ability to:

- Develop a rapport with the child and parent.
- Examine in a structured and systematic manner.
- Complete the task in the time given.
- Summarise the key clinical findings.
- Undertake a discussion around the case.

Being able to demonstrate fluid, systematic and structured clinical skills in a short period of time on children of varied ages requires confidence and a well-honed approach. To reach the standard expected requires practice over time. Undertaking practice individually, with a partner or in small groups will enhance these skills and develop confidence that will help you perform better in stressful situations, such as a clinical examination where you are being directly observed.

When summarising physical findings with the examiner, report on the positive and important negative findings. Always remember that a 'normal' child could be present at the station and don't feel you must 'find' signs to report. If you 'make up' signs that are not present, you will be penalised by the examiner.

Opening statements

Since the potential cases in this station are many and diverse, this book cannot provide a complete list of all the possible cases you may encounter. The RCPCH has published a DCH syllabus and it is essential that all candidates refer to this syllabus when preparing for the examination (please refer to: http://www.rcpch.ac.uk/training-examinations-professional-development/assessment-and-examinations/examinations/syllabus).

Examples of 'opening statements' given by examiners are included below, but will vary depending on the cases the host recruits for that diet.

Sarah is now 10 years old and has just been admitted with her fourth chest infection in the last 6 months. Please examine her respiratory system.

Ben, who is 8 years old, has recently moved into the area and his GP has referred him due to a long-standing heart murmur. Please examine his cardiovascular system.

Emily, who is 6 years old, has needed repeated blood transfusions since she was born. Please examine her abdomen.

Shan, who is 12 years old, was born prematurely and she walks with a limp. Please conduct a neurological examination of her arms and legs.

Lilia, who is 7 years old, is the shortest girl in her class. Please carry out a general examination, reporting any features you may observe.

Managing time in the clinical assessment station

Timing: This is a 9-minute station. A knock will be given at 6 minutes to mark the end of the recommended time for demonstrating clinical skills, and examining the child. The remaining 3 minutes should be dedicated to summarising key clinical findings and undertaking further discussion around the case as directed by the examiner. As each station only allows 6 minutes to complete the clinical examination, it is important to be fluid and systematic in your approach. Failure to complete the task will lead to you being marked down.

When the bell rings: On entering the room, the examiner will take your mark sheet, introduce you to the parent and child, and give you specific instructions about the task in the form of an 'opening statement'. The examiner will then observe your interaction and examination technique. **Listen carefully** to the instructions given in the opening statement and carry out only what has been asked.

How consistency is ensured

Examiners work in pairs, reviewing all children recruited to help in the clinical station. They undertake a process of benchmarking called 'standard setting', where agreement is reached on the physical signs present, the complexity of the case, and what is the appropriate standard to be expected for this station in the examination. Based on these discussions, the examiners agree on an 'opening statement' to introduce each patient and explain the candidate's task. Pass/fail criteria and the questions that will follow in the 'discussion' time are agreed. This process is followed for all college clinical examinations, and provides consistency for the expected standard.

'Mark sheets' are specific for each station and help to guide examiners in their assessment of candidates. The sheets indicate the different areas examiners consider when awarding marks and, as importantly, areas where marks can be lost. Like the other 9-minute stations, this one carries 2 separate scores for each candidate – 1 for demonstrating structured, fluid and systematic clinical examination skills and 1 for the correct interpretation of clinical signs, differential diagnoses and the discussion around management planning (Appendix 5.11).

The RCPCH has developed 'anchor statements' that examiners refer to when deciding on pass/fail criteria during standard setting. They also use these for guidance when marking. Candidates should review these documents to familiarise themselves with the scoring criteria explained in the anchor statements (Appendix 5.12).

Setting the stage

Before you begin your examination, remember the key introductory steps, which can be remembered with the mnemonic WIPE.

Wash hands: Just like in a real-life clinical setting, hand washing remains the mainstay of infection control and is as important in the exam as in day-to-day clinical work. There should be facilities for hand washing or alcohol gel available.

Introduce yourself: It is important to make introductions to the parents as well as to the child. **P**ain, **P**ermission and **P**osition:

Make sure you identify any particularly *painful* areas and leave these areas of the examination until last.

Permission must be sought from the parent, and from the child if they are old enough to consent. This is a good opportunity to briefly explain what you are doing and why. Although the examiners will have explained to the parents and the child what will happen, it is important that you introduce yourself and gain permission to undertake the assessment.

Adequate *positioning* of the patient is important to facilitate a good examination, but these positions can be adapted to the age of the child. If the child is old enough, utilise their maturity and ask them to sit or stand to enable you to get easy access. It is always simpler and less time-consuming if the candidate moves around the child than for the child to move several times. If the child is very young, sitting them on their mother's lap may improve the level of cooperation.

Exposure: It is important to be sensitive to the modesty of the child. Children may respond better if you only expose the area you need to look at without undressing them fully, and if re-dress them upon completion of each stage. You can seek parental help with this to save time. Be aware of when a chaperone is required and of cultural sensitivities.

Technique

Follow the traditional method of ***inspection***, ***palpation***, ***percussion*** and ***auscultation***. It is important, however, to not be too rigid about this depending on the age of the child. Ensure you let the examiner know when and why you are deviating from the traditional technique.

All instructions given to the child should be done quietly, confidently and empathetically. If, for any reason, the child is unwilling to be examined, help can be sought from the mother and sitting the child on the mother's lap may be helpful. If this fails, then the examiner will step in to help or alter the task that has been set for you.

Always undertake the clinical examination from the right side of the patient.

Consider carefully how you will report your clinical findings: whether you will do this as you go along, reporting findings to the examiner, or whether you will wait until you complete the task before doing so. Either way, once you commit to your approach, stick to it. Otherwise, it may reveal lack of practice or clinical confidence. Some systems lend themselves better to one or the other approach and, with practice, you can decide for yourself which approach you prefer.

Be prepared to summarise your clinical findings and undertake further discussion in the 3 minutes before the end of the station. Discussion will be around:

- Differential diagnoses of your findings.
- Investigations that may help make a diagnosis or rule out possible diagnoses.
- Management of the case.

Make sure you thank the parent and child before leaving the room.

Syllabus mapping

Skills

The candidate must:

- Be able to handle babies and children of different age groups comfortably and with confidence.
- Be able to perform a general and systemic physical examination of children of different age groups opportunistically and with empathy.
- Be able to explain, and counsel children and the family on, the conclusions reached.
- Demonstrate good generic communication skills when dealing with children and adolescents.
- Recognise special needs of adolescents during consultation.
- Be able to maintain appropriate interaction with special needs children.

Further reading and references

RCPCH (2015) 'DCH Clinical Examination 2013 Syllabus': http://www.rcpch.ac.uk/training-examinations-professional-development/assessment-and-examinations/examinations/dch-clinical (accessed March 2015).

Appendix 5.11: Mark Sheet (Front and Back): Clinical Assessment Station

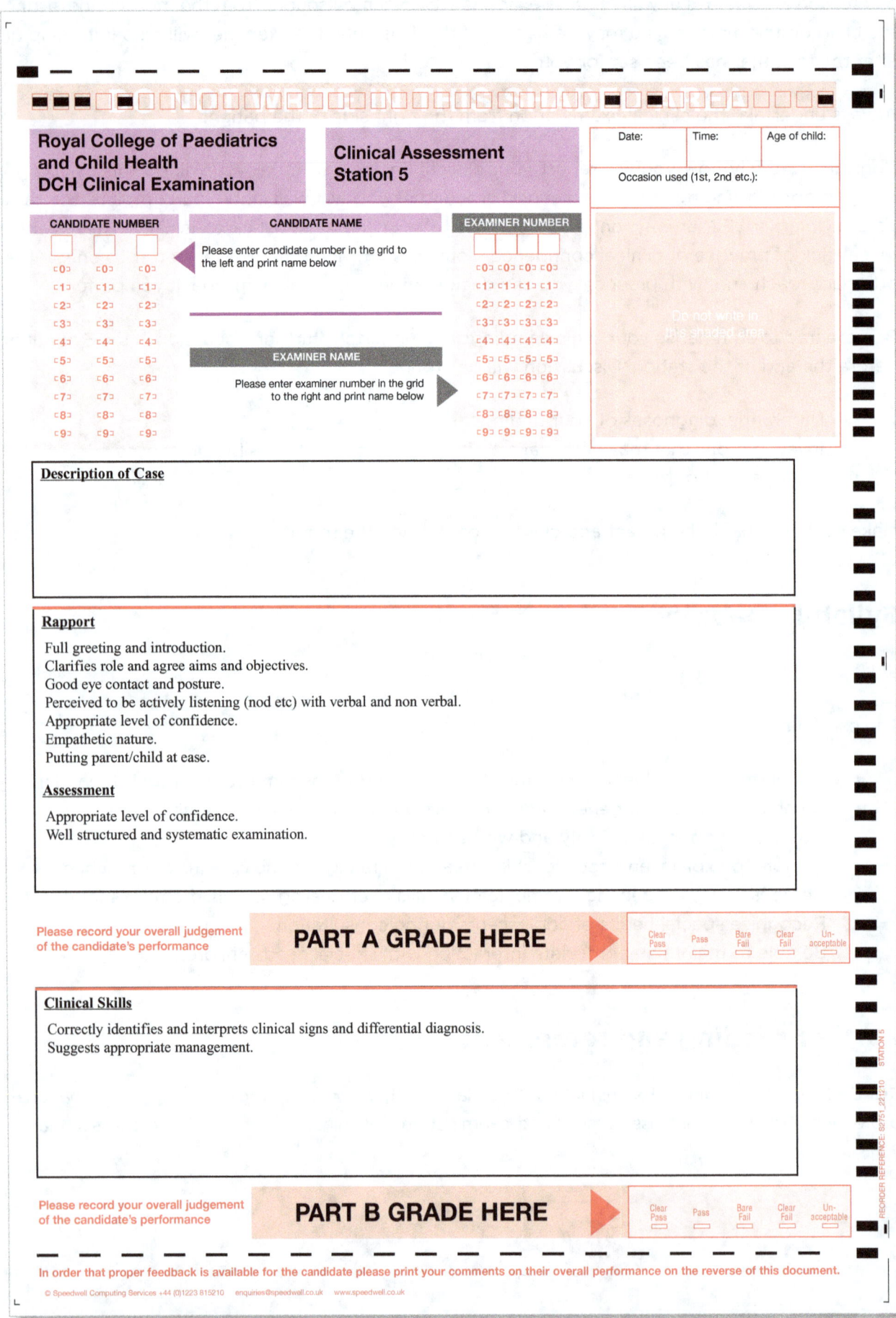

☐ Disorganised and unsystematic approach (please add additional comments)

☐ Missed physical signs / ☐ Found physical signs not present (please add additional comments)

☐ Poor time management (please add additional comments)

☐ Inaccurate assessment/conclusion (please add additional comments)

Please add any additional comments here:

Appendix 5.12: Anchor Statement: Clinical Assessment Station

	Expected Standard/ CLEAR PASS	PASS	BARE FAIL	CLEAR FAIL	UNACCEPTABLE
RAPPORT	Full greeting and introduction. Clarifies role and agrees aims and objectives. Good eye contact and posture. Perceived to be actively listening (nod etc) with verbal and non-verbal. Appropriate level of confidence. Empathetic nature. Putting parent/child at ease.	Adequately performed but not fully fluent in conducting interview.	Incomplete or hesitant greeting and introduction. Inadequate identification of role, aims and objectives. Poor eye contact and posture. Not perceived to be actively listening (nod etc) with verbal and non-verbal cues. Does not show appropriate level of confidence, empathetic nature or putting parent/child at ease.	Significant components omitted or not achieved.	Dismissive of parent/child concerns. Fails to put parent or child at ease.
CLINICAL SKILLS	Appropriate level of confidence. Well-structured and systematic examination. Correctly identifies and interprets clinical signs and differential diagnosis. Suggests appropriate management.	Majority of clinical skills demonstrated accurately eliciting the majority of physical signs correctly. Identifies majority of signs correctly. May need some prompting and may be some lack of fluency.	Too many minor errors. Examination technique not well structured. Non-fluent approach.	Misses several important clinical signs. Slow, uncertain, unstructured, unsystematic examination.	Misses crucial important clinical signs or potentially dangerous interpretation. Rough handling of child. Disregards child's distress or shyness or modesty.

Chapter 5.2: Case Study 1: Respiratory: 10 Year Old with Cystic Fibrosis

Dr Rachel Varughese, Dr Elliott Ridgeon

This station assesses your ability to demonstrate the respiratory examination of a child, interpret the physical findings, and conduct a discussion with the examiner. You will be assessed on the rapport, manner and structure of your examination with the child and parent.

Logistics:

Timing: This is a 9-minute station. A knock at 6 minutes will denote that 3 minutes remain before the end of the station. At this point, it is important to summarise your clinical findings and proceed with the discussion with the examiner.

When the bell rings: On entering the room, the examiner will greet you, take your mark sheet, introduce you to the child and parent, and give you your task. Listen carefully to these instructions.

The examiner will then remain mostly silent during the consultation, as they will be observing your clinical skills, but may provide some direction should it be required. A discussion around the case will be undertaken in the final 3 minutes of the station.

If you finish early, you will be asked to remain in the room until the session has ended.

Candidate role and task:

You are an ST3 GP trainee working in the day unit.

Sarah is 10 years old. She has been admitted with her fourth chest infection in the last 6 months.

Task: You are asked to examine her respiratory system.

The respiratory examination

Inspection

Close and observant inspection is essential to arrive at a diagnosis. This is especially important for infants and young children, where most of the information needs to be gained from inspection and auscultation.

End of the bed

- Judge the severity of the illness. Does the child look well or does she look ill?
- Is the child receiving oxygen or is she connected to monitors? If so, what are the readings?
- Look for respiratory aids. Particular devices to look for are spacers, inhalers and peak flow meters.
- A visual judgement of growth and nutritional status should be made (with a subsequent offer to plot height and weight on the appropriate growth chart).

- Look for signs of respiratory distress.
    - Stridor or wheeze
    - Use of accessory muscles (sternocleidomastoid strain, intercostal recession, use of abdominal muscles, nasal flaring, head bob in an infant)
    - Cyanosis
    - Inability to complete full sentences
    - Grunting
- Take notice of the presence of a cough, and the nature of this (e.g. dry, chesty, barking).
- Count the respiratory rate.
    - Infant: 20-40/min
    - 5 year old: 15-25/min
    - 10 year old: 15-20/min

Top tip!
In older children, it may be helpful to count the respiratory rate at the same time as feeling the pulse. This will save you time, and will not cause the child to be self-conscious and modify their breathing while you count.

Hands and arms

- Count the pulse rate.
- Tremor – This may indicate salbutamol overuse. To elicit this further, you could place a piece of paper on the dorsum of an outstretched hand.
- Clubbing – The most common causes for clubbing in children are cystic fibrosis and congenital cyanotic heart disease. Other gastrointestinal causes (e.g. inflammatory bowel disease) could also be considered.
- Scar on the upper arm from previous percutaneous long lines (PICC lines) – This indicates previous admissions that required extended courses of antibiotics.

Face

- Cyanosis – This is best assessed centrally by asking the child to point their tongue to the ceiling and noting the colour underneath.
- Conjunctival pallor – Gently pull down the lower eyelid (one is enough). Pale conjunctivae indicate anaemia.
- Tracheostomy scar on the lower neck.

Chest

- Chest wall deformity:
    - Pectus excavatum (hollow chest)
    - Pectus carinatum (pigeon chest)
- Symmetry – Asymmetrical in terms of pulmonary fibrosis and pulmonary hypoplasia.
- Hyperinflation – Barrel chest indicates chronic obstructive airway disease, e.g. asthma.
- Harrison's sulcus – Poor asthma control.
- Hickman line or portacath (long-term or repeated courses of antibiotics, e.g. in cystic fibrosis).
- Scars (e.g. chest drain, thoracotomy, sternotomy).

Palpation

Tracheal deviation

- This should only be routinely assessed in the older child, as it can cause discomfort.
- Deviation may occur towards the same side with lung collapse, or away from the side with pleural effusion or tension pneumothorax.

Apex beat

- Feel for the apex beat. Displacement may indicate a mediastinal shift.

Top tip!
Place both of your hands on the sides of the chest to feel the apex – this will help to diagnose dextrocardia, an occasional association with recurrent chest infections due to bronchiectasis.

Chest expansion

- Place thumbs parasternally, wrapping hands around the chest wall and keeping thumbs loose to the chest. Note the movement of thumbs away from the centre; look for symmetry.

Tactile fremitus

- The same principles as with vocal resonance apply. Attempt this only if you have enough time. Place the ulnar border of the hand along an intercostal space, and ask the child to say "99". Compare the character of the vibration felt on the hand symmetrically on both sides of the chest. These vibrations are typically increased over an area of consolidation, and decreased with collapse, or fluid.

Percussion

Compare symmetrically between the 2 lung fields.

Resonant – Normal lung

Dull percussion – *Things that are denser than alveoli filled with air.*

- Pleural effusion, consolidation, collapse, fibrosis

Hyperresonant percussion – *Things that are less dense than alveoli filled with air.*

- Pneumothorax, emphysema

Top tip!
Continue to complete the examination of the front of the chest before moving to the back of the chest. This will avoid discomfort to the child from frequent repositioning.

Auscultation

Compare symmetrically between the 2 lung fields, and describe the quality of breath sounds, commenting on any added sounds (Table 5.21).

Table 5.21: Breath sounds and interpretation	
Breath sounds	**Causes**
Vesicular breathing	Normal
Diminished breath sounds	Collapse, pleural effusion, pneumothorax
Bronchial breathing	Consolidation, fibrosis
Expiratory wheeze	Asthma, foreign body
Crepitations (crackles)	Fine (pulmonary oedema, fibrosis), coarse (consolidation, bronchiectasis)

Vocal resonance

Auscultate all lung fields and ask the child to say "99" while you are auscultating.

- Increased – Consolidation
- Reduced – Collapse, fluid

> *Top tip!*
> Interpreting your auscultatory findings:
>
> To help with recognition of bronchial breathing, listen over the trachea of a healthy patient, as it is simply transmitted sounds of turbulent airflow in large airways.
>
> Bilateral wheezing indicates obstructive airways disease, e.g. asthma. Unilateral wheezing indicates the presence of a mechanical obstruction, e.g. foreign body or mass.
>
> Vocal resonance is the sound of air passing from the airway, via the chest wall, to the stethoscope. Anything that provides a barrier produces decreased resonance, e.g. pleural effusion, pneumothorax, and collapse. Solids transmit sound better than gases, so resonance is increased in consolidation.

> *Thinking time!*
> Once you have auscultated all areas and elicited all signs, keep up the appearance of auscultating while you put all your findings together and get ready to present!

Assimilating the signs

Now that you have conducted a thorough general respiratory examination, you will be expected to assimilate and present your positive clinical findings in order to arrive at a differential diagnosis. Below is a summary of the signs elicited from Sarah, and an example presentation.

End of the bed – Persistent cough, productive of purulent sputum. Respiratory rate is 24/min. Mild intercostal and subcostal recession

Hands – Finger clubbing

Chest – Portacath palpable, scattered coarse inspiratory crepitations

To present...

"Sarah is a 10 year old child who has been admitted with her fourth chest infection in the last 6 months. On examination, she looks comfortable at rest and well grown. However, I would like to confirm that later by plotting her height and weight on the growth chart. She has evidence of finger clubbing; she is not pale or cyanosed. I was able to palpate a portacath device on her upper chest wall. Her respiratory rate is 24/min; she has mild intercostal and subcostal recession. Chest expansion is equal bilaterally, the percussion note is resonant and the breath sounds vesicular, with a few scattered coarse crepitations over both lung fields.

The combination of Sarah's history, presence of finger clubbing, portacath and signs of an intercurrent chest infection raises the probability of a chronic suppurative lung condition, and I would like to consider cystic fibrosis as the most likely diagnosis."

Discussion

Now that you have arrived at a likely diagnosis, there is time for a discussion with the examiner about this condition. Possible questions from the examiner are highlighted below. It is unlikely all of these can be asked within the given time frame.

■ What is the differential diagnosis for a child with repeated chest infections?

These can be listed, as it is unlikely there will be time to undertake a detailed discussion on any of these differentials.

- Cystic fibrosis
- Immune deficiency
- Primary ciliary dyskinesia
- Gastro-oesophageal reflux
- Inhaled foreign body
- Other rarer causes

■ What is cystic fibrosis?

Cystic fibrosis is an autosomal recessive condition involving gene mutations of the cystic fibrosis transmembrane conductance regulator (CFTR) protein – a membrane chloride channel. This leads to abnormalities in the transportation of ions across the epithelial cells lining the airways, leading to a reduction in the availability of surface liquid and consequent viscid secretions. This problem is perpetuated in other organs of the body, notably the gastrointestinal tract, the pancreas and the reproductive organs.

Cystic fibrosis affects 1 in every 2,500 children in the UK, with an asymptomatic carrier rate of 1:25. There are currently 1,900 identified mutations in the CFTR gene linked to the diagnosis of cystic fibrosis. The most common in the Caucasian population is DELTA F508. Cystic fibrosis is a multisystem disorder that can affect several organs of the body. It frequently presents with recurrent chest infections, signs of poor growth and malabsorption. In the developed world, patients under close management due to an early diagnosis may display normal growth with the aid of detailed feeding plans.

■ What organ systems can be affected by cystic fibrosis?

Respiratory tract – The tendency to repeated chest infections that ultimately lead to bronchiectasis is the hallmark of cystic fibrosis. Gene mutations lead to an interruption in the availability of surface liquid and the accumulation of thick, viscid secretions. This affects ciliary function on the epithelial lining of the airways, resulting in impaired mucociliary clearance and repeated chest infections. Sputum cultures or cough swabs over time typically reveal the presence of Staphylococcus aureus, Haemophillus influenzae or Pseudomonas aeruginosa.

Gastrointestinal tract – Thick, viscid meconium can cause meconium ileus in infants and intestinal obstruction in older children. Rectal prolapse occurs in about 10% of patients with cystic fibrosis.

Pancreas – Most children with cystic fibrosis display evidence of pancreatic insufficiency and subsequent malabsorption. Pancreatic duct blockage causes this exocrine insufficiency.

Reproductive tract – Most males are azospermic and infertile as a result. This is due to congenital absence of the vas deferens.

■ What investigations are routinely carried out to support a diagnosis of cystic fibrosis?

Sweat test – The gold-standard diagnostic investigation is the sweat test. This will reliably make the diagnosis for 98% of patients. Patient with cystic fibrosis have an elevated concentration of chloride (60–125 mmol/L) compared to the normal (10–40 mmol/L).

Cystic fibrosis genotype – Diagnosis can be confirmed by identifying CFTR protein gene abnormalities. In spite of there being 1,900 mutations, a cystic fibrosis genotype request usually only screens for the most common 50 mutations, as a large number of the identified mutations are extremely rare.

Faecal elastase – This looks for the presence of the pancreatic enzyme Elastase in the stool. Low levels indicate the presence of pancreatic insufficiency, further supporting the diagnosis of cystic fibrosis.

Neonatal immunoreactive trypsinogen (IRT) screening – In the UK, universal neonatal heel-prick screening tests for IRT. Abnormally raised levels increase the likelihood of cystic fibrosis, and are an indication that further testing is needed to help confirm the diagnosis.

■ What are the broad approaches to the management of children with cystic fibrosis?

The mainstay of management is a multidisciplinary team approach with shared-care cystic fibrosis centres in the UK. Important members of the team include paediatricians, physiotherapists, specialist nurses, dieticians, psychologists, the GP and the family.

Management broadly involves attention towards the respiratory and gastrointestinal tract.

Respiratory management

- Antibiotics – Prophylactic oral antibiotics are prescribed at diagnosis on a continuous basis. The choice of antibiotic can change over time, depending on the respiratory tract culture results. This almost invariably includes nebulised antibiotics over time.
- Additional *oral antibiotics* are often necessary to manage increasing respiratory symptoms, sputum production or a drop in lung function.

- With persistent infective symptoms, admission for *IV antibiotics* is necessary, with a long line often required for ongoing IV access over the length of the hospital admission. A more long-term solution for subsequent IV access if antibiotics are to become regular will need to be considered in the form of a totally implanted central venous access device, such as a portacath.
- Chest physiotherapy – This is routinely recommended twice a day when well, and more often when unwell. Physiotherapists are closely involved with the family, as physiotherapy techniques vary with age and levels of independence and thus change as the child gets older.

Other respiratory treatments

- Dornase alfa (DNase) – DNase is a synthetic enzyme that breaks down neutrophil-derived DNA in sputum, reducing the viscosity and thereby hopefully helping sputum removal. It is now routinely prescribed in some centres for all cystic fibrosis children over the age of 6 years, regardless of their lung function status.
- Hypertonic saline (HS) – HS is used to induce sputum in symptomatic children where a positive culture is needed to guide treatment. It can also be used as part of their regular physiotherapy package. If used, it is usually administered prior to physiotherapy. As HS can cause bronchoconstriction, physiotherapists should oversee its initial administration so that this can be managed effectively with bronchodilators if necessary.
- Lung transplant – In end-stage lung disease, bilateral sequential lung transplantation can be considered.

Gastrointestinal tract

- Nutritional management is essential, with *pancreatic replacement therapy*, replacement *fat-soluble vitamins* and *high-calorie diets* sometimes being supplemented with overnight feeding via a gastrostomy. *Constipation* is treated if and when it presents as per national guidelines.

Disability Living Allowance (DLA)

- All children with cystic fibrosis will be eligible for DLA.

Syllabus mapping

Respiratory medicine with ENT

Knowledge

The candidate must:

- Know and understand the pathophysiology of cystic fibrosis and understand the principles of treatment.

Skills

The candidate must:

- Be able to examine the respiratory system, as well as interpret and discuss physical findings.

Further reading and references

1. Lissauer T et al. *Illustrated Textbook of Paediatrics*, 4th edition. Edinburgh: Mosby, 2012: 17–18.
2. Newell SJ, Darling JC. *Paediatrics Lecture Notes*, 9th edition. Chichester: Wiley-Blackwell: 2014; 19: 186–188.
3. Ratjen F, Döring G. Cystic fibrosis. *Lancet* 2003; 22; 361(9358): 681–9
4. RCPCH (2015) 'DCH Clinical Examination 2013 Syllabus', pp. 29: http://www.rcpch.ac.uk/training-examinations-professional-development/assessment-and-examinations/examinations/dch-clinical (accessed April 2015).
5. Royal Brompton Hospital Paediatric Cystic Fibrosis Team. *Clinical Guidelines: Care of children with Cystic Fibrosis*. Royal Brompton Hospital, 6th edition. 2014.
6. Rudolf M, Lee T, Levene M. *Paediatrics and Child Health*, 3rd edition. Chichester: Wiley-Blackwell, 2011: 66–69.

Video resources

http://learnpediatrics.com/videos/ (accessed April 2015).
https://www.youtube.com/user/MRCPCHRevision (accessed April 2015).

Chapter 5.3: Case Study 2: Abdomen: 7 Year Old with Intermittent Jaundice

Dr Geethika Bandaranayake, Dr Anna Mathew

This station assesses your ability to demonstrate the examination of the abdomen, interpret physical findings and conduct a discussion with the examiner. You will be assessed on the rapport, manner and structure of your examination with the child and parent.

Logistics:

Timing: This is a 9-minute station. A knock at 6 minutes will denote that 3 minutes remain before the end of the station. At this point, it is important to summarise your clinical findings and proceed with the discussion with the examiner.

When the bell rings: On entering the room, the examiner will greet you, take your mark sheet, introduce you to the child and parent, and give you your task. Listen carefully to these instructions.

The examiner will then remain mostly silent during the consultation, as they will be observing your clinical skills, but may provide some direction should it be required. A discussion around the case will be undertaken in the final 3 minutes of the station.

If you finish early, you will be asked to remain in the room until the session has ended.

Candidate role and task:

You are a GP trainee working on the paediatric day unit.

Devika, a 7 year old girl, came for her routine clinic follow-up. She has a past history of intermittent jaundice.

Task: Please examine her abdomen.

The abdominal examination

Inspection

End of the bed

- Judge the severity of the illness. Does the child look well or does she look ill?
- Look around for feeding support – feeding pumps, percutaneous endoscopic gastrostomy (PEG) tubes, etc.
- A visual judgement of growth and nutritional status should be made, with an offer to plot the height and weight on an appropriate growth chart.
- Does she have any dysmorphic features to suggest a syndrome or storage disorder?
- Hands – Look closely at the hands. Search for finger clubbing (chronic liver disease, rarely in inflammatory bowel disease), leuconychia, palmar erythema, flapping tremors (these are all features of chronic liver disease but are rare nowadays, as most of the children are managed well).

- Face – Look at the face. Search for pallor (a sign of chronic haemolytic anaemia), jaundice (chronic liver involvement, acute haemolytic disease).
- Mouth – Inspect the mouth. Search for aphthous ulcers (inflammatory bowel disease), any perioral pigmentation, or large tongue (storage disorders).
- Lymph nodes – Check for any lymphadenopathy.
- Spider naevi – The presence of this is evidence of chronic liver disease. This is usually distributed over the area drained by the superior vena cava, and occurs due to abnormal oestrogen metabolism.

Abdomen

- Abdominal distension
    - Central or generalised
    - Symmetrical or asymmetrical (look from the foot end of the bed)
- Scars – Examine both anterior and posterior abdomen (Figure 5.31).
- Dilated veins – "Evidence of collaterals".
- Scratch marks may signify obstructive jaundice.
- Pigmentation could be due to thalassaemia and iron overload.

Figure 5.31: Common abdominal surgical scars in children (refer to Table 5.31 for details) (Illustration by Dr G Bandaranayake)

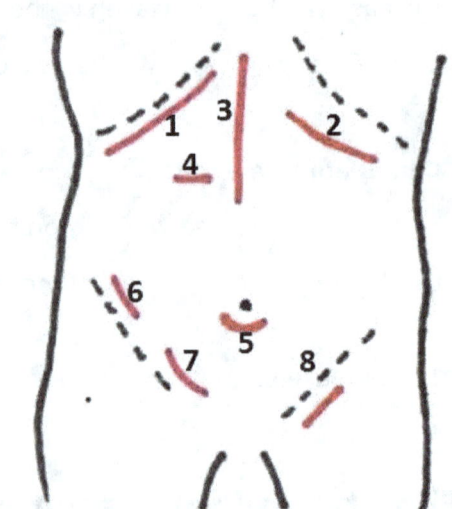

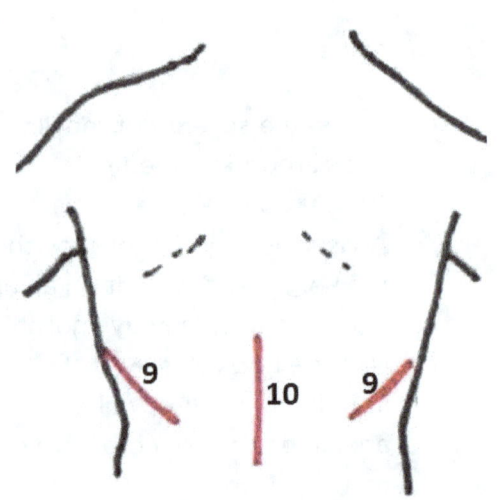

Table 5.31: Common abdominal surgical scars in children (numbers refer to Figure 5.31)
1. Kocher's incision – Liver surgery, surgery for biliary atresia (Kasai procedure)
2. Transverse upper abdominal – Splenectomy, repair of congenital diaphragmatic hernia
3. Upper mid-line – Nissen fundoplication (severe reflux)
4. Right upper transverse – Ramstedt's pyloromyotomy (pyloric stenosis)
5. Subumbilical – Exomphalos or gastroschisis repair
6. Gridiron incision – Appendicectomy
7. Hockey stick scar – Renal transplant
8. Inguinal scar – Inguinal hernia repair
9. Lateral thoracolumbar – Renal surgery
10. Midline (lumbar area) – Neural tube defect repair

Palpation

- Superficial palpation of all the areas of the abdomen is done to assess the presence of any tenderness. Always look at the child's face while doing this, and stop if you are causing pain.
- Deep palpation is undertaken to look for any palpable abdominal masses.
    - Liver – Check the span, presence of tenderness, consistency and percuss for the upper border (Table 5.32).
    - Spleen – Palpate initially in supine position. If unable to palpate, turn the patient onto their side, towards you (Table 5.33).
    - Kidney – Undertake bimanual palpation (ballottement).
    - Any other masses.

Percussion

Tympanic note – Normal abdomen signifying air in the bowel.

Dull note to the percussion – Suggests the presence of a mass/fluid in the abdomen.

- Check for shifting dullness, horse-shoe dullness, and fluid thrill, which suggests the presence of ascites.

Auscultation

- Listen for bowel sounds and renal bruits (e.g. renal artery stenosis).

In addition

- Offer to examine the hernia orifices and anal area (for tags and fistula), and offer a stool examination in an infant if required.

Table 5.32: Causes of hepatosplenomegaly	
Haematological	Thalassaemia, hereditary spherocytosis
Infection	Viral illnesses (glandular fever, EBV [Epstein Barr Virus])
Hepatic	Cirrhosis, biliary atresia, autoimmune hepatitis, all causes of portal hypertension
Malignancy	Leukaemia, lymphoma
Storage disorders	Glycogen storage disorders, mucopolysaccharidoses
Metabolic	Wilson's disease, Alpha-1 antitrypsin deficiency, tyrosinaemia
Connective tissue disorders (rarely)	SLE (Systemic Lupus Erythematosis), juvenile idiopathic arthritis (systemic type)

Thinking time!
Once you have completed the examination and elicited all the signs, put all your findings together and get ready to present.

Assimilating the signs

Now that you have conducted a thorough abdominal examination, you will be expected to assimilate and present your positive clinical findings in order to arrive at a possible diagnosis. Below is a summary of the signs elicited from Devika, and an example presentation.

> "Devika is a 7 year old girl who looks well and comfortable. She is adequately grown for her age but I would like to plot her growth on an appropriate centile chart. She has mild jaundice with subtle pallor. She does not have features of chronic liver involvement, such as palmar erythema, spider naevi or any evidence of portal hypertension. There are no obvious surgical scars and her abdomen is soft and non-tender. There is a 4-cm firm spleen that is palpable. No hepatomegaly or any other masses are felt. To complete my examination, I also looked at her mother and she does not demonstrate any jaundice.
>
> My findings are clinically consistent with uncomplicated haemolytic condition, most likely hereditary spherocytosis. She may benefit from an elective splenectomy."

Discussion

After presenting your clinical findings, you will discuss the case with the examiner. Some possible questions from the examiner are highlighted below. It is unlikely all of these can be asked within the given time frame.

■ *What is the mode of inheritance of hereditary spherocytosis?*

- Autosomal dominant.

■ *What are the common presentations of hereditary spherocytosis?*

- Neonatal jaundice (can occur within the first 24 hours of life)
- Pallor with fluctuating jaundice
- Splenomegaly (later in life)
- Pigment gallstones – Can cause cholecystitis
- Haemolytic crisis following parvovirus B19 infection
- Leg ulcers
- Positive family history

■ *What are the principles of management of hereditary spherocytosis?*

- Confirmation of diagnosis – Full blood count, raised reticulocyte count (evidence of haemolysis) and blood film (look for spherocytes) and liaison with a paediatric haematologist for advice on specific confirmatory test.
- May need blood transfusion in an acute haemolysis.
- Folic acid supplementation.
- Elective splenectomy usually after 7 years of age. The child must be vaccinated against Haemophilus influenzae b, meningitis C and Streptococcus pneumoniae prior to the surgery.
- Ideally, oral penicillin for life following the removal of the spleen to prevent sepsis due to Polysaccharide capsular bacteria (Pneumococcus, Meningococcus and Haemophilus influenzae b).

■ *Why is a splenectomy beneficial in this condition?*

- In hereditary spherocytosis, due to an abnormal red cell membrane protein, the surface area of the cells is reduced. These spherical red cells have decreased deformability and, as such, get destroyed mainly by the spleen. By removal of the site of destruction (splenectomy), the patient improves clinically but the primary condition persists.

■ *Please mention a few causes of haemolytic anaemia.*

- Red cell membrane disorders, e.g. hereditary spherocytosis
- Red cell enzyme disorders, e.g. Glucose-6-phosphate dehydrogenase deficiency
- Haemoglobinopathies, e.g. thalassaemia major, sickle cell disease

Syllabus mapping

Gastroenterology and hepatology

Knowledge

The candidate must:

- Know the causes of neonatal and childhood jaundice and when to refer.

Skills

The candidate must:

- Be able to perform a general and systemic physical examination of children of different age groups opportunistically and with empathy.
- Be able to examine the gastrointestinal system, as well as interpret and discuss physical findings.

Further reading and references

1. Kliegman RM, Stanton BF, St Geme JW et al. *Nelson Textbook of Pediatrics*, 19th edition. Philadelphia: Elsevier, 2015: 1375.
2. Lissauer T, Clayden G. *Illustrated Textbook of Paediatrics*, 4th edition. 2012. Edinburgh: Mosby. pp. 20-22.
3. Newell SJ, Darling JC. *Paediatrics Lecture Notes*, 9th edition. Chichester: Wiley-Blackwell: 2014; 8:76-78
4. RCPCH (2015) 'DCH Clinical Examination 2013 Syllabus', pp 13: http://www.rcpch.ac.uk/training-examinations-professional-development/assessment-and-examinations/examinations/dch-clinical (accessed April 2015).
5. Rudolf M, Lee T, Levene M. *Paediatrics and Child Health*, 3rd edition. Chichester: Wiley-Blackwell, 2011: 66-69.
6. Sidwell R, Thomson M. *Concise Paediatrics*, 2nd edition. CRC Press, 2009: 179, 182, 184-185.

Video resources

http://learnpediatrics.com/videos/ (accessed April 2015).
https://www.youtube.com/user/MRCPCHRevision (accessed April 2015).

Chapter 5.4: Case Study 3: Cardiovascular: 2 Year Old Post Cardiac Surgery
Dr P Venugopalan

This station assesses your ability to demonstrate the cardiovascular examination of a child, interpret physical findings and conduct a discussion with the examiner. You will be assessed on the rapport, manner and structure of your examination with the child and parent.

Logistics:

Timing: This is a 9-minute station. A knock at 6 minutes will denote that 3 minutes remain before the end of the station. At this point, it is important to summarise your clinical findings and proceed with the discussion with the examiner.

When the bell rings: On entering the room, the examiner will greet you, take your mark sheet, introduce you to the child and parent, and give you your task. Listen carefully to these instructions.

The examiner will then remain mostly silent during the consultation, as they will be observing your clinical skills, but may provide some direction should it be required. A discussion around the case will be undertaken in the final 3 minutes of the station.

If you finish early, you will be asked to remain in the room until the session has ended.

Candidate role and task:

You are an ST3 GP trainee working in the paediatric outpatient clinic.

Emily is a 2 year old. She had cardiac surgery at the age of 6 months. She has come for a routine follow-up visit.

Task: You are asked to examine her heart.

The cardiovascular examination

Inspection

End of the bed

- Judge the severity of the illness. Does the child look well or does she look ill?
- Comment on her growth. Offer to measure and plot weight and height on the appropriate growth chart.
- Does she have any dysmorphic features that suggest a syndrome, such as Down's syndrome, William's syndrome, etc.?
- Is the child receiving oxygen or is she connected to monitors? If so, what are the readings?
- Look for signs of heart failure.
    - Shortness of breath
    - Use of accessory muscles – Nasal flaring, sternocleidomastoid strain, intercostal and subcostal recession, and use of abdominal muscles
    - Cyanosis, and offer to check oxygen saturations using a pulse oximeter.

- Count the respiratory rate.
    - Infant: 20-40/min
    - 5 year old: 15-25/min
    - 10 year old: 15-20/min

Top tip!
General examination is important, as it can give clues to the presence of an underlying syndrome, as well as the effect of the heart disease on the growth of the child.

Hands and legs

- Count the pulse rate.
    - Infant: 100-180/min
    - 5 year old: 70-110/min
    - 10 year old: 55-90/min
- Clubbing – The most common cardiac causes for clubbing in children are congenital cyanotic heart disease, and infective endocarditis. Other causes include cystic fibrosis and inflammatory bowel disease.
- Peripheral signs of infective endocarditis – These include Osler's nodes, clubbing, subungual bleeds.
- Scar on upper arm from previous PICC (peripherally inserted central catheter) lines – This indicates previous admissions that required extended courses of antibiotics (e.g. for endocarditis).
- Look for pedal oedema (or sacral oedema in infants)
- Feel for the femoral pulses and also check for radio-femoral delay, after taking permission from the child and/or the parent. In adolescents, request permission from the examiner.

Face

- Cyanosis – This is best assessed centrally by asking the child to point their tongue to the ceiling and noting the colour underneath. Offer to check oxygen saturation using a pulse oximeter at some stage in the presentation.
- Conjunctival pallor – Gently pull down the lower eyelid (one is enough). Pale conjunctivae indicate anaemia, and plethoric conjunctivae indicate polycythaemia (which signify long-standing systemic desaturation). Warn the child that you are going to examine the eyes.
- Healed scars on the sides of the neck – Cannulation for central venous access or for extracorporeal membrane oxygenation (ECMO).
- Tracheostomy scar in the neck – Heart diseases may be associated with tracheo/bronchomalacia, occasionally requiring long-term ventilation.

Chest

- Chest wall deformity:
    - Pectus excavatum (hollow chest)
    - Pectus carinatum (pigeon chest)
- Symmetry – Asymmetrical due to left ventricular hypertrophy, or dextrocardia
- Harrison's sulcus – Long-standing heart failure in infancy
- Hickman line or portacath (long-term or repeated courses of antibiotics, e.g. for endocarditis)

- Scars (Figure 5.41)
    - Thoracotomy – Patent ductus arteriosus (PDA) ligation, repair of the coarctation of the aorta, pulmonary artery banding
    - Sternotomy – Open-heart surgery, and also in babies with low birth weight for cardiac surgery in the place of a thoracotomy
    - Chest drain – Seen in the mid-axillary area, and also in the epigastrium
    - Scars of pacing wires – Usually seen in the epigastrium. These reflect sites of exit of pacing wires that are left on the external surface of the heart for 24 hours following open-heart surgery (to facilitate management of post-op cardiac arrhythmias).

Figure 5.41: Diagrams showing scars on the chest following cardiac surgery. Left-hand diagram (5.41a) shows the front of the chest with a central sternotomy scar and epigastric scars (from chest drains and pacemaker leads). Right-hand diagram (5.41b) shows the back of the chest with right and left thoracotomy scars. (Illustration by Dr G Bandaranayake)

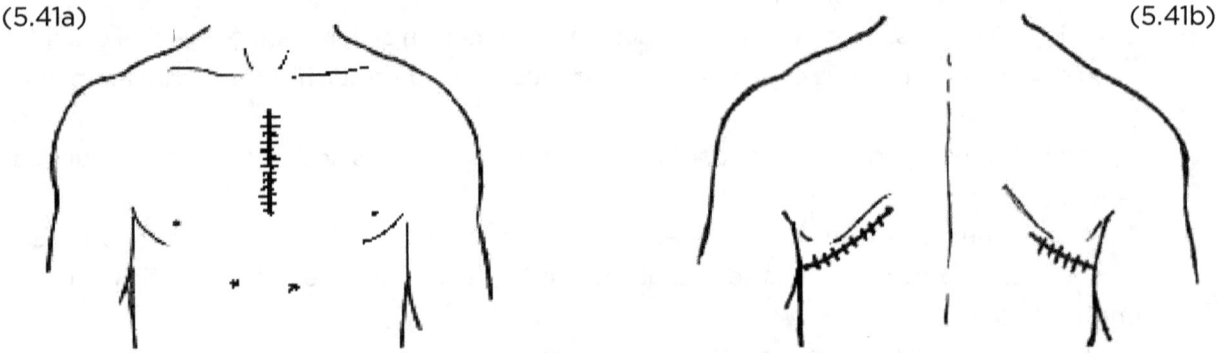

(5.41a)   (5.41b)

Palpation

Apex beat

- Site – Fourth left intercostal space in the mid-axillary line in infants and fifth left intercostal space in older children. Displacement may indicate cardiomegaly.
- Character – Forceful in left ventricular hypertrophy, tapping in right ventricular hypertrophy.

Left parasternal heave

- Place the ulnar border of the hand along the left sternal border and feel for a lift. Left parasternal heave indicates right ventricular hypertrophy.

Palpable second heart sound

- Feel with the flat of the hand over the second, left intercostal space. The second heart sound is palpable in presence of pulmonary hypertension.

Palpable thrills

- Feel with the flat of the hand over the apex, left parasternal areas: lower and upper, aortic area and the carotids in the neck. The presence of an apical systolic thrill is a feature of mitral regurgitation. A lower left parasternal thrill suggests ventricular septal defect (VSD), an upper left parasternal thrill suggests pulmonary stenosis, and a thrill over the carotids in the neck points towards aortic stenosis.

Top tip!
Place both hands simultaneously over both sides of the chest to feel the apex. This will help to diagnose dextrocardia, an occasional diagnosis in the cardiac station.

Percussion

This is not generally helpful in the cardiac examination. It may be performed if you suspect pericardial effusion, in which case the percussed left border is far outside the palpable cardiac apex.

Auscultation

Cardiac auscultation is commenced by applying the bell of the stethoscope over the cardiac apex (to look for a diastolic murmur of mitral stenosis), followed by using the diaphragm over the cardiac apex, lower left parasternal area, upper left parasternal area, upper right parasternal area, neck on both sides and over the back of the chest.

At each site, listen to the heart sounds and murmurs. Most murmurs in children are systolic. Listen for a loud second heart sound and also wide splitting of the second heart sound when auscultating over the pulmonary area.

> *Thinking time!*
> Once you have auscultated all areas, briefly keep up the appearance of auscultating while you put all your findings together and decide what you are going to present!

Assimilating the signs

Now that you have conducted a thorough general and cardiac examination, you will be expected to assimilate and present your positive clinical findings in order to arrive at a differential diagnosis. Below is a summary of the signs elicited from Emily, and an example presentation.

End of the bed – Alert, pleasant young girl, not in distress. She is growing well and is interactive for her age.

General examination – No cyanosis or clubbing, palpable femoral pulses, and no facial dysmorphism.

Chest – Well-healed central sternotomy scar and small scars in the epigastrium. The apex beat is palpable in the fifth left intercostal space in the mid-clavicular line and there are no palpable thrills. Grade 3/6 pansystolic murmur is best heard over the lower left sternal border, with no radiation.

To present...

> "Emily is a 2 year old girl who has come for a follow-up appointment in the cardiac clinic. She had cardiac surgery at the age of 6 months. On examination, she looks comfortable at rest and well grown. However, I would like to confirm this by plotting her height and weight on the growth chart. She is not cyanosed or clubbed, but I would like to check her oxygen saturation with a pulse oximeter. Her femoral pulses are palpable, and I would like to check her blood pressure later. She has a sternotomy scar and small scars in the epigastrium. Her heart is not enlarged and I could hear a grade 3/6 pansystolic murmur best over the lower left sternal border, with no radiation. I would like to listen to the lung fields and palpate the abdomen for hepatomegaly.
>
> Emily's clinical findings are suggestive of a congenital heart disease, operated earlier, and a residual VSD."

Discussion

Now that you have arrived at a likely diagnosis, there is time for a discussion with the examiner about this condition. Possible questions from the examiner are highlighted below.

- **What is the differential diagnosis for the murmur?**

    - Residual pulmonary stenosis – The murmur should be best heard over the upper left sternal border, and may be conducted to the back of the chest.
    - Residual tricuspid regurgitation – The murmur would increase in inspiration, although it would be difficult to elicit this sign at 2 years.
    - Residual aortic stenosis – The murmur would be best heard over the upper right parasternal border and conducted to the neck with a possible thrill over the carotids.

- **What could have been the underlying heart disease to start with?**

    - Large VSD (ventricular septal defect)
    - Severe pulmonary stenosis
    - Tetralogy of Fallot
    - Congenital aortic stenosis
    - Any of the complex heart diseases

- **What further investigations are generally carried out in the cardiac follow-up clinic?**

    - ECG – This would show the right bundle branch pattern that follows open-heart surgery. It would also help to confirm sinus rhythm, and the absence of ventricular hypertrophy.
    - Echocardiogram – It would help to visualise the residual defect, as well as assess its severity and any haemodynamic effect on the heart.

- **What advice will you give parents?**

    - Attention to dental hygiene – Brushing teeth twice a day, and regular dental check-ups. There is no need for antibiotic prophylaxis prior to dental procedures.
    - Avoid tattoos and piercing – These increase the risk of endocarditis.
    - Be aware of the symptoms of endocarditis – Prolonged fever with no obvious focus should alert the family and professionals to consider endocarditis as the cause of the fever.

Additional information

The following tables will help in the clinical assessment of the heart (Tables 5.41, 5.42, 5.43).

- Cyanosis – Indicates cyanotic heart disease such as tetralogy of Fallot, or operated complex heart diseases such as hypoplastic left heart syndrome. In older children, cyanosis may be a feature of Eisenmenger's syndrome (pulmonary hypertension with shunt reversal across a VSD) (Table 5.41).

Table 5.41: Causes of acyanotic and cyanotic heart diseases		
Acyanotic heart diseases		Cyanotic heart diseases
Shunt lesions	Obstructive lesions	
Ventricular septal defect (VSD)	Pulmonary stenosis (PS)	Tetralogy of Fallot (TOF)
Atrial septal defect (ASD)	Aortic stenosis (AS)	Transposition of great arteries (TGA)
Atrioventricular septal defect (AVSD)	Coarctation of the aorta (CoA)	Hypoplastic left heart syndrome (HLHS)
Patent ductus arteriosus (PDA)		Tricuspid atresia or pulmonary atresia
		Total anomalous pulmonary venous drainage (TAPVD)
		Truncus arteriosus (TA)
		Eisenmenger's syndrome

Table 5.42: Interpreting findings on auscultation	
Where is the murmur best heard?	Probable diagnoses
Lower parasternal	Ventricular septal defect (VSD) Tricuspid regurgitation (TR)
Upper parasternal	Pulmonary stenosis (PS) Patent ductus arteriosus (PDA) Atrial septal defect (ASD) Ventricular septal defect (VSD)
Aortic area	Aortic stenosis (AS)
Apical	Mitral murmurs, aortic murmurs

Table 5.43: Interpreting findings on auscultation		
Is the murmur systolic?	Diastolic?	Or continuous?
Ventricular septal defect (VSD) Tricuspid regurgitation (TR) Mitral regurgitation (MR) Pulmonary stenosis (PS) Atrial septal defect (ASD) Patent ductus arteriosus (PDA)	Atrial regurgitation (AR) Pulmonary regurgitation (PR) Mitral stenosis (MS)	Patent ductus arteriosus (PDA) Venous hum Arterio-venous (AV) malformations

Conduction of murmurs over the precordium:

- Aortic stenosis – To the carotids
- VSD – All over the chest
- PDA – To the left clavicle
- Pulmonary stenosis – To the clavicle or back
- Coarctation of the aorta – To the back

Innocent murmurs:

The majority of heart murmurs heard in children are benign or innocent cardiac murmurs. In an asymptomatic child who is discovered to have a murmur, the following features would make it more likely to be an innocent murmur.

- Systolic (except venous hum)
- Small (heard over a small area)
- Soft (low amplitude)
- Short (never pansystolic)
- Single (not accompanied by clicks or gallop)
- Sweet (never harsh)
- Sensitive (to posture or breathing)

Cardiovascular-related symptoms according to age of presentation

It is useful to know that the symptoms children present with can vary according to age of presentation, as listed in the table below (Table 5.44).

Table 5.44: Cardiovascular-related symptoms according to age of presentation	
Symptoms in infants	Symptoms in older children
Breathlessness Poor feeding Excess sweating Blue episodes 'Generally unwell' Not gaining weight Excess weight gain ALTE Positive family history	Exercise intolerance Palpitation Chest pain Syncope Pedal oedema Positive family history

Syndromes and associated cardiac disease risk

Children who present with a syndromic diagnosis often have a predisposition to underlying cardiac disease as listed in the table below (Table 5.45).

Table 5.45: Syndromes and probable associated cardiac diseases	
Syndromes	Associated heart diseases
Down's syndrome (Trisomy 21)	Atrioventricular septal defect (AVSD) Ventricular septal defect (VSD) Atrial septal defect (ASD)
William's syndrome	Supravalvular aortic stenosis (AS) Pulmonary stenosis (PS)
Alagille syndrome	Pulmonary stenosis (PS)
Holt-Oram syndrome	Atrial septal defect (ASD)
22q deletion syndrome	Interrupted aortic arch

Syllabus mapping

Cardiology

Knowledge

The candidate must:

- Be aware of the investigations and management of heart diseases.
- Know common congenital heart disease, including aetiological factors.

Skills

The candidate must:

- Be able to examine the cardiovascular system in children of different ages, as well as interpret and discuss physical findings.
- Be able to identify common congenital heart diseases (ASD, VSD) and know when to refer.
- Be able to identify an innocent cardiac murmur.

Further reading and references

1. Lissauer T, Clayden G. *Illustrated Textbook of Paediatrics*, 4th edition. Edinburgh: Mosby, 2010: 18-19.
2. Rudolf M, Lee T, Levene M. *Paediatrics and Child Health*, 3rd edition. Chichester: Wiley-Blackwell, 2011: 60-63.
3. Venugopalan P, Ranaweera M. Patient Management: Clinical Approach To Heart Murmurs In Children. *Foundation Years Journal* 2014; 8(6): 20.

Video resources

http://learnpediatrics.com/videos/ (accessed April 15).
https://www.youtube.com/user/MRCPCHRevision (accessed April 15).

Chapter 5.5: Case Study 4: Neurology: 12 Year Old with a Limp

Dr Geethika Bandaranayake, Dr Anna Mathew

This station assesses your ability to demonstrate the neurological examination of the lower and upper limbs of a child, interpret physical findings and conduct a discussion with the examiner. You will be assessed on the rapport, manner and structure of your examination with the child and parent.

Logistics:

Timing: This is a 9-minute station. A knock at 6 minutes will denote that 3 minutes remain before the end of the station. At this point, it is important to summarise your clinical findings and proceed with the discussion with the examiner.

When the bell rings: On entering the room, the examiner will greet you, take your mark sheet, introduce you to the child and parent, and give you your task. Listen carefully to these instructions.

The examiner will then remain mostly silent during the consultation, as they will be observing your clinical skills, but may provide some direction should it be required. A discussion around the case will be undertaken in the final 3 minutes of the station.

If you finish early, you will be asked to remain in the room until the session has ended.

Candidate role and task:

You are a GP trainee working on the day unit.

Shan, a 12 year old girl, was born prematurely and walks with a limp.

Task: Please conduct a neurological examination of her arms and legs.

The lower limb neurological examination

Inspection

Top tip!
In order to undertake a proper neurological examination, it is important to expose the limbs being examined as fully as possible. Seek both the parent's and the child's permission to do so soon after the initial introductions are completed.

End of the bed

Inspection will provide vital clues in the neurological examination. Spend a few minutes observing in order to:

- Judge the severity of the illness. Does the child look well or does she look ill?
- Comment on her growth. Offer to measure and plot weight and height on the appropriate growth chart.

- Look for any dysmorphic features that suggest a syndromic diagnosis.
- Look for any mobility or orthotic aids, such as crutches, wheelchairs, and orthotic splints.
- Look for wasting. Ideally, compare both lower limbs.
- Note the resting posture. Any obvious deformities noted?
- Look for scars. These are indicative of corrective surgical intervention for contractures.
- Observe the gait. Ask the parent (and the child, if appropriate): "Can he/she walk independently or with help?" If so, ask the child to walk. An assessment of gait is essential, and provides vital information early in the examination. The observed gait will provide information that guides further assessment of the patient (Table 5.51).

Table 5.51: Types of gait

	Anatomical lesion
Circumduction gait	Upper motor neurone paralysis
Ataxic gait	Cerebellar lesion
High stepping gait	Lower motor neurone paralysis
Wide-based gait	Cerebellar lesion
Antalgic gait	Local pain
Waddling gait	Developmental dysplasia of the hip Myopathies Spastic diplegia

Palpation

Tone

- Assess tone by qualifying the degree of resistance to passive movements. This is best done with the child lying down and gently rocking the limb sideways in the neutral position, with the hands placed on the major joints.
- Look for ankle clonus (avoid patella clonus) – It is always easier to assess clonus soon after assessing tone. Remember to flex and support the knee joint while eliciting ankle clonus. In this position, sharply dorsiflex the foot and observe whether there is a beat response (repeated flexion-extension movements of the ankle against the hand).
- Increased tone and the presence of clonus are usually demonstrated in upper motor neurone lesions.

Power

- Remember to give simple instructions in a kind, empathetic manner and check power across all ranges of movement.
    - Hip – Flexion, extension, abduction and adduction.
    - Knee – Flexion, extension.
    - Foot – Dorsiflexion, plantar flexion, inversion and eversion.
    - Toe – Flexion and extension.

Reflexes

- Check the reflexes – This may need reinforcement techniques (Jendrassik manoeuvre).
- Knee jerk.
- Ankle jerk.

Plantars

- To perform this test, draw fairly firmly along the lateral aspect of the plantar surface of the foot (from the heel to the forefoot) using a pointed yet blunt object. Upward movement and fanning of the toes are positive responses supporting the presence of an upper motor neurone lesion.

Coordination

- Assess the degree of coordination using the heel-shin test.
- Gower's sign – Only positive in proximal myopathies. Ask the child to sit on the floor and then stand up as quickly as possible without using their hands. If this sign is positive, the child will have difficulty rising up and will be noted to use their hands to 'climb' up their legs to achieve the upright position (Table 5.52).

Table 5.52: Causes of proximal myopathy
Duchenne muscular dystrophy
Becker muscular dystrophy
Juvenile dermatomyositis
Spinal muscular atrophy type III

Sensation

- Offer to test sensation – This is rarely tested at the DCH level. It is useful to have a basic idea about the sensory dermatomes. Only light touch with a piece of cotton wool is assessed in children.

The upper limb neurological examination

Inspection

End of the bed

Inspection will provide vital clues in the neurological examination. Spend a few minutes objectively looking for:

- Wasting – Ideally, compare both upper limbs. Ask the child to "hold your arms out straight" and compare both arms. Any involuntary movements can be noted at the same time.
- Resting posture – Any obvious deformities noted?
- Scars – These are indicative of corrective surgical intervention for contractures, commonly over the Achilles tendons.

Palpation

Tone

- Tone – Assess tone by qualifying the degree of resistance to passive movements. In the elbow and wrist, move the limbs passively across the major joints and note the degree of resistance.

Power

- Remember to give simple instructions in a kind, empathetic manner and check power across all ranges of movement.
    - Shoulder – Adduction, abduction
    - Elbow – Flexion, extension
    - Wrist – Flexion, extension
    - Fingers – Abduction, opposition, grip

Reflexes

- Check the reflexes – This may need reinforcement techniques (Jendrassik manoeuvre).
- Biceps jerk
- Triceps jerk
- Supinator jerk

Coordination

- Finger-nose test

Sensation

- Offer to test the sensation – This is rarely tested at the DCH level. It is useful to have a basic idea about the sensory dermatomes. Only light touch with a piece of cotton wool is assessed in children.

> *Thinking time!*
> Once you have completed the examination and elicited all the signs, put all your findings together and get ready to present (Table 5.53).

Table 5.53: Interpretation of neurological signs		
Upper motor neurone lesion	Lower motor neurone lesion	Cerebellar lesion
Hypertonia	Hypotonia	Horizontal nystagmus
Muscle power relatively preserved	Reduced muscle power	Intention tremor
Muscle bulk – Wasting relatively common	Muscle bulk relatively preserved	Muscle bulk preserved
Increased/exaggerated tendon reflexes. Clonus	Reduced/absent tendon reflexes	Dysarthria
Upward plantars	Gower's sign may be present	Romberg's sign. Poor coordination
Circumduction or waddling gait	High stepping gait	Ataxic or wide-based gait

Assimilating the signs

Now that you have conducted a thorough neurological examination, you will be expected to assimilate and present your positive clinical findings in order to arrive at a possible diagnosis. Below is a summary of the signs elicited from Shan, and an example presentation.

To present...

> "Shan is a 12 year old girl who was born prematurely. She walks with a limp. On examination, she looks well and is adequately grown for her age. She walks with a waddling gait and has increased tone in all 4 limbs, but this is more marked in the lower limbs than the upper limbs. I could elicit ankle clonus and brisk reflexes in the lower limbs. There are no visible surgical scars on the limbs and she has grade-4 muscle power in both lower limbs. The shape of her head is long and narrow (scaphocephaly), which is commonly seen in children who were born very prematurely.
>
> My findings are consistent with spastic diplegia, most likely following complications associated with prematurity."

Discussion

After your clinical findings, you will discuss the case with the examiner. Some possible questions from the examiner are highlighted below. It is unlikely all of these can be asked within the given time frame.

■ *What is the definition of cerebral palsy?*

This is a permanent, non-progressive but often changing disorder of posture and movement secondary to lesions or traumatic insults that occur in the early stages of the developing brain. Although the brain lesion is static, the condition develops throughout life due to progressive maturation of the nervous system.

■ *What are the common aetiological factors in cerebral palsy?*

- Antenatal – Intrauterine infections, chromosome abnormalities, cerebral malformations
- Perinatal – Prematurity, birth asphyxia
- Post natal – Infections (neonatal meningitis), hyperbilirubinaemia (kernicterus)

■ *How do you broadly classify cerebral palsy?*

Spastic (pyramidal) (Figure 5.51)

- Hemiplegia – Upper limbs affected more than the lower limbs. Hand manipulation affected.
- Diplegia – Lower limbs are affected more when compared to the upper limbs. Scissoring and toe walking seen in severe cases.
- Quadriplegia – All 4 limbs affected, but the upper limbs are affected more. Learning difficulty is common.

Dyskinetic (extrapyramidal)

- Athetoid movements can be seen. Oro-motor dysfunction common.

Mixed

- A mixed picture can arise, comprising some of the features mentioned above.

Figure 5.51: Common types of spastic cerebral palsy (Illustration by Dr G Bandaranayake)

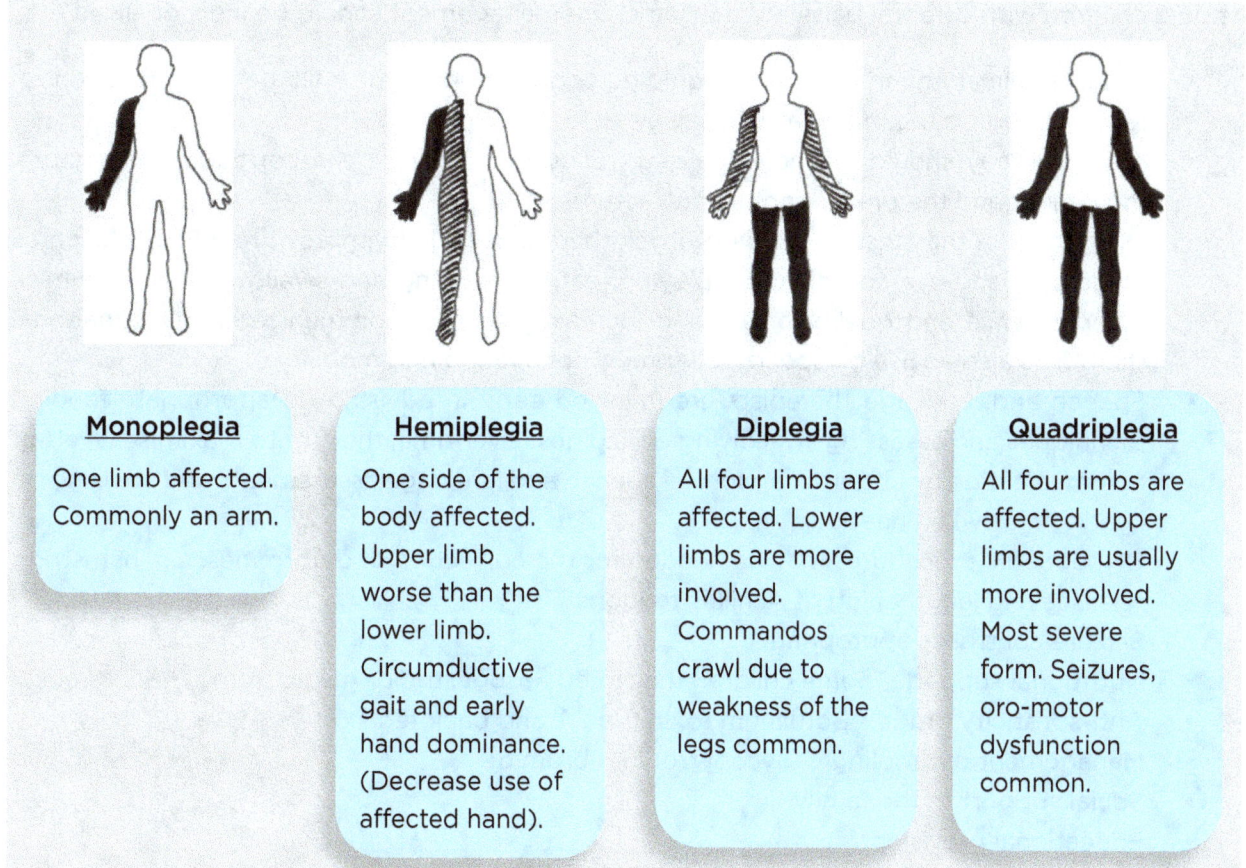

- **What are the associated complications seen in children with cerebral palsy?**

  - Learning difficulties can be seen in up to 75% of children with cerebral palsy
  - Epilepsy can be a complication in up to 15–60% of children with cerebral palsy
  - Visual impairment
  - Hearing impairment
  - Gastro-oesophageal reflux
  - Kyphoscoliosis

- **Suggest some early presenting features of cerebral palsy.**

  - Delayed gross motor milestones, e.g. poor head control
  - Abnormal posturing
  - Feeding difficulties
  - Persistence of primitive reflexes
  - Early hand dominance <1.5 years
  - Lack of response to external stimuli, such as delayed social skills (e.g. smiling)
  - Abnormal gait

■ What are the broad principles of the management of children with cerebral palsy?

As no 2 children with cerebral palsy are the same, the management should be individualised.

- Multidisciplinary team approach should be coordinated by the child development centre.
- Rehabilitation is the mainstay of therapy.
- Physiotherapy should be individualised, focusing mainly on the correction of posture, movement and the prevention of contractures.
- Occupational therapists work with physiotherapists to help improve hand skills, such as grasping, hand-eye coordination, playing, eating, drinking and swallowing, to maximise independence and quality of life and increase levels of communication. Occupational therapists also advise on special equipment for seating and mobility.
- Speech and language therapists are involved early in advising on appropriate feeding techniques and assessing swallowing difficulties. Over time, they try to maximise levels of communication by undertaking formal speech and language assessments and advising on hearing aids when needed.
- Orthopaedic procedures may be needed for the correction of deformities, e.g. hamstring releases and lengthening of Achilles tendons.
- Seizure control as appropriate
- Nutritional support – Some children may need nasogastric or gastrostomy (PEG) feeds.
- Anti-spasticity drugs – Botulinum toxin type A and baclofen
- Management of drooling – Glycopyrronium bromide
- Social support to the family
- Educational provision
- Consideration for DLA

Syllabus mapping

Neurology and neurodisability

Knowledge

The candidate must:

- Understand the definition and concepts of disability, and what this means for the child and family.
- Be familiar with the common causes of disability, disordered development and learning difficulties.
- Understand the need for multidisciplinary team input in the care of the disabled child, and be aware of the work of the child development team and centre.

Skills

The candidate must:

- Be able to examine the nervous system, including examination of cranial nerves, as well as interpret and discuss physical findings.

Further reading and references

1. Kliegman RM, Stanton BF, St Geme JW et al. *Nelson Textbook of Pediatrics*, 19th edition. Philadelphia: Elsevier, 2015: 2061-2065.
2. Lissauer T, Clayden G. *Illustrated Textbook of Paediatrics*, 4th edition. Edinburgh: Mosby, 2012: 22-23.
3. McIntosh N, Helms P, Smyth R et al. *Forfar and Arneil's Textbook of Pediatrics*, 7th edition. Edinburgh: Churchill Livingstone, 2012: 889-896.
4. Rudolf M, Lee T, Levene M. *Paediatrics and Child Health*, 3rd edition. Chichester: Wiley-Blackwell, 2011: 70-75, 236-241.

Video resources

http://learnpediatrics.com/videos/ (accessed April 15).
https://www.youtube.com/user/MRCPCHRevision (accessed April 15).

Chapter 5.6: Case Study 5: 'Other' System: 10 Year Old with Tall Stature

Dr Edward Yates, Dr Jonathan Rabbs

This station assesses your ability to demonstrate the general examination of a child, interpret physical findings and conduct a discussion with the examiner. You will be assessed on the rapport, manner and structure of your examination with the child and parent.

Logistics:

Timing: This is a 9-minute station. A knock at 6 minutes will denote that 3 minutes remain before the end of the station. At this point, it is important to summarise your clinical findings and proceed with the discussion with the examiner.

When the bell rings: On entering the room, the examiner will greet you, take your mark sheet, introduce you to the child and parent, and give you your task. Listen carefully to these instructions.

The examiner will then remain mostly silent during the consultation, as they will be observing your clinical skills, but may provide some direction should it be required. A discussion around the case will be undertaken in the final 3 minutes of the station.

If you finish early, you will be asked to remain in the room until the session has ended.

Candidate role and task:

You are an ST3 GP trainee working in the paediatric outpatient clinic.

Marianne is a 10 year old. Her parents have asked for a referral because she is self-conscious about her appearance and chest shape.

Task: Please carry out a general examination.

The general examination

Inspection

End of the bed

- Judge the severity of the illness. Does the child look well or does she look ill?
- Comment on her growth. Offer to measure and plot weight and height on the appropriate growth chart.
- Does she have any dysmorphic features that suggest a syndrome, such as Down's syndrome, William's syndrome, etc.?
- Note whether she is wearing spectacles/glasses.

Top tip!
General examination is particularly important in this station, as it can offer clues to the presence of an underlying syndrome or underlying genetic or developmental diagnosis.

Hands, feet and limbs

- Ask the patient to stand with shoes and socks off, and assess whether any aspects are abnormal.
    - Body habitus (upper segment/lower segment ratio)
    - Limb length and arm span
    - Limb shape
    - Muscle bulk
- Inspect the joint angles and assess whether they are hyper-extendable.
- Look for pedal oedema and foot arch defects.
- Comment on any rashes or skin markings/scars.
- Inspect the hands and feet:
    - Size and shape of digits (arachnodactyly)
    - Clubbing or nail abnormalities
    - Small joint hypermobility
    - Ask the patient to try to circumvent their wrist with their opposite thumb and fifth finger.
    - Sternberg sign – The thumb adducts fully across the narrow palm.

Head and neck

- Politely inform the child that you are going to look at their face. Look for any dysmorphic features and ensure you also observe the head and neck in profile (specifically the nose, chin and ear shape/site/size).
- Comment on any hairline abnormality or neck deformity.
- Comment on any vision aids/spectacles. Inspect the eyes and each iris and pupil (squint, colour, symmetry, etc.).
- Inspect the mouth:
    - Dentition – Comment on crowded teeth, tooth quality/condition.
    - Palate – Comment on arch size and shape.

Chest and thorax

- Politely ask the patient to undress her torso to the limit of modesty and comfort.
- Are there any skin lesions, specifically striae (stretch marks)?
- Chest wall deformity:
    - Pectus excavatum (hollow chest)
    - Pectus carinatum (pigeon chest)
- Symmetry:
    - Are the nipples normally spaced?
    - Are the shoulders and the scapulae symmetrical and level?
    - Inspect the back – Comment on spine (lordosis, kyphosis) and assess for scoliosis.

Top tip!
Assess for scoliosis by asking the patient to touch their toes while standing. Observe scapular alignment – 1 scapula or side of posterior ribcage will protrude if there is scoliosis present.

At this point, it would be appropriate to tell the examiner that you would like to listen to the heart (as you have observed some features of a connective tissue disease), and palpate the abdomen. The examiner may ask you to proceed. Alternately, the examiner may ask you to examine the musculoskeletal system in more detail.

Cardiovascular assessment

- Palpate for the cardiac apex and any palpable thrills over the praecordium.
- Auscultate while specifically looking for evidence of aortic or mitral incompetence (refer to chapter 5.4 for cardiovascular examination).

Abdomen

- Politely ask patient to expose her abdomen to the limit of modesty and comfort.
- Are there any skin lesions, specifically striae (stretch marks), scars or birthmarks?
- Are there any visible masses?
- Quickly feel for the liver and spleen (refer to chapter 5.3 for abdominal examination).

Musculoskeletal examination

- Appropriate use of pGALS (web link given below), modifying as required.

> *Thinking time!*
> Use the time while auscultating to compose your answer by compiling your findings in a logical manner. You should also formulate a differential diagnosis and the management plan.

Assimilating the signs

Now that you have conducted a thorough general examination, you will be expected to assimilate and present your positive clinical findings in order to arrive at a differential diagnosis. Below is a summary of the signs elicited from Marianne, and an example presentation.

End of the bed – Alert, pleasant young girl who is not in distress and is tall for her age.

General examination – Soft dysmorphic facial features (long, thin face with intermaxillary narrowness) with reduced upper segment/lower segment ratio. There are striae despite not being obese.

Head and neck – High arched palate, dental overcrowding, and her vision corrected with spectacles.
Hands, feet, limbs – Long limbs, hypermobile joints, Sternberg test positive, and collapsed foot arches.

Chest – Pectus carinatum, grade 3/6 apical pansystolic murmur, scoliosis.

To present...

"Marianne is a 10 year old who presents with concerns about her general appearance and chest shape. On observation, she is tall and thin for her age, but I would like to plot her weight and height. She wears glasses and has soft dysmorphic facial features, including a high arched palate and dental overcrowding.

Limb examination reveals hypermobile joints with a positive Sternberg sign. Foot arches are collapsed bilaterally and there is evidence of incidental striae. Examination of the torso reveals pectus carinatum and scoliosis.

Auscultation reveals normal heart sounds with a grade 3/6 pansystolic murmur, loudest at the mitral area and radiating to the axilla, which is suggestive of mitral regurgitation.

In conclusion, there are soft, dysmorphic features with evidence of connective tissue abnormalities and mitral valve regurgitation in a very tall girl. I would like to exclude Marfan's syndrome by referring her for a genetic assessment, and would like to make a referral to a cardiologist to assess the mitral valve disease."

Discussion

Now that you have arrived at a likely diagnosis, there is time for a discussion with the examiner about this condition. Possible questions from the examiner are highlighted below.

■ *What is the differential diagnosis?*

- Klinefelter syndrome
- Gigantism/acromegaly/pituitary disorder
- Constitutional tall stature
- Ehlers-Danlos syndrome or other connective tissue disorders
- Mitral valve syndrome
- Loeys-Dietz syndrome
- Ectopia lentis syndrome

■ *What are the other features of Marfan's syndrome?*

- Dysmorphic features:
    - Dolichocephaly – Long and narrow head
    - Downward slanting palpebral fissures
    - Enophthalmos – Recession of the eyeball within the orbit
    - Retrognathia – A receding chin
    - Malar hypoplasia
    - Tall body habitus – Reduced upper segment/lower segment ratio (dolichostenomelia)
    - High arched palate
    - Striae not related to a physical cause
    - Musculoskeletal
    - Hypermobility
    - Arachnodactyly
    - Scoliosis
    - Pectus carinatum or pectus excavatum
    - Foot arch collapse later in life

- Ocular
  - Ectopia lentis (lens dislocation)
  - An abnormally flat cornea
  - An increased axial length of the eyeball (as measured by an ultrasound)
  - Myopia caused by hypoplastic ciliary muscles or iris
- Cardiovascular
  - Aortic regurgitation
  - Dissection of the ascending aorta
  - Mitral valve prolapse
  - Dilatation of the main pulmonary artery
  - Calcification of the mitral valve annulus
  - Abdominal aortic dilatation or dissection
- Respiratory
  - Spontaneous pneumothorax due to apical blebs

■ **What information and advice will you give parents, and what referrals will you make?**

- Marfan's syndrome is an autosomal dominant disorder with an incidence of approximately 1 among 5,000. A proportion of cases (30%) are new mutations but there may be a family history of the syndrome.
- It is caused by an FBN1 (Fibrillin 1) gene mutation on chromosome 15q. Usually, diagnosis is on clinical grounds using the revised Ghent criteria but mutation analysis testing can be done in some cases.
- Inform the parents that you will send Marianne to see both a geneticist and a cardiologist. Share information about warning signs of aortic dissection and visual loss, and state that if these occur to see a doctor urgently.

■ **What do you say if the parents ask how this will affect her future?**

- Marfan's syndrome is a genetic disorder affecting the FNB1 gene. It is not curable and is an autosomal dominant condition; therefore, there is a 50% chance she will pass on the gene to her offspring. Variable severity and phenotype presentations occur. This means that the complications that Marianne will develop are not certain despite having the mutation, and may be different from other affected family members.
- The most significant complications that could occur are posterior retinal detachment and aortic arch dilatation (which can lead to aortic dissection in the most severe and uncontrolled cases). Therefore, it is important that the family are aware of the possible symptoms of these complications, and they will need to seek medical help should they occur.
- Aortic dilatation will be present in 50% of children, but can be managed with medication.
- Inform the family that there are useful websites and support groups with good reference material where they can seek further information, as well as the official patient information literature about Marfan's syndrome.

■ **What is the clinical score for joint hypermobility?**

- Beighton score – This is a clinical score on 5 components, and each component is marked 0 if negative and 1 if positive, for each side (left and right limb/joint) and finally 0–1 for trunk flexibility. The total is then added and a score from 0–9 is given. The exact threshold for hypermobility is controversial, but it can be used as a guide to assessment (Table 5.61).

Figure 5.61: Beighton score for hypermobility (Illustration by Dr G Bandaranayke)

Test	Right	Left	
While standing forward bending you can place palms on the ground with legs straight	0-1		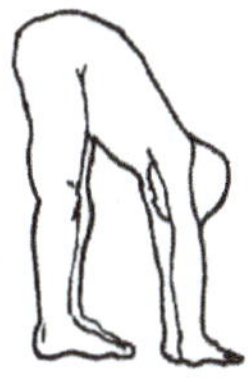
Elbow that bends backwards	0-1	0-1	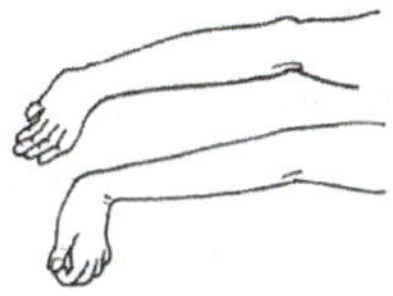
Knee that bends backwards	0-1	0-1	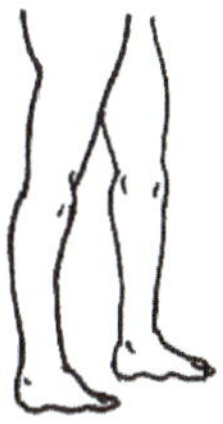
Thumb that touches the forearm when bent backwards	0-1	0-1	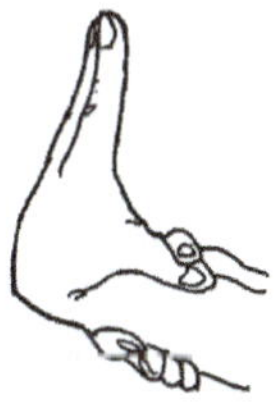
Little finger that bends backwards beyond 90 degrees	0-1	0-1	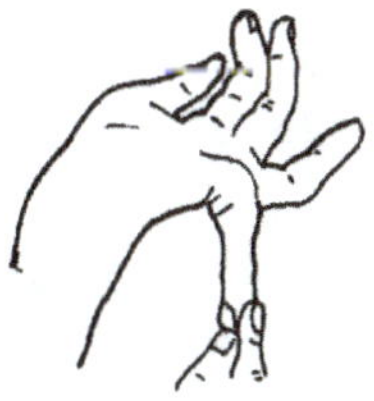
Total	/9		

Syllabus mapping

Growth and development

Skills

The candidate must:

- Be able to identify common clinical syndromes associated with short or tall stature.

Further reading and references

1. Kliegman RM, Stanton BF, St Geme JW et al. *Nelson Textbook of Pediatrics*, 20th edition. Philadelphia: Elsevier, 2015; 693:2440-2446
2. Smits-Engelsman B, Klerks M, Kirby A. Beighton score: A valid measure for generalized hypermobility in children. *The Journal of Pediatrics* 2011; 158(1): 119-23
3. Sponseller PD, Erkula G, Skolasky RL et al. Improving Clinical Recognition of Marfan Syndrome. *J Bone Joint Surg Am* 2010; 92: 1868-75
4. Talley NJ, O'Connor S. *Clinical Examination: A Systematic Guide to Physical Diagnosis*, 7th edition. Churchill Livingstone, 2013.
5. Van der Giessen LJ, Liekens D, Rutgers KJ et al. Validation of Beighton score and prevalence of connective tissue signs in 773 Dutch children. *Journal of Rheumatology* 2001; 28(12): 2726-30.

Video resources

http://www.arthritisresearchuk.org/health-professionals-and-students/video-resources/pgals.aspx (accessed June 2015).

http://learnpediatrics.com/videos/ (accessed April 2015).

https://www.youtube.com/user/MRCPCHRevision (accessed May 2015).

SECTION 6:
THE FOCUSED HISTORY AND MANAGEMENT PLANNING STATION

Chapter 6.1: Introduction
Dr P Venugopalan, Dr Anna Mathew

The first step in any clinical assessment is to enquire about the patient's current status and identify important contributory factors. In the accident and emergency department, this process may be very brief and executed at the same time as an urgent examination and intervention. This is in contrast to an outpatient setting, where a full history should be elicited. The information obtained will identify relevant issues and problems, help assess their impact on the child and family, guide physical examination and investigation, and ultimately lead to the formulation of an effective management plan.

The DCH focused history and management planning station is designed to test communication, history taking and management planning skills. Physical examination and other skills are tested elsewhere in the circuit. Usually, the task centres on reviewing chronic disease management with a parent and child or a role player. Although it is less likely, you could be presented with a child who has acute problems.

What to expect

While waiting to enter the station, you will be presented with brief background information on a child who typically will have a common chronic paediatric problem. For example, the information provided may be in the form of a referral letter from the GP to the outpatient clinic, stating that the child has just moved into the area and asking the hospital to provide ongoing management of a pre-existing condition. It is impossible within the remit of this book to state all the conditions that could present, but examples of common paediatric problems include asthma, constipation, diabetes, eczema, enuresis, epilepsy, migraines or recurrent abdominal pain. As the amount of time to take the history is brief, you should focus on the areas outlined in the background information.

You will be required to undertake and direct an interview with the parent and child or role player. Your task would be to ask relevant questions in order to gather the maximum amount of information in the time available. If the parent, child or role player asks questions during the consultation, it would be appropriate to answer these. However, during standard setting with the examiners beforehand, parents are discouraged from asking candidates any questions about the management of their child's condition.

When you enter the station, the examiner will greet you and introduce you to the parent and child, or the role player. Your task in this station is to take a focused history, so you will not be required to examine the patient. After taking the history, you will discuss a management plan with the examiner.

The examiner will assess your ability to:

- Conduct an interview.
- Display effective skills in history taking.
- Demonstrate the ability to interpret the information given to formulate a differential diagnosis and management plan.

In doing so, you should demonstrate:

- Effective skills in 3-way consultation.
- An understanding of effective communication and interpersonal skills with children of all ages.
- Empathy, sensitivity and skills in engaging the trust of, and receiving consent from, children and their families.
- An understanding of equality and diversity in paediatric practice.
- Ethical personal and professional practice.
- Effective skills in paediatric assessments.
- Skills in formulating an appropriate differential diagnosis in paediatrics.
- Knowledge of any pertinent investigations.
- Effective initial management of ill health and clinical conditions in paediatrics, seeking additional advice and opinion as appropriate.
- Knowledge of common and serious paediatric conditions and their management.

Being able to demonstrate fluid, systematic and structured history taking in a short period of time on children of varied ages requires confidence and a well-honed approach. To reach the standard required necessitates frequent practice and the identification of areas where you can improve your skills. Undertaking practice individually, with a partner or in small groups will help you to develop the confidence needed to perform well under the stress of direct observation encountered in an examination situation.

You are expected to summarise key aspects of the history for the examiner at the beginning of the discussion time. It is important at this stage to be concise and precise, and present the main positive and important negative aspects of the history. If the diagnosis was not obvious at the beginning, it would be good to end the summary with your probable diagnosis or differential diagnoses, and list the reasons for your conclusion. Most often, the discussion to follow will centre on management planning.

The examiner may choose to ask about a particular aspect of the diagnosis. This could include physical examination findings that would aid the differential diagnosis, investigations that you may require, and the formulation of a management plan. You may also be asked questions on the disease itself, including aetio-pathogenesis, recent advances in management, etc. Do not forget to discuss the provision of a holistic approach, taking into account the family and community support available.

Managing time in the focused history and management planning station

Timing: This is a 9-minute station. A knock at 6 minutes will mark the end of the recommended time for history taking. The remaining 3 minutes should be dedicated to summarising your clinical history and undertaking further discussion around the case.

As only 6 minutes is allowed to complete the history-taking task, it is important to be fluid and systematic in your approach. Failure to complete the task will lead to you being marked down. Your initial presentation summary to the examiner must be concise, because if adequate time is not left for discussion, more marks may be lost.

How consistency is ensured

Examiners work in pairs to review all children and parents or the role players helping in the station. They undertake 'standard setting', where an agreement is reached on the salient facts to be obtained by the candidate while taking the history and the questions to be asked during the discussion time. Based on these deliberations, examiners decide on a number of pass/fail criteria to be applied consistently to every candidate.

'Mark sheets', individualised for each station, help to guide examiners in their assessment. These sheets indicate the different areas examiners consider when awarding marks and, as importantly, areas where marks will be deducted. Like the other 9-minute stations, this one carries 2 separate scores for each candidate – 1 for the history taking and 1 for management planning (Appendix 6.11).

The RCPCH has developed 'anchor statements' that examiners refer to when deciding on pass/fail criteria during standard setting. They also use these for guidance when marking. You should review these documents to familiarise yourself with the scoring criteria explained in the anchor statements (Appendix 6.12).

Setting the stage

Before you begin taking the history, remember the key introductory steps.

Introduce yourself. It is important to introduce yourself to the child and parent or role player.

Permission must be sought from the parent or role player, and from the child if they are old enough to consent. This is a good opportunity to briefly explain the purpose of your interaction.

Position yourself in such a way that you are audible to the parent and child or role player. As in the communication station, your posture must be a neutral one, not too close or too leisurely.

Make sure you thank the parent and child or the role player before leaving the room.

Technique

You should ask open-ended questions, and direct further questioning towards the area of the expected discussion if the parent, child or role player deviates from the subject. Generally, the parent, child or role players are instructed to answer the questions asked, and desist from asking questions themselves. Involve the child as much as possible, both by verbal and non-verbal communication. This is especially important if 'the child' is a teenager.

While the importance of listening very carefully to the historian cannot be emphasised enough, you can take notes intermittently if you feel that it will help you to summarise and discuss better. This station is also a test of your communication skills, and the examiner will be watching how you interact with the parent and child or role player, especially if they ask you a question.

When gathering the history, follow the usual method of identifying the main complaint and how it has affected the child and family. Then, move on briefly to cover other past medical history, birth history, immunisation, development, diet, and family and social history. Remember that it is important to focus on the areas mentioned in the background information. You should pay attention to any aspects of the history that the parent brings up and, at the end, ask further questions to complete your task.

Be prepared to summarise your clinical findings and undertake a discussion with the examiner in the 3 minutes before the end of the station. The discussion will be around:

- Your assessment of the problem with a differential diagnosis where relevant (most parents can tell you the diagnosis).
- Further investigations that may be helpful.
- Management of the case, with emphasis on the specific issue that you are asked to address or that you identify as relevant.

The summary that you provide will set the trend for further discussion, and the examiner will also be guided by the standard setting and anchor statements.

Further reading and references

1. DCH clinical syllabus: http://www.rcpch.ac.uk/training-examinations-professional-development/assessment-and-examinations/examinations/syllabus (accessed March 2015).
2. MRCP Foundation of Practice syllabus: http://www.rcpch.ac.uk/sites/default/files/page/FoundationofPracticeSyllabus.pdf (accessed March 2015).

Appendix 6.11: Mark Sheet (Front and Back): Focused History and Management Planning Station

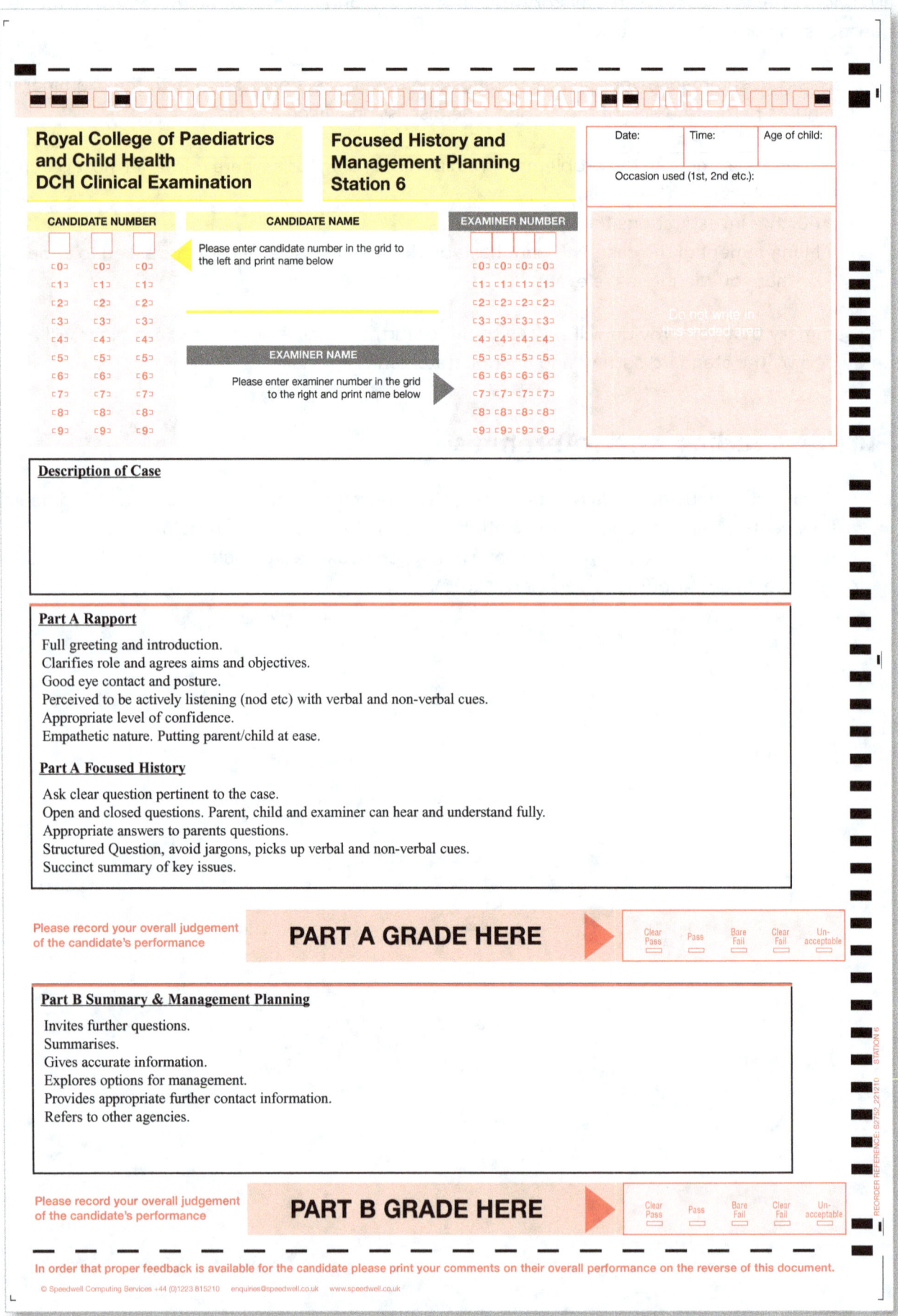

☐ Poor approach & unstructured consultation (please add additional comments)

☐ Lacking in sensitivity - failed to address parental concerns (please add additional comments)

☐ Failed to elicit adequate focussed history (please add additional comments)

☐ Failed to develop management plan along lines of best practice (please add additional comments)

Please add any additional comments here:

Appendix 6.12: Anchor Statement: Focused History and Management Planning Station

	Expected Standard/ CLEAR PASS	PASS	BARE FAIL	CLEAR FAIL	UNACCEPTABLE
PART A: RAPPORT	Full greeting and introduction. Clarifies role and agrees aims and objectives. Good eye contact and posture. Perceived to be actively listening (nod etc) with verbal and non-verbal cues. Appropriate level of confidence. Empathetic nature. Putting parent/child at ease.	Adequately performed but not fully fluent in conducting interview.	Incomplete or hesitant greeting and introduction. Inadequate identification of role, aims and objectives. Poor eye contact and posture. Not perceived to be actively listening (nod etc) with verbal and non-verbal cues. Does not show appropriate level of confidence, empathetic nature or putting parent/child at ease.	Significant components omitted or not achieved.	Dismissive of parent/child concerns. Fails to put parent or child at ease.
PART A: FOCUSED HISTORY	Ask clear question pertinent to the case. Open and closed questions. Parent, child and examiner can hear and understand fully. Appropriate answers to parents questions. Structured Question, Avoid jargons, picks up verbal and non-verbal cues. Succinct summary of key issues.	Question reasonable and covers essential issues but omits occasional essential points. Overall approach structured. Appropriate style of questioning. Main points summarised.	Misses relevant information, which would make a difference to management if known. Excessive use of closed question. Occasional use of jargon. Summary incomplete.	Ask irrelevant questions, poorly understood by parent and child. Excessive use of jargon. Does not seek the view of parent/child. Very poor summary.	Questions totally unrelated to the problem presented. Shows no regard to the child/parent. No summary.
PART B: SUMMARY, MANAGEMENT PLANNING AND CLOSURE	Invites further questions. Summarises. Gives accurate information. Explores options for management. Provides appropriate further contact information. Refers to other agencies.	Summarises most of the important points and suggests **best** management strategy. Provides some information about other services and future plan. Deals with uncertainty in diagnosis or management.	Incomplete summary of problems and inadequately planned management. Does not relate management to child/parents needs or concerns. Inadequate attempt to determine child/parent understanding.	Poor exploration of parent's or child's views or desires about treatment. Poor use of referral to other agencies.	Abrupt ending. Inaccurate information given. Lack of regard for safe, ethical and effective treatments. Poor arrangements for future contact.

Chapter 6.2: Case Study 1: 7 Year Old with Asthma

Dr Benita Morrissey, Dr Arvind Shah, Dr Anna Mathew

This station assesses your ability to take a focused history from a child and family, and undertake a discussion based on this. As the candidate, you will be asking most or all of the questions, but if parents or role players do ask questions during the consultation, it will be appropriate to answer these.

You will be assessed on your communication with the child and parent, and the rapport, structure and manner of your interview. During the discussion, the examiner will focus on your understanding of chronic disease management.

Logistics:

Timing: This is a 9-minute station. You will have up to 2 minutes before the start of this station to read the candidate sheet and prepare yourself.

When the bell rings: On entering the room, the examiner will greet you, take your mark sheet, and introduce you to the child and parent. The examiner will then remain silent during the consultation.

You will have 6 minutes to conduct your consultation. A knock at 6 minutes will indicate that 3 minutes remain before the end of the station. At this point, it is important to summarise the history and proceed with the discussion with the examiner.

If you finish early, you will be asked to remain in the room until the session has ended.

Candidate role and task:

You are an ST3 GP trainee working in the outpatient clinic.

Tom is 7 years old. He has recently moved into the area and has a diagnosis of asthma.

Task: The GP has referred him to the clinic for further assessment and ongoing management.

Top tip!
Always ensure you greet the parent and child at the beginning. Examiners will assess your ability to include Tom in the consultation, and to put him at ease.

Before entering the station

As there are only 6 minutes to take the history, utilise the time before entering the station to:

- Decide on which areas of the history you want to focus on and where examiners will expect detail.
- Consider what the differential diagnosis for the presenting condition may be.
- Consider how the condition is managed, and how treatment could be escalated if the response is inadequate.
- Make notes around these thoughts if that will help.

On entering the station

Greet the examiner and hand in your mark sheet. Then turn to the mother and child, introduce yourself, and greet them both before sitting down.

Clarify your role and agree aims and objectives of the consultation with Tom's mother.

Taking the history

If you feel you want to gather the history from the mother, tell Tom you will be asking the mother some questions but that you would be happy to listen if he wanted to help with the answers.

- *Chronology of symptoms* – Proceed with taking a structured and fluent history around Tom's asthma. Ask about when his symptoms first started (and when the diagnosis of asthma was made), how often he experiences the symptoms of asthma (difficulty in breathing, wheeze, chest tightness or cough) and any triggers to these symptoms.
- *Background asthma control* – Ask about interval symptoms, particularly symptoms at night, symptoms with exercise and the need for rescue salbutamol.
- Ask about *prior hospitalisations* with acute wheeze, including any previous admissions to the paediatric high dependency unit (HDU) or intensive care unit (ICU).
- Ask about *prior visits to the GP or emergency department* with acute asthma and the number of courses of systemic steroids he has needed in the last 6 months.
- You could also ask about the *number of repeat prescriptions* he has had for salbutamol inhalers – *A need for more than 1 prescription per month of salbutamol may be a marker of poor control.*
- Discover *coexisting medical conditions*, particularly allergic rhinitis, hay fever, eczema and allergies.
- Ask about the number of *school days missed* due to asthma.
- *Background regular treatment for asthma*, including dosages of medications, delivery and frequency of use – *Always ask children and families how they are taking/giving the inhalers. Are they using a spacer? If they are on regular preventer medication, consider compliance. How many days a week do they forget to take the medication?*
- Take a *family and social history* (including a family history of atopy, smokers at home, housing and pets).
- Use of *complementary therapies* for asthma.
- Take an *immunisation history*, including flu vaccine (if appropriate).
- Take a *birth history*, including any prematurity.
- If you are seeing a young person or adolescent, ask them if they smoke and, if they do, signpost them to local National Health Service (NHS) smoking cessation services. Ask about symptoms of anxiety and depression. These are significantly more prevalent in young people with asthma.
- In addition, throughout the history, consider whether there are any clues that suggest an alternative diagnosis to asthma (Table 6.22).

Top tips!
Ask a range of *open-ended and closed questions*. Ensure the questions are clear and avoid jargon. Practise *active listening* throughout the consultation.

Assimilating the information

Now that you have taken a focused history, you will be expected to assimilate and present the most salient points to the examiner. Below is a summary of the history obtained from Tom's mother, and an example presentation.

To present...

> "Tom is a 7 year old boy who has recently moved into the area with a diagnosis of asthma made at the age of 3. He has presented to his GP several times over the years with recurrent wheeze and a nocturnal cough, and his GP has gradually increased his asthma medication over that time. He was admitted to the ward with an acute exacerbation last month, his second admission this year. He received oral steroids on both occasions. He is currently receiving beclometasone 200 micrograms twice a day and salbutamol when needed, both via a spacer. His GP has treated Tom for chest infections on a few occasions. The mother is concerned that Tom is still coughing at night and seems breathless with exercise. She is using the salbutamol almost every day. Tom has 1 sister, 6 years old, and she suffers with eczema. The mother has hay fever. The family owns a dog. I believe Tom's asthma is not adequately controlled."

Discussion

Now that you have arrived at a likely diagnosis, you will spend the remainder of the 3 minutes discussing aspects of this condition with the examiner. Possible questions from the examiner are highlighted below. It is unlikely all of these can be asked within the given time frame.

■ ***What do you think the current problem is and what would you do next?***

Tom has poorly controlled asthma. When assessing a child with poorly controlled asthma, you should consider the following before changing the drug therapy:

- Is the diagnosis correct? In Tom's case, there are no features in the history that suggest an alternative diagnosis. Tom also has a strong family history of atopy, which makes a diagnosis of asthma more likely.
- Are there modifiable triggers? Cigarette smoke exposure is associated with a higher prevalence of asthma symptoms in children, so you should ask about this.
- Does the child have allergic rhinitis? If they do, treating this may help asthma control.
- Is there good adherence with existing therapy and, if not, why?
- Is the inhaler technique good? Check that the inhalers are being given through a spacer and, if time permits, ensure the family knows how to care for the spacer.

Top tip!
The aim of asthma treatment is to control symptoms so that children experience no daytime symptoms and no night-time awakening due to asthma, there is no need for rescue medication, no limitations on activities (including exercise) and no exacerbations.

If you have identified no clear reversible or treatable factor, it is appropriate to move up a step on the asthma treatment guidelines, if Tom's asthma is poorly controlled.

The British Thoracic Society (BTS) guidelines suggest a step-wise approach to asthma treatment in children. Children should start at the step most appropriate to the initial severity of their asthma. If a child has poorly controlled asthma, and you have excluded other possible factors, you should step up his treatment, as shown in Table 6.21.

Table 6.21: BTS step-wise asthma treatment in children over 5 years	
Severity of asthma	Treatment
Step 1 – Mild intermittent asthma	Add inhaled short-acting beta-agonist as required
Step 2 – Regular preventer therapy	Add inhaled steroid* at 200–400 micrograms per day. Start at a dose appropriate to the severity of the disease.
Step 3 – Add-on therapy	Add an inhaled long-acting beta-agonist. Assess response. If there is no response or if control is still inadequate, stop long-acting beta-agonists and consider: Trial of other therapies, including leukotriene receptor antagonists (montelukast); OR Increasing the dose of inhaled steroids to 400 micrograms per day*.
Step 4 – Persistent poor control	Increase inhaled steroid* up to 800 micrograms per day.
Step 5 – Frequent use of oral steroids	Refer to the respiratory paediatrician.

* Beclomethasone dipropionate

Due to Tom's frequent interval symptoms (nocturnal cough, breathlessness on exertion), it would be appropriate to move him up to step 3. This would necessitate adding in a long acting beta 2 agonist along to his inhaled steroid therapy. To aid concordance, it is best to use a combination inhaler of steroid plus salmeterol (seretide) or formoterol (symbicort).

■ Are there any side effects from inhaled corticosteroids in children?

Side effects from inhaled corticosteroids are rare in children. The inhaled medicine (if used through a spacer) will work predominantly on the airways, where it is needed, and systemic absorption is minimal. Children can get a sore tongue or throat, hoarseness of the voice and oral candidiasis; these side effects can be prevented by ensuring children rinse their mouth after using a steroid inhaler.

High doses of inhaled corticosteroids have the potential to cause impaired growth, adrenal suppression, decreased bone mineral density, skin thinning, bruising and cataract, but these are rare. Children who are on high doses of inhaled corticosteroids should be monitored closely, especially for growth. You should remember that severe asthma by itself could lead to growth failure, if left untreated.

> *Top tip!*
> You should explore the child and parent's understanding of the disease and the treatment options, as well as their expectations and concerns.

■ What is the differential diagnosis of asthma in children?

Asthma is a clinical diagnosis in children. It causes the recurrent respiratory symptoms of wheeze, cough, difficulty in breathing, and chest tightness due to variable airway obstruction. Asthma is more likely if wheezing is frequent and recurrent, worse at night and early in the morning, and worse with exercise or precipitated by other triggers such as exposure to pets, cold or damp air, or with emotional upset. Presence of interval symptoms in between acute exacerbations is also highly suggestive. An atopic tendency is often forthcoming in the history, such as eczema, allergic rhinitis or other allergies. A family history of asthma or other atopy also favours asthma.

However, all that wheezes is not asthma. Table 6.22 lists the differential diagnoses and clues to alternative diagnoses.

Table 6.22: Pointers to an alternative diagnosis in wheezy children	
Clinical clue	Alternative diagnoses to consider
Symptoms present from birth or neonatal period	Congenital lung abnormality, cystic fibrosis, chronic lung disease of prematurity, ciliary dyskinesia
Family history of respiratory disease	Cystic fibrosis, immunodeficiency, neuromuscular disorder
Severe upper respiratory tract disease	Ciliary dyskinesia, immunodeficiency
Excessive vomiting	Gastro-oesophageal reflux disease
Breathlessness with light-headedness and peripheral tingling	Hyperventilation/panic attacks
Persistent moist cough	Cystic fibrosis, bronchiectasis, recurrent aspiration, ciliary dyskinesia, immunodeficiency
Inspiratory stridor	Tracheal or laryngeal disorder
Abnormal voice or cry	Laryngeal problem
Focal signs in the chest	Inhaled foreign body, congenital abnormality, bronchiectasis, pneumonia
Finger clubbing	Cystic fibrosis, bronchiectasis
Failure to thrive	Cystic fibrosis, immunodeficiency, gastro-oesophageal reflux
Focal or persistent CXR changes	Congenital abnormality, cystic fibrosis, recurrent aspiration, bronchiectasis, tuberculosis
Tachypnoea without wheeze	Severe acidosis – e.g. diabetic ketoacidosis, renal failure
New onset of wheeze in older child +/- orthopnoea	Mediastinal mass

■ *Is there any further information you want to give Tom?*

You should provide Tom with a *personalised and written asthma plan*. This plan should include details of his regular medications (preventers), guidance on how to know if his symptoms get worse, and what the family should do about it. It will also inform Tom and his parents regarding what to do in an emergency if he has a severe exacerbation of wheeze. You may also want to give Tom a *peak flow meter and diary*, if he is able to use it correctly.

■ *How often should Tom see his GP about his asthma?*

This depends on Tom's asthma control. If you make a change to his asthma treatment, Tom should see his GP in the next month to assess the efficacy of the change you have made. If his asthma is well controlled for 3 months, he should see his GP to discuss whether his medication can be reduced. All children with asthma should have a yearly asthma review at their GP practice. Children who have been admitted with an acute exacerbation of asthma should see their GP or practice nurse ideally within 48 hours of discharge to assess their recovery and reinforce asthma education. Many GP surgeries have asthma specialist nurses who follow up with these children regularly.

■ What is the asthma control test?

The asthma control test is a validated tool to check asthma control in children. It can be used in the GP and outpatient setting. More details of the test can be obtained from the reference mentioned below.

Syllabus mapping

General competence

The candidate must:

- Demonstrate good generic communication skills when dealing with children and adolescents.

Respiratory medicine

The candidate must:

- Be able to discuss the assessment and management of children with acute asthma and plan long-term management (BTS guidelines for management of asthma).
- Be aware of the long-term complications of medications used for asthma.
- Be able to teach and assess inhaler technique, as well as teach care of spacer.

Further reading and references

1. Asthma Plans. http://www.asthma.org.uk/advice-asthma-and-me (accessed June 2015).
2. British guidelines on the management of asthma. British Thoracic Society (BTS) and Scottish Intercollegiate Guidelines Network Clinical Guidelines. London and Edinburgh, 2012. http://www.brit-thoracic.org.uk/document-library/clinical-information/asthma/btssign-guideline-on-the-management-of-asthma/ (accessed June 2015).
3. Bush A, Fleming L. Diagnosis and management of asthma in children. *BMJ* 2015; 350: h996. doi: 10.1136/bmj.h996
4. Childhood Asthma Control Test. http://www.asthma.com/resources/childhood-asthma-control-test.html (accessed June 2015).
5. Hedlin G, Konradsen J, Bush A. An update on paediatric asthma. *Eur Respir Rev* 2012; 21: 175–85. doi: 10.1183/09059180.00003212
6. Itchy, Sneezy, Wheezy. http://www.itchysneezywheezy.co.uk (accessed June 2015).
7. Paton J. Asthma: Standards of care. *Arch Dis Child* 2013; 98: 928–9. doi: 10.1136/archdischild-2012-303141

Chapter 6.3: Case Study 2: 5 Year Old with Chronic Constipation
Mr M De La Hunt

This station assesses your ability to take a history that is focused on a child's chronic condition and, subsequently, undertake a discussion based on this. As the candidate, you will be leading the consultation, and parents or role players should normally desist from asking questions. If they do, it is appropriate to answer them.

You will be assessed on the rapport, manner and structure of your interview with the child and parent. During the discussion, the examiner will focus on your understanding of chronic disease management.

Logistics:

Timing: This is a 9-minute station. You will have up to 2 minutes before the start of this station to read the candidate sheet and prepare yourself.

When the bell rings: On entering the room, the examiner will greet you, take your mark sheet, and introduce you to the child and parent. The examiner will then remain silent during the consultation.

You will have 6 minutes to conduct your consultation. A knock will be given at 6 minutes to indicate that 3 minutes remain before the end of the station. At this point, it is important to summarise the history and proceed with the discussion with the examiner.

If you finish early, you will be asked to remain in the room until the session has ended.

Candidate role and task:

You are an ST3 GP trainee working in a GP surgery.

Alice is 5 years old. She suffers from chronic constipation. She has recently started having accidents at school with incontinence of stool.

Task: The mother has come to the surgery requesting a referral to the hospital.

Top tip!
Always ensure you greet the parent and child at the beginning. Examiners will assess your ability to include the child in the consultation and to put the child at ease.

Before entering the station

As there are only 6 minutes to take the history, use the time before entering the station to:

- Decide on which areas of the history you want to focus on and where the examiners will expect detail.
- Consider what the differential diagnosis for the presenting condition may be.
- Consider how the condition is managed and how treatment could be escalated if response is inadequate.
- Make notes around these thoughts if that will help.

On entering the station

Greet the examiner and hand in your mark sheet.
Turn to the mother and child, introduce yourself, and greet them both before sitting down.
Clarify your role and agree aims and objectives of the consultation with Alice's mother.

Taking the history

While taking the history for this scenario, you should aim to:

- Establish the diagnosis and underlying causes
- Look for potentially serious underlying problems
- Assess the severity and impact of the problem
- Explore the best way to manage the problem

You will need to take most of the history from Alice's mother, but it is very important to consider Alice in the process, particularly relating to her symptoms and perceptions, and in forming a realistic management plan. This is a complex clinical situation, and you will need to remain very focused in taking the history. A complete history will lead you to the cause. Remain focused and use all the verbal and non-verbal clues provided by both parent and child.

> *Top tip!*
> Examiners will assess your ability to include the child in the consultation.

Assimilating the history

Now that you have taken a focused history, you will be expected to assimilate and present the most salient points to the examiner. Below is a summary of the history obtained from Alice's mother, and an example presentation.

To present...

> "Alice is a 5 year old girl who has had problems with constipation from the age of 1 year and began soiling since she started at a new school 3 months ago. There were no earlier concerns about her bowel function or delay in passing meconium, and her growth and development have otherwise been normal. She has been taking Movicol for 1 year and her stooling pattern has improved from passing a massive painful stool every 6 to 7 days to soft stools every 1 to 2 days. For the past month, she has been soiling once or twice a week with quite large volumes, enough to need a change of clothes. This happens only at school. Her mother is concerned that this could result in teasing or bullying. Alice has never liked passing stool anywhere other than at home."

> *Top tip!*
> Once you have gathered the history, summarise this with the mother. Don't be tempted to repeat the whole history.

Discussion

Now that you have arrived at a likely diagnosis, you will spend the remainder of the 3 minutes discussing aspects of this condition with the examiner. Possible questions from the examiner are highlighted below. It is unlikely all of these can be asked within the given time frame.

■ *What do you think is the underlying problem?*

- The above history would suggest long-standing retentive constipation with some degree of stool withholding, but now is reasonably well controlled with her current treatment. The new problem is her soiling, which occurs only at school. This suggests a problem adjusting to school life or an underlying psychological cause. Overflow soiling associated with faecal impaction is usually low volume and continuous. Alice has been passing a soft stool every 1 to 2 days and her soiling is heavy when it occurs.
- There could be a more generalised psychological problem relating to a toilet phobia. Normal bowel function up to 1 year of age makes it unlikely that there is any serious underlying anatomical problem or Hirschsprung's disease.

■ *What advice would you offer Alice's mother?*

- Explain the factors that contribute to constipation and soiling, and discuss the principles behind management options. This enhances compliance and improves outcomes.
- It is important to maintain regular soft stools with adequate doses of laxatives (Movicol) to prevent a large build-up with the passage of a hard, painful stool. This should continue until it is reasonably certain that Alice is able to pass regular soft stools without laxatives and is not afraid of passing stool or trying to delay defaecation.
- It is important to maintain a healthy diet and high fluid intake. Encourage regular, unhurried toileting.
- It is also important to try to defuse tensions arising in the household relating to constipation. The family may be concerned that constipation can result in a burst bowel, absorption of toxins or cancer. They should be reassured that, although distressing, primary idiopathic constipation very rarely causes any serious or life-threatening complications. Strenuous stool withholding is often misinterpreted by the family as unsuccessful straining and struggling to pass stool. In this situation, there is also often a history of only passing stool into a nappy after being unable to do so on the toilet. It is important to stress that, even if Alice is trying to delay or withhold stool, this does not mean that she is being naughty, bad or lazy. At the age of 5 years, children are not mature enough to rationalise these issues in the same way as an adult. Patience with an encouraging approach is needed.
- This could take a long time to correct. Until a normal stool pattern is established, it is better to err on the side of giving too much rather than too little Movicol.
- The history does not suggest a serious underlying problem with bowel function, but we still cannot absolutely exclude a problem with the ability to pass stool normally, such as an abnormal defaecation reflex or acquired megarectum (when the bowel has been stretched by chronic constipation and can take a long time to return to normal).
- Careful follow-up is needed until Alice's bowel function has returned to normal.

■ **Is there anything more you might need to do to exclude any serious underlying conditions?**

In taking the history, the important 'amber/red flags' you need to explore are:

- Delayed passage of meconium or severe constipation from birth, particularly if associated with abdominal distension and vomiting
- Faltering growth
- History of previous perineal trauma or surgery
- Spinal problems
- Any suspicion of abuse or neglect

If any red flags are present, or the constipation and soiling fail to improve with treatment, you will need to consider referral for further investigation and treatment. This may involve physiological studies (e.g. bowel transit, anorectal manometry), rectal biopsy if there is any suspicion of Hirschsprung's disease, or surgery for anatomical problems (e.g. ectopy or stenosis).

Top tip!
Presence of a 'red flag' should initiate a referral to secondary/tertiary care.

■ **What is the role of the Bristol stool chart in the diagnosis and management of idiopathic constipation in children?**

- The Bristol stool form scale (Figure 6.31) helps patients and parents or carers to describe their stools without embarrassment. The chart helps in the diagnosis and follow-up of chronic constipation. The scale was developed by researchers at the Bristol Royal Infirmary. Hard or impacted stools are of types 1, 2 and 3, while normal stools are types 4 and 5. Loose stools are type 6 and diarrhoea gives rise to type 7 stools.

Additional Information

Constipation is very common. Depending on the criteria used, it affects 5–30% of children and young people, and becomes chronic in about one third of these.

There are many definitions of constipation, but most would make the diagnosis when the frequency, consistency or passage of stools causes distressing symptoms. Constipation may also be associated with flatulence, abdominal discomfort and distension, overflow soiling, reduced appetite, irritability or general malaise. Painful anal fissures can exacerbate stool withholding, leading to a worsening cycle of constipation and soiling. Most childhood constipation will be primary or idiopathic. This is defined as constipation that cannot be explained by any anatomical, physiological, radiological or histological abnormalities.

Soiling may be the result of overflow secondary to constipation. This is usually characterised by continuous leakage of small volumes of stool. You will need to consider other causes if the constipation is very mild, or if the soiling does not directly relate to the stooling pattern.

There may still be many important causative or precipitating factors that you will need to explore while taking the history.

- **Social and lifestyle**
    - Onset associated with changes in diet and fluid intake (e.g. weaning, travel, intercurrent illness) or other medication
    - Social and family changes, such as starting at nursery or a new school, moving house, changes in the family
    - Problems with toilet access at school

- **Psychological/behavioural**
    - Stool avoidance due to painful defaecation, with or without anal bleeding (e.g. acute or chronic fissure)
    - Toilet avoidance, toilet phobias and deliberate stool withholding
    - Encopresis – Deliberate inappropriate defaecation
    - Neurodevelopmental problems (e.g. cerebral palsy, autistic spectrum disorders, severe learning difficulties)

- **Physiological**
    - Slow bowel transit
    - An abnormal defaecation reflex (failure of sphincter relaxation, 'anorectal achalasia')
    - Metabolic and endocrine (e.g. hypothyroidism, hypercalcaemia)
    - Hirschsprung's disease
    - Neurological (spinal dysraphism and other spinal cord lesions interfering with motility or defaecation)

- **Anatomical**
    - A history of congenital gastrointestinal abnormalities
    - Previous abdominal, pelvic or perineal surgery
    - Congenital or acquired spinal problems

It is important to look for red flag features in the history and examination (Table 6.31), although, in the context of the focused history and management planning station, you will not be examining the child. Furthermore, you may be able to elicit potential serious causes or underlying conditions that can cause or exacerbate constipation (Table 6.32).

Table 6.31: Red flags in the history and physical examination (modified from NICE 2010)	
Key component	Red flags
Onset of constipation	From birth or first few weeks of life Delayed passage of meconium (more than 48 hours from birth)
Stool pattern	'Ribbon' or narrow stools
Growth and general health	Faltering growth, features of neglect or abuse
Abdomen	Abdominal distension, vomiting, palpable mass (other than faecal), recurrent enterocolitis in infancy
Examination of the perineum	Abnormal position or calibre/patency of anus Anal fistulae, fissures, bruising Abnormal anal tone (patulous or spastic) Absent anocutaneous reflex
Spine/lumbosacral region	Asymmetry or flattening of the gluteal muscles, sacral agenesis, discoloured skin, naevi or sinus, hairy patch, lipoma, scoliosis
Lower limb neuromuscular examination	Abnormal neuromuscular signs, deformity or locomotor delay

Table 6.32: Serious causes of chronic constipation	
Cause	Suggestive clinical findings
Hirschsprung's disease	Delayed passage of meconium (>24 hours) Can present with life-threatening enterocolitis (abdominal distension, with explosive diarrhoea, rapid dehydration sepsis and collapse) Constipation from birth Chronic abdominal distension and vomiting Family history of Hirschsprung's disease Faltering growth
Neurological/neurodevelopmental or genetic conditions (e.g. trisomy 21, autistic spectrum disorders, cerebral palsy, spinal anomalies)	Delayed development Neurological deficits (e.g. cerebral palsy) Behavioural problems Dysmorphic features
Psychiatric conditions and encopresis	Suggestive history
Severe dysmotility, visceral myopathies, chronic pseudo-obstruction, congenital megarectum	Persistent abdominal distension Poor response to treatment May be associated with urinary tract dysmotility
Anatomical or structural abnormalities (e.g. ectopia or stenosis of the anus, pelvic masses)	History of an earlier surgical correction of congenital abnormalities or abnormality on clinical examination
Urinary problems (wetting, urine infection)	May coexist Can occur as a consequence of severe constipation or have the same underlying cause
Child abuse or neglect	Adverse social circumstances Failure to thrive Other signs of neglect or physical abuse

Assess the severity and impact of the problem

Establish how much of a problem this really is causing:

- The soiling – The severity (from small stains on the underwear to large volumes), the frequency and times, and the situations in which it occurs (e.g. only at school)
- The constipation – The chronicity, stool frequency and consistency. The Bristol stool chart is a very useful clinical tool for documenting and monitoring stool consistency (Figure 6.31).
- The level of distress caused by passing massive stools or painful defaecation
- Associated urinary problems
- Impact on daily life, school activity and social exclusion
- Impact on the rest of the family and home

Explore the best way to manage the problem

- Treatment and care should take into account the child's and the family's needs, preferences and circumstances. Education through a clear and appropriate explanation of the situation improves outcomes.
- Establish what treatments or strategies have already been tried and the likely degree of compliance with your recommended treatment plan.
- It is important to assess all children and young people with idiopathic constipation for faecal impaction, by using a combination of history taking and physical examination. Digital rectal examination can be extremely distressing and counterproductive in many situations. Thus,

it should be performed only with very clear indications and by healthcare professionals fully trained to interpret the subtlety of the findings. When faecal impaction is suspected, NICE 2010 recommends treatment using a disimpaction regimen. This is initiated with polyethylene glycol 3350 and electrolytes (Movicol Paediatric) using an escalating dose regimen until there is passage of a large amount of stools. Another laxative (e.g. Sodium Picosulfate, Senna, Bisacodyl or Docusate sodium) may be tried in resistant cases.

- Once emptying is achieved, it is important to maintain regular soft stools with adequate doses of laxatives (Movicol) to prevent a large build-up with the passage of a hard painful stool. This should be done until it is reasonably certain that the patient is able to pass regular soft stools without help, and is not afraid of passing stool or is trying to delay defaecation. This can take a long time to resolve and a maintenance dose of medication may need to be continued for many months and sometimes years. Until a normal stool pattern is established, it is better to err on the side of giving too much rather than too little Movicol.
- Recommend good fluid intake and healthy diet.
- Encourage a regular healthy toileting pattern. Encouraging stooling after a warm breakfast recruits the gastrocolic reflex and this can also be augmented by individualising the timing of taking laxatives to achieve the maximum effect.
- Positive reinforcements alone should be used, and no form of punitive measures will help in the long-term management. Avoid conflict or blame.
- Address psychological issues.
- Seek help through the school (teachers and school nurse) or other relevant agencies.
- Specialist referral may be needed for severe chronic symptoms, treatment failure or any suspicion of more complex pathology (see amber/red flags).
- Surgical approaches will be needed if there is an underlying anatomical abnormality or for failure of medical treatment. Depending on the diagnosis, these include sphincter Botox injections, sphincterotomy, exteriorisation of the appendix to enable antegrade colonic enemas, and excision of dysfunctional, grossly dilated segments of bowel. Stomas (temporary or even permanent) may be needed only when all other treatments have failed.
- Prolonged support may be needed for many children and young people who experience social, psychological and educational consequences.

Figure 6.31: The Bristol stool form scale (Illustration by Dr G Bandaranayake)

Stool type	Description	Diagram
Type 1	Separate hard lumps, like nuts (hard to pass)	
Type 2	Sausage-shaped but lumpy	
Type 3	Like a sausage, but with cracks on the surface	
Type 4	Like a sausage or snake, smooth and soft	
Type 5	Soft blobs with clear cut edges (passed easily)	
Type 6	Fluffy pieces with ragged edges, a mushy stool	

Syllabus mapping

General competence

The candidate must:

- Demonstrate good generic communication skills when dealing with children and young adults.

Gastroenterology

The candidate must:

- Be familiar with the diagnosis and management of constipation (NICE 2010).

Further reading and references

1. Bae SH. Diets for constipation. *Pediatr Gastroenterol Hepatol Nutr* 2014; 17: 203-8
2. Lewis SJ, Heaton KW. Stool form scale as a useful guide to intestinal transit time. *Scand J Gastroenterol* 1997; 32: 920-4
3. National Institute for Health and Care Excellence. (CG99) - Constipation in children and young people. Diagnosis and management of idiopathic childhood constipation in primary and secondary care. London, 2010. https://www.nice.org.uk/guidance/cg99 (accessed July 2015).
4. Paré P, Fedorak RN. Systematic review of stimulant and nonstimulant laxatives for the treatment of functional constipation. *Can J Gastroenterol Hepatol* 2014; 28: 549-57
5. Russell KW, Barnhart DC, Zobell S et al. Effectiveness of an organized bowel management program in the management of severe chronic constipation in children. *J Pediatr Surg* 2015; 50: 444-7

Chapter 6.4: Case Study 3: 6 Year Old with Communication Problems
Dr Abdul Razak Sheik

This station assesses your ability to take a focused history from a child and family, and undertake a discussion based on this. As the candidate, you will be asking most or all of the questions, but if parents or role players do ask questions during the consultation, it will be appropriate to answer these.

You will be assessed on your communication with the child and parent, and the rapport, structure and manner of your interview. During the discussion, the examiner will focus on your history-taking skills and the management of behavioural problems in children.

Logistics:

Timing: This is a 9-minute station. You will have up to 2 minutes before the start of this station to read the candidate sheet and prepare yourself.

When the bell rings: On entering the room, the examiner will greet you, take your mark sheet, and introduce you to the child and parent. The examiner will then remain silent during the consultation.

You will have 6 minutes to conduct your consultation. A knock at 6 minutes will indicate that 3 minutes remain before the end of the station. At this point, it is important to summarise the history and proceed with the discussion with the examiner.

If you finish early, you will be asked to remain in the room until the session has ended.

Candidate role and task:

You are an ST3 GP trainee working in a GP surgery.

You have an appointment to meet Mrs Clarke and her 6 year old son, Charlie Clarke.

Task: Charlie Clarke is a 6 year old boy in Year 1 at Round Tree Infant School. Mrs Clarke has come to see you on the advice of her son's class teacher. The teacher has expressed concerns to Charlie's mother about his immature communication skills, lack of friends in school and his general behaviour with other children. She has suggested the mother should contact his GP regarding the possibility of autistic spectrum disorder.

Top tip!
Always ensure you greet the parent and child at the beginning. Examiners will assess your ability to include Charlie in the consultation.

Before entering the station

As there are only 6 minutes to take the history, utilise the time before entering the station to:

- Decide on which areas of the history you want to focus on and where the examiners will expect detail.
- Consider what the differential diagnosis for the presenting condition may be.
- Consider how the condition is managed and how treatment could be escalated if response is inadequate.
- Make notes around these thoughts if that will help.

On entering the station

Greet the examiner and hand in your mark sheet.

Then turn to the mother and Charlie, introduce yourself and greet them both before sitting down. Clarify your role and agree aims and objectives of the consultation with Charlie's mother.

Taking the history

If you feel you want to gather the history from the mother, tell Charlie you will be asking the mother some questions, but that you would be happy to listen if he wanted to help with the answers.

- Ask Charlie's mother an open-ended question about her concerns.
- Focus your questions on Charlie's general day-to-day activities, including enquiring about his eating habits and sleep routines, Charlie's response to changes in routine, possible repetitive stereotypic behaviour, and sensory sensitivity (touch, taste, smell and noise).
- Enquire about communication and interaction with parents, siblings and while in a group.
- Explore his non-verbal communication – i.e. facial expression, eye contact, gestures, awareness of personal space, voice modulation, and how he shows emotions.
- Assess Charlie's understanding of abstract language (e.g. similes, metaphors). Does he interpret language literally?
- Assess the use of expressive language (vocabulary, echolalia, and use of formal adult-like language during interaction, monotonous or mechanical speech quality).
- Explore patterns of play – i.e. pretend play, taking turns, special interest in particular types of toys or specific approach to playing.
- Note the display of any extraordinary knowledge (numbers, maps, roads, etc.).
- Enquire about his behaviour as a baby (social smile, irritable or placid baby, development of speech, his response to his name).
- Undertake a quick check on the birth history and development.
- Ask about the family and social history.

Top tip!
Once you have gathered the history, *summarise* this with the mother and the examiner. Don't be tempted to repeat the whole history to the examiner.

Assimilating the history

Now that you have taken a focused history, you will be expected to assimilate and present your positive findings. Below is a summary of the history obtained from Charlie's mother, and a sample presentation.

To present...

> "Charlie is a 6 year old boy whose schoolteacher has concerns related to communication difficulties.
>
> Charlie was born at term by normal delivery and did not suffer from any neonatal problems. He has normal motor development. However, he has speech delay, with normal hearing. He likes his daily routines and gets upset even with minor deviations. He likes to play on his own and enjoys arranging dinosaurs and cars in a straight line. He does not have any friends at school. Charlie prefers to eat bland non-sticky foods such as toast, crisps, chips, rice and pasta without cheese, and has had a dietetic review. He does not initiate conversation on his own. Today, he gave limited responses when spoken to, and did not show any eye contact. He has a 3 year old brother who has better communication skills.
>
> This history is suggestive of an autistic spectrum disorder."

Discussion

Now that you have arrived at a likely diagnosis, you will spend the remainder of the 3 minutes discussing aspects of this condition with the examiner. Possible questions from the examiner are highlighted below. It is unlikely all of these can be asked within the given time frame.

■ *What do you think the problem is?*

Charlie functions abnormally in both social interaction and communication, and demonstrates stereotypic patterns of behaviour and interest. The most likely diagnosis is autistic spectrum disorder.

The term 'autism' describes qualitative differences and impairments in reciprocal social interaction and social communication, combined with restricted interests and rigid and repetitive behaviours (NICE 2011). The condition is now thought to occur in at least 1% of children. The mild end of the spectrum is Asperger syndrome, where children do not have a delay in language development or cognitive difficulties. In contrast, at the severe end of the spectrum, children have significant cognitive and learning difficulties and significant sensory sensitivity issues. Children with autistic spectrum disorder may have difficulties with processing information, predicting the consequences of actions, understanding the concept of time, and executive function.

■ *Who would you like to involve in helping the family and child to arrive at a diagnosis?*

Each area has a local pathway for recognition, referral and diagnostic assessment of possible autism. Teachers could initiate referral to the autistic spectrum services after obtaining parental consent (the educational psychologist is the usual professional who does the initial assessment with school referrals). Alternately, it could be GP due to parental concerns.

A multidisciplinary team assessment of the child should be undertaken by a:

- Paediatrician and/or child and adolescent psychiatrist who will take a detailed history, assess the child and involve the rest of the multidisciplinary team.
- Speech and language therapist who does a detailed assessment of the communication skills of the child.
- Clinical psychologist who is involved if the child is of preschool age, or an educational psychologist, who is involved if the child goes to school.
- Occupational therapist who is involved if sensory sensitivity is a significant problem.

After analysing the reports from various professionals, the paediatrician discusses the findings with the parents. If the assessments are inconclusive, these children will have a more detailed specialised autism assessment called Autism Diagnostic Observation Schedule (ADOS) (NICE 2011).

■ *What is the NICE recommendation for autism diagnostic assessment in children and young people?*

Start the autism diagnostic assessment within 3 months of the referral to the autism team. A case coordinator should be identified for every child or young person who is to have an autism diagnostic assessment.

The autism case coordinator should:

- Act as a single point of contact for the parents or carers and, if appropriate, the child or young person being assessed, through whom the child and the parents can communicate with the rest of the autism team.
- Keep parents or carers and, if appropriate, the child or young person, up to date about the likely time and sequence of assessments.
- Arrange for the provision of information and support for parents, carers, children and young people as directed by the autism team.
- Gather information relevant to the autism diagnostic assessment, i.e. seek a report from the preschool or school if one has not already been made available, and gather any additional health or social care information, including results from hearing and vision assessments.

■ *What differential diagnoses should be considered in this situation?*

Several diseases, including neurodevelopmental issues and epileptic disorders, can mimic autistic spectrum disorder. Table 6.41 lists some helpful pointers towards a differential diagnosis.

Table 6.41: Disorders simulating autistic spectrum disorder (ASD)	
Disorders simulating autistic spectrum disorder	**Helpful hints**
Neurodevelopmental disorders • Specific language delay	No difficulties in social interaction or concerns with stereotypical behaviour patterns
• Intellectual disability or global developmental delay	Obvious from the early infantile period compared to autistic spectrum disorder
Mental and behavioural disorders • ADHD • Anxiety disorder • Attachment disorders	Differentiated by the age-appropriate language and social interaction skills
Conditions in which there is developmental regression • Rett syndrome	Onset at 6–18 months of age Slowing of development, followed by regression of language and motor milestones Acquired deceleration of head growth resulting in microcephaly Affects females almost exclusively
• Epileptic encephalopathy	Clear history of epileptic seizures Previous status epilepticus
Miscellaneous • Maltreatment (emotional neglect)	Lack of emotional bonding and stimulus for development

■ *What advice would you offer the mother and the school?*

- Early intervention can often reduce challenges associated with autism, lessen disruptive behaviour, and provide some degree of independence.
- Management has to be individualised depending on the needs of the child, and the severity of the manifestations. In most cases, a combination of different treatment modalities is helpful and recommended.
- Visual timetables and supports – Verbal discussion may need to be complemented with appropriate pictures, written lists, calendars and real objects to enable carers/children to understand what is going to happen and when.
- Colours can be used to indicate the importance or significance of tasks (and therefore help to prioritise tasks and work through them in a logical sequence).
- Contact details for:
    - Local and national support organisations (who may provide, for example, an opportunity to meet other families with experience of autism, or information about specific courses for parents and carers and/or young people).
    - Organisations that can provide advice on welfare benefits.
    - Organisations that can provide information on educational support and social care.

■ *What causes autistic spectrum disorder? What investigations would you perform to confirm the diagnosis?*

The aetiology of autistic spectrum disorder is multifactorial, involving several complex genetic and environmental factors. In some children, an underlying neurologic disease may contribute to autistic spectrum disorder.

In the past, some people believed that the measles, mumps and rubella vaccine (MMR) caused autistic spectrum disorder, but this has been investigated extensively in a number of major studies around the world, involving millions of children, and researchers have found no evidence of a link between the MMR vaccine and autistic spectrum disorder.

Autistic spectrum disorder is a clinical diagnosis, and does not warrant any routine investigations for the diagnosis. Selected children may require an EEG (if epilepsy is suspected) or genetic investigations such as microarray or specific genetic tests (in the presence of specific dysmorphic features, congenital anomalies and/or evidence of intellectual disability).

Syllabus mapping

General competence

The candidate must:

- Demonstrate good generic communication skills when dealing with children and young adults.

Behavioural problems

The candidate must:

- Be able to discuss the assessment and management of children with suspected autistic spectrum disorders (NICE 2011).
- Be able to look at behaviour as a form of communication, and to take this into account when interviewing, examining and assessing children.

Further reading and references

1. National Institute of Health and Care Excellence. (CG128) – Autism diagnosis in children and young people. Recognition, referral and diagnosis of children and young people on the autism spectrum. London, 2011. https://www.nice.org.uk/guidance/cg128 (accessed July 2015).
2. Hirtz DG, Wagner A, Filipek PA. Autistic spectrum disorders. *Swaiman's Pediatric Neurology*, 5th edition. Elsevier Saunders, 2012: 638–63. ISBN 13:9781437704358
3. *Diagnostic and statistical manual of mental disorders*, 5th edition. American Psychiatric Association: Washington DC, 2013:50-59. http://dx.doi.org/10.1176/appi.books.9780890425596

Chapter 6.5: Case Study 4: 13 Year Old with Diabetes

Dr S Kanumakala, Dr P Venugopalan

This station assesses your ability to take a focused history from an adolescent with a chronic condition and his family, and undertake a discussion based on this. As the candidate, you will be asking most or all of the questions, but if parents or role players do ask questions during the consultation, it will be appropriate to answer these.

You will be assessed on your communication with the patient and parents, and the rapport, structure and manner of your interview. During the discussion, the examiner will focus on your understanding of chronic disease management.

> **Logistics:**
>
> *Timing:* This is a 9-minute station. You will have up to 2 minutes before the start of this station to read the candidate sheet and prepare yourself.
>
> *When the bell rings:* On entering the room, the examiner will greet you, take your mark sheet, and introduce you to the child and parent. The examiner will then remain silent during the consultation.
>
> You will have 6 minutes to conduct your consultation. A knock at 6 minutes will indicate that 3 minutes remain before the end of the station. At this point, it is important to summarise the history and proceed with the discussion with the examiner.
>
> If you finish early, you will be asked to remain in the room until the session has ended.

> **Candidate role and task:**
>
> **You are an** ST3 GP trainee working in a GP surgery.
>
> Connor is 13 years old. He developed type 1 diabetes mellitus 6 years ago. Recently, his blood sugars have been running high and his glycosylated haemoglobin (HbA1c) – checked 2 days ago – is high at 90 mmol/mol (10.4%). He has also failed to attend 2 appointments with the children's diabetes team at the district hospital.
>
> **Task: Connor has come to the surgery with his mother. The purpose of this visit is to request a repeat prescription of insulin.**

Top tip!
Always ensure you greet the parent and child at the beginning. Examiners will assess your ability to include Connor in the consultation and to put him at ease.

Before entering the station

As there are only 6 minutes to take the history, utilise the time before entering the station to:

- Decide on which areas of the history you want to focus on and where the examiners will expect detail.
- Consider the factors contributing to poor diabetes control, and explore what options are acceptable to achieve better control.
- Consider how to optimise diabetes management appropriately for this patient and family.
- Make notes around these thoughts if that will help.

On entering the station

Greet the examiner and hand in your mark sheet.

Then turn to the mother and Connor, introduce yourself and greet them both before sitting down. Clarify your role and agree on the aims and objectives of the consultation.

Taking the history

Take as much detail as possible from Connor. If you feel you want to gather the history from the mother, tell Connor you will be asking the mother some questions but that you would be keen to listen if he wanted to help with the answers.

- *Chronology of symptoms* – Proceed with taking a structured and fluent history around Connor's diabetes. Ask about when his symptoms first started (and when the diagnosis of diabetes was made), how often he experiences any symptoms of high or low sugars (hypo/hyperglycaemic episodes), any triggers to these, and if he is able to recognise and manage them easily.
- *Background diabetes control* – Ask about previous HbA1c measurements, the need for using additional insulin for high sugars, dietary knowledge and his carbohydrate and correction ratios (insulin sensitivity factor). In addition, ask about any problems when doing the corrections (i.e. overcorrection or undercorrection).
- Ask about *prior visits to the GP or emergency department (hospitalisations)* with severe hypoglycaemia (unconsciousness or seizures, etc.) or with diabetic ketoacidosis (including any previous admissions to paediatric HDU or ICU.
- You could also ask about the *number of repeat prescriptions* he has had for insulin in the last 3 months. Fewer *prescriptions of insulin requested may be a marker of insulin omission and poor control or poor compliance*.
- Ask about *coexisting medical conditions*, particularly coeliac disease and compliance with a gluten-free diet and hypothyroidism and its management
- Enquire about the number of *school days missed* due to diabetes.
- *Background regular treatment for diabetes*, including dosages of different insulins and their timings – Always ask children and families how they are giving the injections. Are they rotating the injection sites? Enquire if they are taking insulin with all snacks and meals, if they are on a basal bolus regimen, and if the injections are taken prior to eating rather than afterwards. Consider compliance, blood sugar testing prior to meals and frequency of missing insulin doses. What percentage of meals and snacks are taken without appropriate insulin?

- *Family and social history* (including a family history of diabetes and other autoimmune disorders) – These include any challenging social factors (child protection, separated parents, learning difficulties, visual difficulties) that could impact on the care of diabetes.
- *Immunisation history*, including flu vaccine (if appropriate).
- If you are seeing a young person or an adolescent, ask them if they smoke personally and, if they do, signpost them to local NHS smoking cessation services. Ask about symptoms of anxiety, depression and eating disorders. These are significantly more prevalent in young people with diabetes.

Top tip!
Ask a range of open-ended and closed questions. Ensure questions are *clear* and avoid jargon. Practise *active listening* throughout the consultation.

Once you have gathered the history, *summarise* this with the mother and invite any further questions. Don't be tempted to repeat the whole history. The examiner will be listening!

Assimilating the information

Now that you have taken a focused history, you will be expected to assimilate and present the most salient points to the examiner. Below is a summary of the history obtained from Connor and his mother, and an example presentation.

To present...

> "I have seen Connor, a 13 year old with type 1 diabetes mellitus on replacement therapy for the last 6 years. He initially presented with ketoacidosis, and required inpatient treatment. Subsequently, he has been on a basal bolus regimen with NovoRapid and Levemir. He adjusts his insulin based on his meals using carb-counting techniques. The current issues relate to his poor compliance with treatment, and have resulted in suboptimal control of his diabetes. His HbA1c is high at 10.4%. Connor is reluctant to take insulin injections, especially in the presence of peers, and he also has some degree of needle phobia. In the past, he has had a hypoglycaemic episode leading to a fear of hypoglycaemia. This poor control, along with his adolescent behaviour, contributes to the difficulty of engaging with the diabetic team at the hospital, leading to frequent non-attendance at the clinic."

Discussion

Now that you have arrived at a likely diagnosis, you will spend the remainder of the 3 minutes discussing aspects of this condition with the examiner. Possible questions from the examiner are highlighted below. It is unlikely all of these can be asked within the given time frame.

■ ***What do you think the main problem is?***

Connor has suboptimal control of his diabetes – secondary to compliance issues. Contributing factors include reluctance to inject insulin in the presence of friends, some degree of needle phobia, fear of hypoglycaemia and adolescence-related behaviour.

Useful questions to consider at this point would be:

- Is the insulin regimen appropriate for this child?
- Is the child following this insulin regimen?
- Are there any local factors that interfere with insulin absorption?
- Are there any social/family factors that interfere with diabetes care?

■ How will you assess him for good diabetes control?

HbA1c is the gold standard for long-term control assessment. Regular low values (below 7.5%, or <58 mmol/mol) should be achieved (Table 6.51). In addition, it is important that the child does not suffer hypoglycaemic symptoms, and that he has a good quality of life despite the demands of diabetes care.

Table 6.51: Indicators for good diabetic control

Parameter	How this is assessed?	Standards
High blood glucose levels (>8 mmol/L)	Diary record of blood sugars, pre-meal and postprandial values	4-8 mmol/L <50% of all tests show high value - Good control <25% of all tests show high value - Excellent control
Low blood glucose levels (hypos) (<4 mmol/L)	Diary records of blood sugars, symptom recognition, hypo unawareness, need for assistance	<10% of all tests No hypos needing assistance
HbA1c	Finger prick or venous blood test once in 3 months	<7.5% or <58 mmol/mol - Excellent control
Impact on lifestyle	History, school attendance, social life	Aim for normal life standards

■ What is your management plan for this child?

- Suggestions to improve insulin intake with meals and snacks.
  - Discuss that the body needs insulin. Not taking insulin is not helpful, both in the short and in the long term. Consider alarms on the mobile phone to serve as a reminder to take injections and consider insulin-free foods (refers to foods that have very little or no carbohydrates, such as tomatoes, cucumber, or protein-rich foods such as cheese and ham).
  - Help with anxiety and fear - Consider referral to a psychologist.
  - Appropriate expert advice - Encourage the child to attend the diabetes clinics at the hospital.
- Issue the necessary prescription.
- Make a further appointment in the near future to discuss the progress and consider further action as needed.
- Do not increase the dose of insulin. This is not the answer at this point.
- Liaise and share the information with the hospital diabetes team.

Top tip!
Management decisions should be taken around the needs and aspirations of the child and family. Do not try to adjust the child and family to your management plan; adjust the management plan so that the child and family are likely to follow (concordance).

■ Do you think this child will benefit from an insulin pump?

The insulin pump is an option here that needs to be discussed with the child and the family. However, this has its own challenges and, in this case, this is the appropriate time to make that decision.

A decision to start a child on the insulin pump is a joint decision between the child, the family and the healthcare team. There are increased care requirements around the use of the pump from both the child and the family. The child and the family should be proactive and reactive to glycaemic control, and often many children and families find this challenging. The healthcare team is responsible for assessing the appropriateness of insulin pump management and to train the family in its effective usage. There are many indications for its benefits in this child, and some limitations.

- Indications for using the insulin pump in this child:
    - Suboptimal control of diabetes
    - Reluctance with injections (needle phobia)
    - Fear of hypoglycaemia
    - Reluctance to inject in the presence of peers (insulin by pump is more discrete)
    - He is already carb counting, so training to switch to a pump is easier.

- Limitations:
    - Necessitates increased care input from the child and family. This might not happen.
    - Risk of failure – If the pump is subsequently found to be ineffective, Connor is at risk of perceiving this as a personal failure, with psychological implications.
    - Cost factor – A pump costs the NHS approximately £2,500 per year, over and above the costs for a child on insulin injections.

Top tip!
Any decision to commence a child on an insulin pump should not be taken lightly and in haste. Full preparation (which includes a discussion on the pros and cons and the child's and the family's abilities to manage this in the short and the long term) should guide the decision.

■ What are the symptoms of new onset of diabetes?

- Classical symptoms include polyuria, polydipsia, weight loss, and lethargy or tiredness.
- Polyuria can present as nocturia and bed-wetting.
- Less commonly, infections – Thrush may be the presenting symptom.
- The progressive nature of symptoms with each passing week. If unrecognised, these can progress to diabetic ketoacidosis. Younger children progress more rapidly to develop ketoacidosis.
- Abdominal pain and vomiting are related to the ketoacidosis, and hasten the clinical deterioration.
- Children and young adults generally have a shortened period of symptoms, often 2–4 weeks. Often, these symptoms are attributed to other causes in the first instance, partly because these are non-specific and new diabetes is an uncommon diagnosis. As many as 25–30% of children present with ketoacidosis.

■ **What are the principles of management in a patient with diabetic ketoacidosis?**

- Diabetic ketoacidosis is a medical emergency. Always consider airway, breathing and circulation first. Consider and ask for help from seniors, sooner rather than later.
- Fluid resuscitation is important, as many children are dehydrated; however, excessive fluid administration can cause cerebral oedema, a serious complication in diabetic ketoacidosis.
- Correct dehydration gradually over 48 hours, after the initial fluid resuscitation. Always use isotonic solutions such as normal saline with potassium. Add glucose as appropriate.
- Initiate low dose continuous intravenous insulin infusion. Please take extra precautions with calculations, as prescription errors are well recognised.
- Assess, explore and investigate for any underlying or precipitating factors triggering the diabetic ketoacidosis.
- Correct any electrolyte disturbances by adjusting or altering the intravenous fluids.
- Monitor clinical parameters and blood glucose levels, electrolytes, blood gases, and blood ketones as frequently as the clinical situation dictates. More frequent assessments may be needed in severe diabetic ketoacidosis. Continue close monitoring until acidosis and ketosis resolve completely, or at least for the first 24 hours after presentation.
- Consider other supportive measures (including the need for respiratory support), if the patient is unconscious or has a severely depressed Glasgow Coma Scale.
- Consider the need for hypertonic saline and supportive measures for cerebral oedema if there is a sudden deterioration in the patient's condition.
- Patient can be allowed to eat and drink during the recovery phase, if they are conscious and not vomiting, even though their acidosis may not have completely resolved.
- Switch the patient to their usual subcutaneous insulin regimen when they have completely recovered from both acidosis and ketosis. Always allow for a short overlap period and stop the insulin infusion 15–30 minutes after administering the subcutaneous insulin injection.
- Explore the need for any further education and re-education with the patient.

Top tip!
Urgent hospital referral is mandatory when diabetic ketoacidosis is suspected. Delay in appropriate emergency management can endanger the patient's life.

■ **Tell us something about the different types of insulin and insulin regimens.**

- Based on source – Animal insulin, human insulin and synthetic (analogue) insulin (very similar to human insulin)
- Based on onset, peak and duration of action – Rapid-acting, short-acting, medium-acting, long-acting and ultra-long-acting insulins
- Mixtures and pre-mixed insulins
- Insulin regimens – 2, 3 and 4 insulin injections a day
- Insulin pump – Continuous subcutaneous insulin infusion

Table 6.52: The different types of insulin				
Type of insulin	Example	Onset of action	Peak action	Duration of action
Rapid-acting	Lispro, aspart insulin, glulisine	Immediate	15-30 minutes	Up to 4 hours
Short-acting	Soluble insulin	20-30 minutes	1 hour	Up to 4 hours
Medium-acting	Isophane insulin	2-3 hours	4-6 hours	Up to 12 hours
Long-acting	Glargine, detemir	4-6 hours	8-12 hours	Up to 24 hours
Ultra-long-acting	Degludec	30-90 minutes	No peak action	Up to 72 hours

Top tip!
Regular rotation of the injection sites prevents lipohypertropy and atrophy, both of which can delay absorption and action of insulin.

■ **Is there any further information you want to give Connor?**

Provide a personalised diabetes plan that he is able to follow.

- Type and dosage of insulin
- Dose adjustment based on meals and snacks (carbohydrate count)
- Frequency of sugar testing and correction if required
- Low sugars – Prevention and management
- Actions in an emergency situation:
    - Severe hypoglycaemic episode
    - Persistent high blood sugars
    - Ketones in the urine/blood
- Requirement of a blood sugar diary to document progress

Syllabus mapping

General competence

The candidate must:

- Demonstrate good generic communication skills when dealing with children and adolescents.

Diabetes and endocrinology

The candidate must:

- Be able to recognise the early features of a child or young adult presenting with diabetes and know the principles of management.
- Be able to discuss the assessment and long-term management of children with type 1 diabetes mellitus and plan long-term management.
- Be aware of potential complications related to diabetic ketoacidosis and understand the principles of treatment.
- Be able to discuss blood glucose monitoring.

Further reading and references

1. Danne T, Bangstad H-J, Deeb L et al. A Consensus Statement from the International Society for Pediatric and Adolescent Diabetes: Insulin treatment in children and adolescents with diabetes. *Pediatric Diabetes* 2014; 15: 115-34
2. Ragnar H. *Type 1 Diabetes in Children Adolescents*. 6th edition. Class Publishing Ltd: London, 2015.
3. Rewers MJ, Pillay K, de Beaufort C et al. ISPAD Clinical Practice Consensus Guidelines 2014. Assessment and monitoring of glycemic control in children and adolescents with diabetes. *Pediatr Diabetes* 2014; 15: 102-14. doi: 10.1111/pedi.12190
4. Wolfsdorf JI, Allgrove J, Craig ME et al. ISPAD Clinical Practice Consensus Guidelines 2014. Diabetic ketoacidosis and hyperglycemic hyperosmolar state. *Pediatr Diabetes* 2014; 15: 154-79. doi: 10.1111/pedi.12165

Chapter 6.6: Case Study 5: 13 Year Old with Headaches

Dr Ingran Lingam

This station assesses your ability to take a focused history from an adolescent with a chronic condition and his family, and undertake a discussion based on this. As the candidate, you will be asking most or all of the questions, but if parents or role players do ask questions during the consultation, it may be appropriate to answer these.

You will be assessed on your communication with the adolescent and his parent, and the rapport, structure and manner of your interview. During the discussion, the examiner will focus on your understanding of chronic disease management.

Logistics:

Timing: This is a 9-minute station. You will have up to 2 minutes before the start of this station to read the candidate sheet and prepare yourself.

When the bell rings: On entering the room, the examiner will greet you, take your mark sheet, and introduce you to the child and parent. The examiner will then remain silent during the consultation.

You will have 6 minutes to conduct your consultation. A knock at 6 minutes will indicate that 3 minutes remain before the end of the station. At this point, it is important to summarise the history and proceed with the discussion with the examiner.

If you finish early, you will be asked to remain in the room until the session has ended.

Candidate role and task:

You are a GP trainee working in a GP practice.

Tyler is a 13 year old boy who has attended the practice with his mother. He is under treatment at the local hospital for long-standing headaches and has come in for a repeat prescription. Tyler has had headaches over the last 5 years, and his symptoms are not improving. His mother is concerned and has several questions to ask.

Task: Take a focused history and discuss your management plan with the examiner.

Top tip!
Always ensure you greet the parent and child at the beginning. Examiners will assess your ability to include Tyler in the consultation and to put him at ease.

Before entering the station

As there are only 6 minutes to take the history, utilise the time before coming into the station to:

- Decide on which areas of the history you want to focus on and where the examiners will expect detail. Examples include how his symptoms impact on daily activities, what treatments have been previously tried, and how effective they have been.
- Consider what the differential diagnosis for the presenting condition may be.
- Consider how the condition is managed and what symptoms and signs warrant referral to secondary care.
- Make notes around these thoughts if that will help.

On entering the station

Greet the examiner and hand in your mark sheet. Then turn to Tyler and his mother to introduce yourself and greet them both before sitting down.

Clarify your role, and agree on aims and objectives of the consultation with Tyler's mother.

Taking the history

It is important to involve Tyler as much as possible in the consultation. If you find Tyler is not able to give you the required details, tell Tyler you will be asking his mother some questions but that you would be happy to listen if he wanted to help with the answers.

Headache

Gathering details of the headache may be challenging in younger children, and encouraging them to draw pictures of how the headache feels may help. Parental descriptions of the child's behaviour during the headache are also valuable. Reviewing a headache diary, if available, is a useful tool to understanding the frequency, duration and severity of headaches, as well as monitoring the effectiveness of prior interventions.

A detailed and structured approach is essential when characterising a headache.

- Quality (pressure/tightening, pulsatile/throbbing, sharp/burning)
- Location (unilateral, bilateral, orbital, temporal)
- Severity (consider using a pain score)
- Onset (sudden vs gradual)
- Timing (morning vs evening, school days vs holidays)
- Frequency (how often per day or month)
- Duration (few hours vs days)
- Exacerbating factors (trigger factors, worsened by routine activities or stress)
- Relieving factors (impact of simple analgesia, sitting in dark and quiet room)
- Associated symptoms (aura, gastrointestinal symptoms, photophobia, autonomic symptoms)

Previous treatments used

Determining what treatments have been used in the past will help guide further management. Have any prophylactic treatments been used? Is medication overuse contributing to the headache?

Impact on daily activities

How often does his headache prevent him from attending school or playing sports? Has he ever been admitted to hospital due to the severity of the headache?

Past medical history

Has Tyler sought medical attention for any other reasons? Is there a history of recurrent illnesses or periodic syndromes?

It is also important to establish if Tyler has any underlying systemic disorders presenting as headaches. Has Tyler ever had renal problems or hypertension? Has he ever had a visual acuity test performed? Does Tyler have a history of obstructive sleep apnoea?

Family history

A positive family of history of migraines may help support a diagnosis of migraine.

Social history

Try to ask sensitively about symptoms of stress, anxiety and depression, which may exacerbate or be causing the headaches. When assessing an adolescent, it may be valuable to ask about smoking, drugs and alcohol use, but constraints on time will not allow you to interview him alone (as is the usual practice in real-life situations).

Assimilating the information

Now that you have taken a focused history, you will be expected to assimilate and present the most salient points to the examiner. Below is a summary of the history obtained from Tyler and his mother, and an example presentation.

To present...

> "Tyler is a 13 year old boy who has attended the clinic with his mother today. He has been experiencing severe headaches intermittently for the last 5 years. He describes them as a throbbing pain on the top of his head and there is no prior aura or symptoms of nausea or vomiting. He has a previous history of recurrent abdominal pains, which have resulted in hospital admissions. His mother suffers from migraines.
>
> Tyler's symptoms are worsening, resulting in frequent school absences and missing playing football for his team. His symptoms are suggestive of migraine without aura, and I would consider starting him on a prophylactic medication."

Discussion

Now that you have arrived at a likely diagnosis, you will spend the remainder of the 3 minutes discussing aspects of this condition with the examiner. Possible questions from the examiner are highlighted below. It is unlikely all of these can be asked within the given time frame.

What are the possible differential diagnoses?

The differential diagnosis includes migraines, tension headaches and cluster headaches (Table 6.61). It is also important to carefully consider the possibility of medication overuse headaches. The most likely diagnosis in this child is migraine.

Migraines are relatively common, affecting 3–10% of children. The mean age of onset is 7.2 years in boys and 10.9 years in girls; however, this may be a reflection of the difficulty in diagnosis in younger children. The diagnosis is primarily clinical, characterised by recurrent headaches lasting from 1–72 hours that may occur with or without an aura. Acute attacks are usually severe and disrupt routine physical activity. The child often has to rest in a darkened room or sleep during episodes. Younger children tend to present with bilateral headaches, whereas adolescents commonly experience unilateral pain. Associated symptoms include nausea, vomiting, phonophobia and photophobia. The latter symptoms are difficult to identify in young children, though may be inferred by their behaviour (e.g. irritability, crying, seeking a darkened room). Aura is rare in preschool children, but tends to appear during adolescence.

Tension-type headaches are usually milder and feel like a tight band around the head. They may last from 30 minutes to up to a week. They do not have any associated symptoms.

Cluster headaches are rare in young children. They are brief (15 minutes to 3 hours) and unilateral, often presenting as pain behind the eye. These severe episodes of pain occur multiple times in a day and this process may continue for weeks to months before subsiding.

Medication overuse headache is an important health and social burden, occurring often in children taking medication for a primary headache disorder. The NICE guidelines (CG150, September 2012) recommend that a diagnosis of medication overuse should be considered in children whose headaches have developed or worsened while taking triptans, paracetamol or non-steroidals alone or in combination for 3 months or more.

Headaches can also be a symptom of secondary pathological processes, such as intracranial pathologies (tumours, vascular lesions, infection), refractive errors, infections and cervical spine disorders. It is also important to consider more general causes, such as inadequate hydration, obstructive sleep apnoea, psychological/stress factors and hypertension (e.g. due to undiagnosed renal disease).

Table 6.61: Differentiating migraines from tension headaches and cluster headaches (adapted from the NICE guidelines CG150)

Headache feature	Migraines (with or without aura)	Tension headaches	Cluster headaches
Location of pain	Unilateral or bilateral	Bilateral	Unilateral (around the eye, above the eye and along the side of the head/face)
Quality of pain	Pulsating (throbbing or banging in young people aged 12-17 years)	Pressing/tightening (non-pulsating)	Variable (can be sharp, boring, burning, throbbing or tightening)
Intensity of pain	Mild or moderate	Mild or moderate	Severe or very severe
Duration of pain	4-72 hours in adults 1-72 hours in young people aged 12-17 years	30 minutes-continuous	15-180 minutes
Effect on activities	Aggravated by, or causes avoidance of, routine activities	Not aggravated by routine activities	Restlessness or agitation
Other symptoms	Unusual sensitivity to light and/or sound or nausea and/or vomiting Aura and/or pins and needles and/or speech disturbance	None	On the same side as the headache: red and/or watery eye, nasal congestion and/or runny nose, swollen eyelid, forehead and facial sweating, constricted pupil and/or drooping eyelid

International Headache Society (IHS) diagnostic criteria

For migraines without aura:

At least 5 attacks fulfilling the following criteria:

- Headaches lasting 4-72 hours
- Headaches with at least 2 of the following characteristics: unilateral; pulsating; moderate to severe intensity; aggravation by, or causing avoidance of, routine physical activity
- Associated with at least 1 of the following symptoms: nausea, vomiting, photophobia, phonophobia

For migraines with aura:

Two attacks of headaches with the following features:

- Fully reversible aura symptoms (e.g. focal cortical, brainstem dysfunction)
- One aura symptom that develops gradually over more than 4 minutes or multiple aura symptoms occurring in succession
- No aura symptom lasting more than 60 minutes

Top tip!
A detailed description of the headache with particular attention to red flag features and systemic symptoms will help differentiate between the otherwise wide differential diagnoses.

What are the clinical features associated with intracranial lesions (red flags)?

The possibility of intracranial lesions is a source of anxiety for parents and clinicians alike. However, it is possible to exclude brain tumours with a thorough clinical assessment and avoid the need for imaging studies (Table 6.62).

Table 6.62: Red flag features associated with headaches	
Headache	Worse at night or early morning Worse on straining or coughing Early age at presentation (<3 years) Increasing frequency and severity
Associated signs/symptoms	Nausea/vomiting (especially in the morning) Worsens with exercise, coughing, sneezing, straining New cognitive dysfunction or neurological deficit (seizures, impaired consciousness, difficulty in coordination, squints, visual disturbances, etc.) Deteriorating school performance Change in personality Faltering growth Rapidly increasing head circumference

Top tip!
Although headaches may be a presenting feature of a brain tumour, it is extremely unlikely in the absence of 'red flag' symptoms or neurological signs.

What is the significance of the history of recurrent abdominal pain?

The recurrent abdominal pain with vomiting is likely to be abdominal migraines. These are characterised by severe central abdominal pain, pallor and lethargy. Episodes last from hours to days. Abdominal migraines and other childhood periodic syndromes (e.g. cyclical vomiting, benign paroxysmal vertigo of childhood) may be precursors to migraines.

Top tip!
Periodic syndromes may be precursors to migraines and have a combined prevalence of 5% in the paediatric population. However, they are often underdiagnosed.

What is your management plan?

General management

Provide individualised information and support. It is important to explain the diagnosis to the child and parent, taking care to reassure them that other pathology has been excluded. It is important to recognise that headache is a valid medical disorder with a significant impact on the patient as well as their family or carers.

It may be helpful to provide written information about the headache disorder, including appropriate support organisations. It is also important to explain the risks of headaches from medication overuse in patients using frequent acute treatments.

Management of an acute migraine

- Early treatment at the onset of symptoms.
- Consider combination therapy (oral triptan and non-steroidal anti-inflammatory drug (NSAID) or oral triptan and paracetamol).
- Consider nasal triptans in children aged 12–17 years.
- For patients who prefer monotherapy, consider using an oral triptan, NSAID, aspirin (900 micrograms) or paracetamol. Studies have demonstrated intranasal sumatriptan to be effective in relieving headaches and it is licensed for children over 12 years of age. Oral sumatriptan can be given to children over 6 years of age; however, there is limited data on its efficacy.
- Anti-emetics (domperidone or prochlorperazine) may be helpful even in the absence of nausea and vomiting.

Prophylaxis

- Reassure the child and carer to allay fears of more sinister diagnoses.
- Identify and avoid trigger factors when possible. Common triggers in childhood include sleep deprivation, stress, dehydration/warm weather, missed meals and prolonged periods spent playing video games.
- Maintaining a regular routine with meals and sleeping times may help reduce the frequency of attacks. During an acute episode, children should be encouraged to lie in a cool, dark and quiet room and sleep.
- Medication – Migraine prophylaxis is rarely indicated in paediatrics (NICE 2012); however, it should be considered in children with frequent episodes or if the headache impacts the child's daily activities. Prophylactic agents include topiramate or propranolol. Adolescent girls of childbearing age should be advised that topiramate is associated with foetal malformations and may also impair the effectiveness of the oral contraceptive pill.
- The NICE guidelines do not advocate the use of neuroimaging solely for the purpose of reassurance. However, if the headache changes in nature or 'red flag' symptoms develop, then the family should be advised to return for further assessment.

Table 6.63 Criteria for referral to a hospital

Acute admission	Paediatric OPD
1. Acute admission is indicated if there are any symptoms/neurological findings suggestive of intracranial pathology. 2. Migraines that have persisted beyond 72 hours (status migrainous).	1. Diagnosis unclear 2. Poor response to treatment 3. Chronic migraines necessitating prophylaxis

Top tip!
Prophylactic medication is rarely indicated and is reserved for severe and frequent migraines that are impacting on the child's school attendance and social life. These medications have a limited evidence base, and should be initiated following a review by a paediatrician.

Syllabus mapping

General competence

The candidate must:

- Demonstrate good generic communication skills when dealing with children and adolescents.

Neurology and neurodisability

The candidate must:

- Be able to discuss common causes of headaches and head injury, including their management.

Further reading and references

1. Barnes NP, Jayawant S. Best Practice: Migraine. *Arch Dis Child Educ Pract Ed* 2005; 90: 53-57
2. Headache Classification Committee of the International Headache Society (IHS). The International Classification of Headache Disorders, 3rd edition. *Cephalalgia* 2013; 33: 629-808
3. HeadSmart. Be brain tumour aware. www.headsmart.org.uk (accessed January 2016).
4. McCrea N, Howells R. Fifteen minute consultation: Headache in children under 5 years of age. *Arch Dis Child Educ Pract Ed* 2013; 98: 181-5
5. National Institute of Health and Care Excellence Headaches. (CG150) – Diagnosis and management of headaches in young people and adults. London, 2012. https://www.guidance.nice.org.uk/cg150 (accessed July 2015).
6. Ryan S. Pharmacy Update: Medicines for Migraine. *Arch Dis Child Educ Pract Ed* 2007; 92: ep50-ep55

SECTION 7:
THE CHILD DEVELOPMENT STATION

Chapter 7.1: Introduction
Dr Kate Fisher, Dr Lucy Killian

Trainees often feel that child development is unfamiliar territory when, in actual fact, they perform an informal developmental assessment every time they interact with a child in order to engage with and examine them. Observing a child playing and chatting in the waiting room and watching them walk to the consulting room provides a great deal of developmental information.

When preparing for clinical examinations, there is the danger that child development becomes a dry list of milestones in relation to the age range in which they should be achieved. This, then, requires rote learning. However, a structured approach, an understanding of the interrelationship between the developmental domains, and an enjoyment in engaging children can satisfy the child, the candidate and the examiners.

To simplify the assessment of many complex processes, developmental skills are frequently grouped into 'umbrella' domains such as:

- **Gross motor skills** – Using large groups of muscles to sit, stand, walk, run, maintain balance and change position
- **Fine motor skills** – Using hands to be able to eat, draw, dress, play, and write
- **Speech and language** – Speaking, using non-verbal language and gestures, communicating, and understanding what others say
- **Cognition** – Learning, understanding, problem-solving, reasoning, and remembering
- **Social and play** – Interacting with others, having relationships with family, friends, and teachers, cooperating and responding to the feelings of others, and playing

Hearing is often grouped with language, and vision with fine motor skills. However, sensory information facilitates all aspects of development, including cognition, locomotion and social communication. A child may be delayed in all domains – global developmental delay – or have an isolated delay (e.g. in speech and language).

All developmental skills essentially involve sensory, cognitive and motor input. Walking is seen as a motor skill with lower limb movements enacting a step, but also requires eye and head movements to plan a route and avoid obstacles. Cognitive elements contribute by way of intellectual interest in moving towards (or away from) a stimulus, and realising that the individual can direct himself or herself as they wish. From a sensory perspective, sufficient vision is required to plan the route and proprioceptive and kinaesthetic feedback from the trunk and legs control lower limb movement.

What to expect

In the child development station, you will be given a task. It is likely you will be asked to examine *an area* of development in order to allow you to complete your assessment. This quite frequently falls into 3 groups, as outlined below.

Examples include:

- Assessment of a child's gross motor skills
- Assessment of a child's fine motor skills
- Assessment of a child's speech, language and communication skills

It cannot be emphasised enough that it is important to listen very carefully to the examiner's instructions and undertake only what has been asked. If uncertain, it is important to clarify this, as the examiner would be happy to repeat the 'opening statement' given.

Once instructions have been given, the examiner will mostly observe your ability to:

- Develop a rapport with the child and parent.
- Examine in a structured and systematic manner.
- Complete the task in the time given.
- Summarise key clinical findings.
- Undertake a discussion around the case.

Opening statements

It is impossible within the remit of this book to provide a complete list of all the possible cases that could present in this station. The RCPCH has published a DCH syllabus, and it is essential that all candidates refer to this syllabus when preparing for the examination: http://www.rcpch.ac.uk/training-examinations-professional-development/assessment-and-examinations/examinations/syllabus

Examples of 'opening statements' given by examiners are noted below. These will vary depending on the cases chosen for that diet.

Jasmine is 4 years old and has had difficulty walking. Please assess her gross motor skills and estimate her developmental age in this area.

Michael was born at 28 weeks gestation and has difficulty writing. Please assess his fine motor skills and estimate his developmental age in this area.

Samy is nearly 3 and mother is worried that he will not cope in nursery. Please assess his speech and language skills, and estimate a developmental age in this area.

Managing time in the child development station

Timing: This is a 9-minute station. A knock at 6 minutes will mark the end of the recommended time for demonstrating the child's developmental skills. The remaining 3 minutes is for summarising key clinical findings and undertaking further discussion around the case. As this station only allows 6 minutes to complete the task, it is important to be fluid and systematic in your approach. Failure to complete the task will lead to you being marked down.

When the bell rings: On entering the room, the examiner will take your mark sheet, introduce you to the parent and child, and give you your instructions with the 'opening statement'. The examiner will then observe your interaction and examination technique. **Listen carefully** to the instructions and carry out only what has been asked.

How consistency is ensured

Examiners work in pairs to review all children helping in the station. They undertake 'standard setting', where agreement is reached on physical signs present, the complexity of the case and whether the case is of an appropriate standard for this examination. Based on these discussions, examiners decide on an 'opening statement' to introduce each patient and explain the candidate's task. Pass/fail criteria and the questions to follow during the 'discussion' time are agreed upon to provide consistency.

'Mark sheets', individualised for each station, help to guide examiners in their assessment of candidates. Mark sheets can inform candidates of the different areas examiners consider when awarding marks and, as importantly, areas where marks can be lost. It is worth noting that the final score represents the examiner's overall judgement reflecting the candidate's performance at the station (Appendix 7.11).

The RCPCH has developed 'anchor statements' that examiners refer to when deciding on pass/fail criteria. They use these as further guidance during standard setting and marking. Candidates should review these documents to familiarise themselves with the scoring criteria explained in the anchor statements (Appendix 7.12).

Setting the stage

Tips for developmental assessment:

- Wash hands – Just like in a real-life clinical setting, washing hands remains the mainstay of infection control. There should be facilities for hand washing or alcohol gel available.
- Permission to undertake a developmental assessment must be sought from the parent, and from the child if they are old enough to consent. This is a good opportunity to briefly explain what you are doing and why.
- All instructions given to the child should be done quietly, confidently and empathetically. If, for any reason, the child is unwilling to cooperate, help can be sought from the mother, as frequently sitting the child on the mother's lap may be helpful.
- Guess the rough age of the child and start at a slightly easier than age-appropriate level of the task. If it is too hard for them, then quickly give them an easier task to keep them interested. Children like to please and enjoy succeeding. Then progress sequentially through the tasks to estimate their developmental age. Examiners will be noting whether you undertake a systematic approach.
- Start by sitting the child at a small table and completing performance tasks. They are less likely to want to sit after they have been allowed to jump and run around the room!
- Arrange your room so that the carer sits behind and to the side of the child, so that they do not easily distract the child.
- Introduce *1* task at a time to the table in performance tasks to prevent distraction and to engage the child as much as possible. Clear each task away before introducing the next task.
- Be clear and concise in your instructions to the child, demonstrating what is required first before asking the child to repeat the task.
- If the child is shy, you may need to ask carers to help, either by sitting the child with them or asking the carer to perform motor tasks to demonstrate them.
- It is very common for the child to be unwilling to cooperate in such an unfamiliar setting, especially if there are distractions around them. Don't despair! Use these situations to observe the child from a distance and take a brief developmental history from their carer (after getting the examiner's permission). The child may start to comply with tests if not scared off initially.
- Remember that a young toddler's attention span is limited, so move through tasks as quickly as you can!
- While you undertake your assessment, and certainly before finishing, observe whether there are any obvious features that the child may have that are not directly related to the task given to you, as these might help in the discussion that follows.

Be prepared to summarise your clinical findings and undertake further discussion in the 3 minutes before the end of the station. This discussion will be around:

- Differential diagnosis based on the reasons for any developmental delay.
- Investigations that might be necessary.
- Management of the case, considering the health, social and educational consequences affecting the child.

Make sure you thank the mother and the child before leaving the room.

Syllabus mapping

Neurology and neurodisability

Knowledge

The candidate must:

- Understand the definition and concepts of disability and what this means for the child and family.
- Be familiar with the common causes of disability, disordered development and learning difficulties.
- Be able to take a neurodevelopmental history.
- Know the causes of speech and language delay, and know when to refer to a specialist.
- Be aware of local services/disability allowances.
- Understand the need for multidisciplinary team input in the care of the disabled child, and be aware of the work of the child development team and centre.
- Understand the need to work with other services as required, including education, social services, child protection, and respite care facilities.
- Be aware of how agencies work together to address how children with health and medical needs are managed at school.
- Be able to recognise presenting features of visual or hearing impairment, and know when and how to refer for further assessment.

Skills

The candidate must:

- Be able to perform a reliable assessment of neurodevelopmental status at key stages, including the newborn period, the first year of life, nursery age and school entry.

Further reading and references

1. Bedford H, Walton S, Ahn J. Measures of Child Development: A Review. *Policy Research Unit in the Health of Children, Young People and Families* 2013.
2. Denver Developmental Materials Inc. *DENVER II*. http://www.denverii.com/home.html (accessed March 2015).
3. GL assessment. *Schedule of Growing Skills*. http://shop.glassessment.co.uk/home.php?cat=360 (accessed March 2015).
4. Seal A, Robinson G, Kelly A, Williams J. *Children with neurodevelopmental disabilities: The essential guide to management*. MacKeith Press, 2013.
5. Sharma A, Cockerill H, Sheridan MD. *From Birth to Five Years: Children's Developmental Progress*. Abingdon, Oxon: Routledge, 2014.

Appendix 7.11: Mark Sheet (Front and Back): Child Development Station

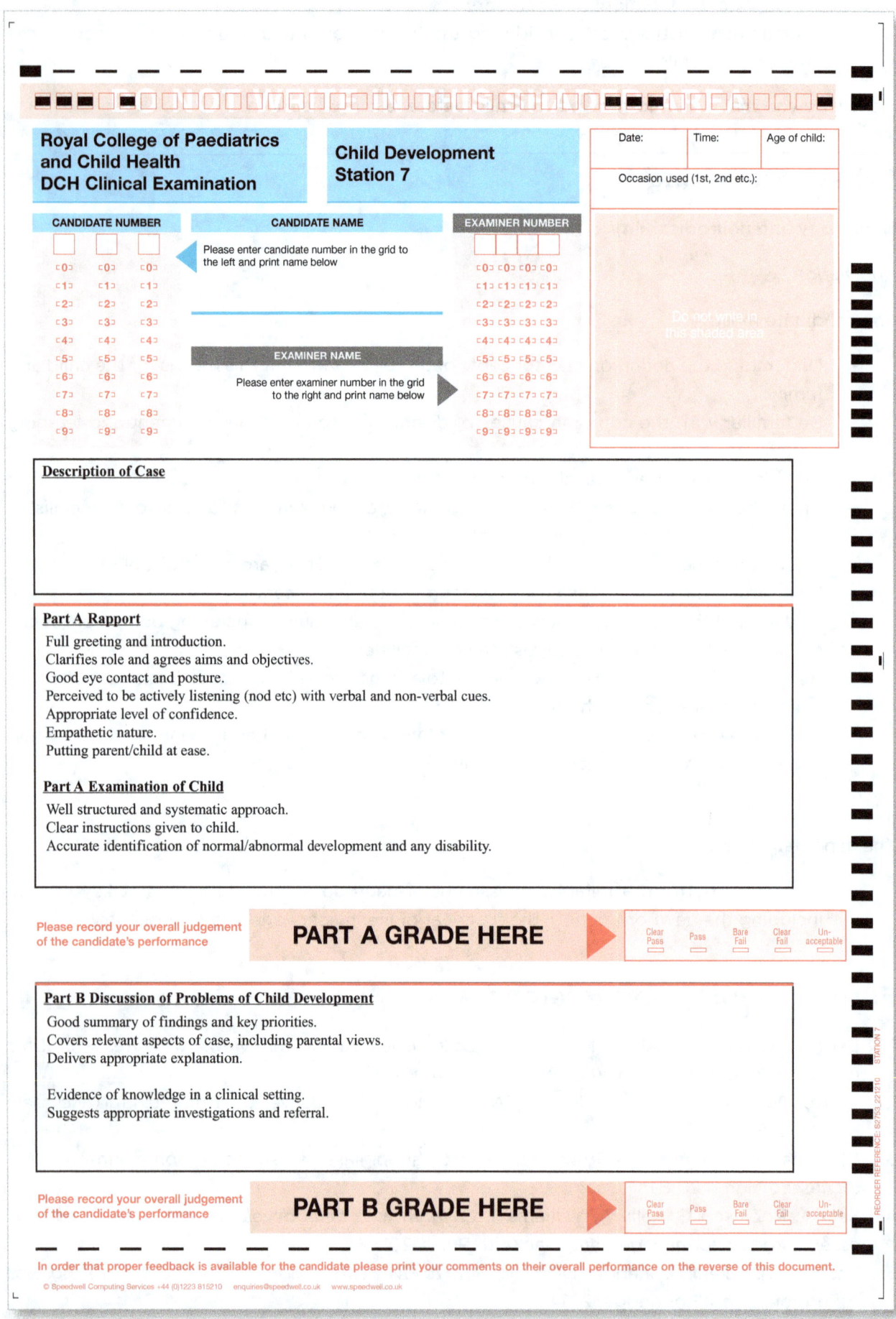

Clinical Cases in Paediatrics: DCH Clinical Examination

☐ Disorganised and unsystematic approach (please add additional comments)

☐ Inappropriate use of tools/assessment aids (please add additional comments)

☐ Poor time management (please add additional comments)

☐ Inaccurate assessment/conclusion (please add additional comments)

Please add any additional comments here:

Appendix 7.12: Anchor Statement: Child Development Station

	Expected Standard/ CLEAR PASS	PASS	BARE FAIL	CLEAR FAIL	UNACCEPTABLE
PART A: RAPPORT	Full greeting and introduction. Clarifies role and agrees aims and objectives. Good eye contact and posture. Perceived to be actively listening (nod etc) with verbal and non-verbal cues. Appropriate level of confidence. Empathetic nature. Putting parent/child at ease.	Adequately performed but not fully fluent in conducting interview.	Incomplete or hesitant greeting and introduction. Inadequate identification of role, aims and objectives. Poor eye contact and posture. Not perceived to be actively listening (nod etc) with verbal and non-verbal cues. Does not show appropriate level of confidence, empathetic nature or putting parent/child at ease.	Significant components omitted or not achieved.	Dismissive of parent/child concerns. Fails to put parent or child at ease.
PART A: EXAMINATION OF CHILD	Well structured and systematic approach. Clear instructions given to child. Accurate identification of normal/abnormal development and any disability.	Reasonably systematic approach. Identifies features of normal development.	Hesitant examination covering main points but leaves out important tasks.	Poorly organised, inappropriate developmental examination. Poor organisation of child. Unable to recognise relevance of normal/abnormal signs.	Completely unstructured assessment with slow hesitant approach. Failure to demonstrate to child. Serious inadequacy in developmental skills.
PART B: DISCUSSION OF PROBLEMS OF CHILD DEVELOPMENT	Good summary of findings and key priorities. Covers relevant aspects of case, including parental views. Delivers appropriate explanation. Evidence of knowledge in a clinical setting. Suggests appropriate investigations and referral.	Adequate though not complete summary of findings and key priorities. Covers main relevant aspects of case and delivers adequate explanation. Appropriate investigations and referral.	Incorrect conclusion. Some identification of further investigation, referral or treatment, but evidence of muddled thinking.	Incorrect explanation. Little clinical knowledge. Poor identification of possible problems. Lack of clarity of future planning.	Unable to interpret findings. Serious deficiencies in knowledge and understanding of child development assessment.

Chapter 7.2: Case Study 1: 3 Year Old with Gross Motor Skills Delay

Lucy Killian, Kate Fisher

This station assesses your ability to demonstrate a developmental assessment of gross motor skills in a child, interpret the findings and conduct a discussion with the examiner. You will be assessed on the rapport, manner and structure of your examination with the child and parent. Always introduce yourself to the child and their carer.

> **Logistics:**
>
> *Timing:* This is a 9-minute station. A knock at 6 minutes will note that 3 minutes remain before the end of the station. At this point, it is important to summarise your clinical findings and proceed with the discussion with the examiner.
>
> *When the bell rings:* On entering the room, the examiner will greet you, take your mark sheet, introduce you to the child and parent, and give you your task. Listen carefully to these instructions.
>
> The examiner will then remain mostly silent during the consultation, as they will be observing your clinical skills, but may provide some direction should it be required. A discussion around the case will be undertaken in the final 3 minutes of the station.
>
> If you finish early, you will be asked to remain in the room until the session has ended.

> **Candidate role and task:**
>
> **You are an** ST3 GP trainee working in a child development centre.
>
> Ben is 3 years old. He was born with transposition of the great arteries and underwent a switch procedure shortly after birth. He sat unsupported at 11 months and walked independently at 22 months. Ben is now using 4-word sentences and asking lots of questions. His vision and hearing have been assessed recently and are within the normal range.
>
> **Task: You are asked to assess Ben's gross motor development.**

The gross motor assessment

Observation

As with other developmental domains, gross motor issues can be the presenting feature of a more global problem. Always look for indicators of a more global problem – e.g. dysmorphic features, squint, mobility or orthotic equipment.

Observing the child yields a great deal of information regarding motor function.

- Consider the quality of their posture and movements. Are they symmetrical? Are there any uncontrolled movements, such as dystonia (involuntary, abnormal muscle tone) or athetosis (involuntary writhing movements)?

- Consider skills in various positions: prone, supine, sitting, standing.
- Consider motor skills. Is the child walking independently? Does he need to be supported in sitting? What about head control?

Of course, assessment needs to be tailored to the developmental level of the child. Walking, running, hopping and jumping can be made into a game. Ask the child to rise to standing from supine (Gower's manoeuvre). If the child turns prone and walks his hands up his thighs, this is indicative of proximal muscle weakness and is commonly seen in Duchenne muscular dystrophy.

Top tip!
Remember to look around the patient for clues to the child's level of mobility:
- Splints – Ankle-foot orthoses (AFOs)
- Lycra suits/splints – Made-to-measure garments that improve proximal stability, often enhancing functional abilities
- Mobility aids – Wheelchairs, walkers
- Evidence of feeding devices – Nasogastric or gastrostomy tube may indicate associated difficulties with feeding and swallowing.
- Hearing aids

Motor milestones

The timing of the acquisition of motor skills varies tremendously between normal individuals. The table below is a guide to the ages by which commonly assessed motor skills are usually achieved (Table 7.21).

Table 7.21	
Gross motor milestones	**Normal age achieved**
Ventral suspension • Head drops below the plane of the body • Head held in the same plane as the body	Birth By 6 weeks
Prone • Attempts to lift head • Raises head and chest, propping up on forearms • Lifts head and chest, supports with extended arms and flattened palms	By 1 month By 3 months By 6 months
Primitive reflexes • E.g. Moro, asymmetric tonic neck reflex, palmer (grasp) reflex	Disappeared by 6 months
Rolling – Front to back/back to front	By 7 months
Protective reflexes • Downward parachute (held vertically and rapidly lowered, legs extend and abduct, feet flat) • Sideward protective reflex (puts arms out to save themselves if tilted off balance) • Forward parachute/protective reflex (arms and hands extend on forward descent)	Present by 6 months Present by 6 months Present by 8 months
Sitting • Held in sitting position, with a curved back • Supported, with a straight back and head • Steady, unsupported	By 3 months By 6 months By 9 months

Table 7.21 continued...

Table 7.21: continued	
Gross motor milestones	Normal age achieved
Stands alone	By 14 months
Walks	By 18 months (bottom shufflers later)
Jumps	2.5–3 years
• Balances on 1 foot momentarily • Hops	3 years 4 years
• Up stairs – 1 foot per step; down stairs – 2 feet per step • Up and down stairs – 1 foot per step	3 years 4 years

As well as recognising and remembering normal milestones, it is also important to recognise when development is significantly disordered, prompting the clinician to seek timely assessment by experts in neurodisability, neurology and the wider multidisciplinary team (Table 7.22).

Table 7.22: Red flags that suggest that development is significantly disordered, requiring prompt assessments by paediatricians in neurodisability, neurology and the multidisciplinary team

Any child who has:
- Lost developmental skills at any age
- Parental/professional concerns about vision, fixing or following (seek ophthalmology review)
- Significant hearing loss at any age (seek audiological/ENT review)
- No speech at 18 months, especially if not communicating by any other means (urgent hearing test)
- Suspected clinical diagnosis of cerebral palsy
- Head circumference above the 99.6th centile, below the 0.4th centile, or has crossed 2 centile lines up or down on the appropriate growth chart

Any child who is not able to:
- Sit unsupported by 12 months
- Walk by 18 months (boys) or 2 years (girls)
- 'Walk' other than on tiptoes
- Run by 2½ years
- Hold an object placed in their hand by 5 months of age (corrected for gestation)
- Reach for objects by 6 months of age (corrected for gestation)
- Point at objects to share interest with others by 2 years

Adapted from: Horridge KA. *Arch Dis Child Educ Pract Ed* (2010). doi: 10.1136/adc.2009.182436

Neurological examination

Gross motor assessment is closely linked with neurological examination. See the chapter on neurological examination.

In the DCH clinical examination, it is unlikely that you will be asked to do a neurological examination in this station, due to the time constraints that exist. However, as a candidate, you should state that, to complete your assessment, you would also like to do a neurological examination.

Assimilating the signs

Now that you have conducted a thorough gross motor skills assessment, you will be expected to assimilate and present your positive clinical findings in order to arrive at a possible diagnosis. Below is a summary of your assessment elicited from Ben, and an example presentation.

History – Cardiac surgery as a neonate, delayed independent sitting and walking. No vision or hearing problems.

Observation – Ben has a lycra splint on his left hand and an ankle foot orthosis on his left ankle. He rose to stand easily, but has an asymmetrical gait. On running, the asymmetry is exaggerated and the left arm comes up into flexion.

Motor development – Ben is able to walk well, beginning to jump but not quite able to get 2 feet off the ground and is not able to balance on 1 leg.

Neurology – Ben has increased tone in both the left upper and lower limb. He has reduced power on his left. He has increased biceps, triceps, supinator, knee and ankle reflexes on the left. His plantar response is upgoing on the left. Ben has a satisfactory range of movements in his hips and knees bilaterally, but there is a catch at his left ankle that can just be passively stretched to 90°.

To present...

> "Ben is a 3 year old boy with a history of heart surgery as a neonate. He has increased tone in his left upper and lower limbs and wears a lycra splint on his left wrist and an ankle foot orthosis on his left ankle. His reflexes are increased on the left. These findings are consistent with a left hemiplegia. Nevertheless, he demonstrated steady walking and jumping, but not balancing or hopping. He has difficulties kicking a ball. This would place his motor development at between ages 2.5-3 years."

Discussion

■ **What is the most likely cause of Ben's hemiplegia?**

Adverse neurological outcomes are a risk after neonatal heart surgery. Ben is likely to have sustained an insult to the brain, which has resulted in a picture typical of cerebral palsy.

■ **What do you understand by the term 'cerebral palsy'?**

Cerebral palsy is defined as "a group of permanent disorders of movement and posture causing limitation of activities and which are attributable to a non-progressive disturbance that occurred in the development of the brain. The motor disturbances are often accompanied by disturbances of vision, sensation, perception, cognition, communication and behaviour, epilepsy and secondary musculoskeletal problems" (Rosenbaum, 2007).

Approximately 1-2 per 1,000 live-born children are diagnosed by the age of 5 years, and approximately half of these were born prematurely.

■ **What are the causes of cerebral palsy?**

The causes of cerebral palsy can be divided into the time of the insult to the developing brain:

- *Prenatal* (hypoxic injury, intrauterine infection, toxins, chromosomal defect)
- *Perinatal* (hypoxic injury, intracerebral haemorrhage, bilirubin encephalopathy)
- *Postnatal* (hypoxic injury, meningitis, encephalitis)

While the underlying brain lesion is not progressive, its physical manifestations can change as the child grows and develops.

■ What are the considerations when describing cerebral palsy?

The definition captures a huge range of conditions. Some of these may have only a minimal effect on the child and their family, and others affect every aspect of their lives and are associated with profound learning difficulties. Describing a unilateral or bilateral spasticity, dyskinesia or ataxia is useful. However, in recent years, the emphasis has shifted to classification systems that focus on function and participation.

Functional classification systems include:

- Gross Motor Function Classification System (GMFCS)
- Manual Ability Classification system (MACS)
- Communication Function Classification System (CFCS)
- Eating and Drinking Ability Classifications System (EDACS)

The most commonly used classification is the GMFCS, scored from 1 (independently mobile) to 5 (full assistance with mobility).

■ What are the mainstays of managing cerebral palsy?

Effective management and prevention of secondary problems is based on a multidisciplinary team approach.

Management of motor disorder:

- Regular physiotherapy aims to strengthen and stretch the muscles, improve function, and work towards individual goals.
- Occupational therapy assessments, often performed jointly with physiotherapy, aim to improve posture and function. A child may require orthotics (rigid splints) to improve posture, most commonly for the ankle. Equipment will be considered during this assessment, such as adapted seating that may be required for certain activities (feeding and toileting).
- More rarely, other medical therapies can be considered to improve comfort and functional ability, including muscle relaxants and anti-dystonic medications, as well as surgical procedures.

Management of comorbidities:

- Coordination of care and management with adjuvant therapies will be managed by community and/or general paediatricians and a GP (with input from other specialists to manage comorbidities).
- Feeding difficulties require dietician and speech and language therapy input, with appropriate specialist advice for drooling, reflux and constipation.
- Regular speech and language therapy will assess verbal and non-verbal communication abilities. A young person may require communication aids – for example, standardised communication books and voice output communication aids (VOCA).
- Regular dental care is important and specialist dentists may be needed.
- Hearing and vision should be checked

- Other specialist opinions may be needed, including:
    - Orthopaedic involvement for scoliosis and contractures
    - Epilepsy and/or other neurological management
    - Respiratory care
    - Specialist nurse assessment for suspected bladder problems

After 19 years of age, the young person will transition to adult services. Care is coordinated by a GP, and different specialists may be required depending on the individual's needs. An adult rehabilitation team may look after the young person.

It is important to consider the impact of the young person's disability on their education and family. Their educational needs will be variable, and they may require a school for special needs or levels of support within a mainstream setting. Families can gain support and advice about local services from social services (e.g. respite care available). Families are entitled to financial support, such as Disability Living Allowance (DLA).

Syllabus mapping

Neurology and neurodisability

Knowledge

The candidate must:

- Understand the definition and concepts of disability and what this means for the child and family.
- Be familiar with the common causes of disability, disordered development and learning difficulties.
- Be able to take a neurodevelopmental history.
- Be aware of local services/disability allowances.
- Understand the need for multidisciplinary team input in the care of the disabled child, and be aware of the work of the child development team and centre.
- Understand the need to work with other services as required, including education, social services, child protection, and respite care facilities.
- Be aware of how agencies work together to address how children with health and medical needs are managed at school.
- Be able to recognise presenting features of visual or hearing impairment, as well as know when and how to refer for further assessment.

Skills

The candidate must:

- Be able to perform a reliable assessment of neurodevelopmental status at key stages, including the newborn period, the first year of life, nursery age and school entry.

Further reading and references

1. Andropoulos DB, Easley RB, Brady K et al. Changing expectations for neurological outcomes after the neonatal arterial switch operation. *Ann Thorac Surg* 2012; 94(4): 1250-6
2. Coghill JE, Simkiss DE. Do lycra garments improve function and movement in children with cerebral palsy? http://www.bestbets.org/bets/bet.php?id=1993 (accessed 20 March 2015).
3. Denver Developmental Materials Inc. *DENVER II*. http://www.denverii.com/home.html (accessed 20 March 2015).
4. Horridge KA. Assessment and investigation of the child with disordered development. *Arch Dis Child Educ Pract Ed* 2010; 96(1): 9-20
5. Rosenbaum P et al. A report: the definition and classification of cerebral palsy. *Dev Med Child Neurol* 2007; 109: 8-14
6. SCPE Collaborative Group. Surveillance of Cerebral Palsy in Europe: A collaboration of Cerebral Palsy surveys and registers. *Dev Med Child Neurol* 2000; 42: 816-24
7. Seal A, Robinson G, Kelly A, Williams J. *Children with neurodevelopmental disabilities: The essential guide to management*. MacKeith Press, 2013.
8. Sharma A, Cockerill H, Sheridan MD. *From Birth to Five Years: Children's Developmental Progress*. Abingdon, Oxon: Routledge, 2014.
9. Sonksen PM. Developmental Assessment: Theory, practice and application to neurodisability. *Clinics in Developmental Medicine Series*. In Press. MacKeith Press, London.

Chapter 7.3: Case Study 2: 4 Year Old with Down's Syndrome and Fine Motor Skills Delay
Dr Kate Fisher

This station assesses your ability to demonstrate a developmental assessment of fine motor skills in a child with a common chromosomal disorder, interpret physical findings and conduct a discussion with the examiner. You will be assessed on the rapport, manner and structure of your examination with the child and parent. Always introduce yourself to the child and their carer.

Logistics:

Timing: This is a 9-minute station. A knock at 6 minutes will note that 3 minutes remain before the end of the station. At this point, it is important to summarise your clinical findings and proceed with the discussion with the examiner.

When the bell rings: On entering the room, the examiner will greet you, take your mark sheet, introduce you to the child and parent, and give you your task. Listen carefully to these instructions.

The examiner will then remain mostly silent during the consultation, as they will be observing your clinical skills, but may provide some direction should it be required. A discussion around the case will be undertaken in the final 3 minutes of the station.

If you finish early, you will be asked to remain in the room until the session has ended.

Candidate role and task:

You are an ST3 GP trainee working in a child development centre.

Alice is 4 years old. She is being seen for a review of her developmental progress.

Task: You are asked to assess her fine motor skills.

Observation

Although you have been requested to examine 1 developmental domain, remember that there may be global developmental issues. Always look for indicators of a more global problem, e.g. dysmorphic features, squint, mobility or orthotic equipment.

Observing the child yields a great deal of information, so look for:

- Dysmorphic features
- Hearing aids
- Visual symptoms – e.g. nystagmus, squint, glasses
- Signs of a motor disorder such as cerebral palsy
- Play and interaction skills

Top tip!
Fine motor skills in this age group are easier to assess if the child sits at a table.

Observe the child's play. Is she manipulating objects easily?

Introduce a task playfully that the child should find easy – for example, picking up a small object to show a pincer grasp. Move on to pencil tasks and the manipulation of bricks. A selection of fine motor skills and the age range at which they are achieved should be noted (Table 7.31).

Table 7.31	
Fine motor milestone	**Age range**
Hands together	2–4 months
Palmar grasp	4–6 months
Transfers object from hand to hand	6 months
Rakes a raisin	5–7 months
Pincer grip	7–10 months
Scribbles	12–16 months
2-brick tower	13–19 months
6-brick tower Copies a line	19–30 months 2–3 years
3-brick bridge Copies a circle, later a cross	3 years
Copies a square Makes 3 steps out of 6 bricks	4 years
Copies a triangle Draws a person with 6 parts	5 years

As with all developmental tasks, there are 3 elements to fine motor tasks:

- Cognitive (understanding what is required and how to do it)
- Motor (power and movement control)
- Sensory elements (hear the instructions, see and feel the equipment, and understand
- how they relate to themselves and each other).

Top tip!
Hand dominance does not emerge until 2 to 4 years, and then does not become firmly established until 4 to 6 years. Early hand dominance may indicate an underlying neurological cause. Observe BOTH hands. For example, when building a brick tower, place the cubes one by one on the table alternately to the right and the left side of the base brick. Say and gesture "put it on the top". This gives the best opportunity to observe the levels of grasp, manipulation and release for each hand.

Pencil grasp

Young children make marks using whole arm movements. As their strength and control develop, the process of writing will move from the whole arm to the wrist, and finally to the fingertips. Initially, they use a palmar supinate grasp (fisted grip) between about 1 and 2 years. They go on to develop a digital pronate grip (all fingers) at around 2 to 3 years. Transition to an immature and static tripod grasp (thumb, index and middle fingers) occasionally occurs as early as 2½ years, but more typically between 3 and 4 years. Mature tripod grips typically develop around 5 years of age.

> *Top tip!*
> Be careful of children who are developmentally at the stage where they explore objects by mouthing them. For typically developing children, this phase can last up from 18 to 24 months. Introducing a small object, such as a peg, to demonstrate a mature pincer grasp will not impress the examiners if the child then chokes on it.

Vision and cognitive interest

In the first year of life, a baby's vision matures considerably and this will affect the objects she can manipulate. A 5 month old will show visual interest in a 2-cm square brick, but not a smaller item. A 6 month old will show interest in a 1 cm item and a 9 month old in a 1-mm item. Success in picking up the latter is limited until the baby's pincer grasp is fully mature.

As well as recognising and remembering normal milestones, it is also important to identify when development is significantly disordered, prompting the clinician to seek timely assessment by experts in neurodisability, neurology and the wider multidisciplinary team (Table 7.32).

Table 7.32: Red flags that suggest that development is significantly disordered, requiring prompt assessments by paediatricians in neurodisability, neurology and the multidisciplinary team

Any child who has:
- Lost developmental skills at any age
- Parental/professional concerns about vision, fixing or following (seek ophthalmology review)
- Significant hearing loss at any age (seek audiological/ENT review)
- No speech at 18 months, especially if not communicating by any other means (urgent hearing test)
- Suspected clinical diagnosis of cerebral palsy
- Head circumference above the 99.6th centile, below the 0.4th centile, or has crossed 2 centile lines up or down on the appropriate growth chart

Any child who is not able to:
- Sit unsupported by 12 months
- Walk by 18 months (boys) or 2 years (girls)
- 'Walk' other than on tiptoes
- Run by 2½ years
- Hold an object placed in their hand by 5 months of age (corrected for gestation)
- Reach for objects by 6 months of age (corrected for gestation)
- Point at objects to share interest with others by 2 years

Adapted from: Horridge KA. *Arch Dis Child Educ Pract Ed* (2010). doi: 10.1136/adc.2009.182436

Assimilating the signs

Now that you have conducted a thorough fine motor skills assessment, you will be expected to assimilate and present your positive clinical findings in order to arrive at a possible diagnosis. Below is a summary of your assessment elicited from Alice, and an example presentation.

Observation – Prominent epicanthic folds, down sloping palpebral fissures, brachycephaly, single palmar creases. No hearing aid; no glasses.

Manipulation – 4-brick tower, neat pincer grasp

Pencil skills – Copies a line, prefers scribbling

To present...

> "Alice is 4 years of age. On examination, she has features as consistent with a diagnosis of Down's syndrome. She does not wear glasses. She uses both hands equally. She uses a palmar pencil grasp and scribbles. She is just able to copy a vertical line. She built a tower of 4 bricks and enjoyed knocking them over. I am not sure this is the limit of her ability in this task. Alice's fine motor skills are delayed at an approximately 2-year level. I would like to assess the rest of her development to ascertain whether she has globally delayed development in line with her diagnosis."

Discussion

■ *What are the key elements of managing a child with Down's syndrome?*

A holistic, child-centred, multidisciplinary approach is advocated. Developmental progress is supported by:

Occupational therapists who help children develop play and self-care skills such dressing, eating, washing and toileting. They help children achieve their potential in school by developing their fine motor and coordination skills.

Speech and language therapists who support communication, interaction and language development. This may involve sign language, such as Makaton.

Physiotherapists who provide input and advice regarding gross motor development and physical activities.

Dieticians who provide advice on food and drink intake, nutrition and weight monitoring.

Paediatricians who coordinate medical care while monitoring for complications of Down's syndrome (see below). They interact with professionals involved with Alice to provide a holistic package of care and support.

The child will be followed up in a child development centre at least annually.

■ *Given Alice's diagnosis and developmental delay, what educational support should be instigated?*

Alice should be referred for a statutory assessment of her educational needs. The child development team often undertakes this for preschool children, but families and other professionals involved with the child may undertake the referral. If this is agreed, local educational psychologists undertake an assessment with contributions from therapists, the nursery, the paediatrician and parents.

Children with learning difficulties, disabilities or special educational needs have a legal right to appropriate extra help and support in nurseries, schools and colleges. In September 2014, the government replaced statements of special educational needs and learning difficulty assessments with a single education, health and care plan (EHCP) for children and young people with complex needs. The EHCP aims to place more emphasis on personal goals, and describes the support a child will receive while they are in education or training. A significant change is a 0 to 25 year focus. The paediatrician and therapists involved in Alice's care are legally obliged to provide reports to help inform her EHCP.

■ **What support is available to Alice and her family?**

'Portage' is a home-visiting educational service for preschool children with additional support needs, and their families. Portage home visitors are employed by local authorities and charities to support the development of play, communication, relationships, and learning for young children within the family. Different areas have similar schemes for home-based learning with varying names.

DLA is for children who have extra care needs due to their illness or disability. It is not means-tested. All children with Down's syndrome will eventually be eligible for DLA. Applications can be made from when the child is 3 months old, if they need more help and support than a child of the same age with no difficulties. DLA has 2 parts: the care component and the mobility component. The mobility component is available for children who are at least 3 years old.

Social care – Some children with Down's syndrome qualify for support from the Childhood Disability Team in social services.

Local and national support groups exist, such as the Down's Syndrome Association.

■ **What medical problems are more common in children with Down's syndrome?**

Atlantoaxial instability

This condition presents as a very small risk throughout the patient's life.

Symptoms of cord compression include: neck pain, restricted neck movement, unsteadiness in walking, and deterioration in bowel and bladder control. These symptoms warrant urgent medical attention. There is no screening procedure that can predict those at risk. X-rays are not useful. The annual physical examination should include a check for signs of cord compression. Children with Down's syndrome should not be barred from sporting activities, except vigorous trampolining, intensive horse riding and high diving. When undergoing any treatment requiring anaesthesia, a collar should be used to keep the neck stable.

Hypothyroidism

This affects between 10% and 20% of people with Down's syndrome, the prevalence increasing with age. Newborn babies have a neonatal screen for hypothyroidism using the Guthrie test. At the first birthday, and then every 2 years throughout their lives, thyroid function and antibodies should be checked.

Congenital cardiac defects

About 1 in 3 children born with Down's syndrome will have a congenital cardiac defect, with atrioventricular septal defects being the most common (1 in 6). Echocardiography is recommended even if the cardiac examination is normal in order to facilitate prompt referral to paediatric cardiologists and, if necessary, cardiac surgeons.

Hearing loss

Over 50% of children and adults with Down's syndrome will have a significant hearing impairment, which may be mild, moderate or severe. Conductive hearing loss is more prevalent in this population, with an above average incidence of glue ear, as the eustachian tube can be particularly narrow. Infections should be treated promptly and hearing aids introduced early if necessary. The Down Syndrome Medical Interest Group recommends the following schedule for hearing screening in Down's Syndrome:

- All babies in the UK are screened as part of the newborn hearing screening programme (NHSP).
- Full audiological assessment should be conducted between 6 and 10 months of age.
- There should be yearly reviews until the child reaches the age of 5.
- There should be 2 yearly reviews throughout life (more frequently if problems exist).

Vision

Over 90% of children and adults with Down's syndrome have some type of problem with vision. Refractive errors and/or squint (strabismus) may be present from an early age. Check-ups should be conducted every 1-2 years. Children with no obvious defect should have a further ophthalmological review at around 4 years, and then at least every 2 years throughout life.

Syllabus mapping

Neurology and neurodisability

Knowledge

The candidate must:

- Understand the definition and concepts of disability, and what this means for the child and family.
- Be familiar with the common causes of disability, disordered development and learning difficulties.
- Be able to take a neurodevelopmental history.
- Be aware of local services/disability allowances.
- Understand the need for multidisciplinary team input in the care of the disabled child, and be aware of the work of the child development team and centre.
- Understand the need to work with other services as required, including education, social services, child protection, and respite care facilities.
- Be aware of how agencies work together to address how children with health and medical needs are managed at school.
- Be able to recognise presenting features of visual or hearing impairment, as well as know when and how to refer for further assessment.

Skills

The candidate must:

- Be able to perform a reliable assessment of neurodevelopmental status at key stages, including the newborn period, the first year of life, nursery age and school entry.

Further reading and references

1. Dennis J. The Down Syndrome medical interest group: Guidelines for essential medical surveillance. 2012. http://www.dsmig.org.uk/publications/guidelines.html (accessed February 2015).
2. Down Syndrome Association. Disability Living Allowance. 2015. http://www.downs-syndrome.org.uk/for-families-and-carers/benefits-and-financial-help/disability-living-allowance/ (accessed March 2015).
3. Hall M, Hill P. *The Child with a Disability*. Blackwell, Oxford, 2014.
4. Horridge KA. Assessment and investigation of the child with disordered development. *Arch Dis Child Educ Pract Ed* 2010; 96(1): 9–20
5. National Portage Association. http://www.portage.org.uk/ (accessed March 2015).
6. Timpson E. New arrangements for supporting children and young people with special educational needs and disabilities. 2014. https://www.gov.uk/government/uploads/system/uploads/attachment_data/file/301837/SEND_reforms_-_letter_for_parents.pdf (accessed March 2015).

Chapter 7.4: Case Study 3: 3 Year Old with Language and Communication Skill Difficulties

Dr Kate Fisher

This station assesses your ability to demonstrate a developmental assessment of a child's language and communication skills and conduct a discussion with the examiner. You will be assessed on the rapport, manner and structure of your examination with the child and parent. Always introduce yourself to the child and their carer.

Logistics:

Timing: This is a 9-minute station. A knock at 6 minutes will note that 3 minutes remain before the end of the station. At this point, it is important to summarise your clinical findings and proceed with the discussion with the examiner.

When the bell rings: On entering the room, the examiner will greet you, take your mark sheet, introduce you to the child and parent, and give you your task. Listen carefully to these instructions.

The examiner will then remain mostly silent during the consultation, as they will be observing your clinical skills, but may provide some direction should it be required. A discussion around the case will be undertaken in the final 3 minutes of the station.

If you finish early, you will be asked to remain in the room until the session has ended.

Candidate role and task:

You are an ST2 trainee working in GP practice.

Cameron is 3 years old. His mother is concerned as she feels his speech is delayed compared with his cousin, who is the same age. He is not yet joining words into short phrases. His mother estimates he has a vocabulary of approximately 20–30 words.

Task: You are asked to assess his speech and language development.

The speech and language assessment

Observation

Although you have been requested to examine 1 developmental domain, remember that speech and language delay can be the presenting feature of more global developmental issues. Observing the child yields a great deal of information, so look for:

- Dysmorphic features
- Hearing aids
- Signs of a motor disorder, such as cerebral palsy
- Play and interaction skills (e.g. pretend play)

> *Top tip!*
> Establish a rapport with the child safely on mother's lap. If the child is playing happily with some toys, get down to their level and show interest in their play. Gently introduce books or objects as suggested below.

Language has 2 elements:

1. **Receptive Language** – Understanding, decoding, integrating and organising what is heard
2. **Expressive language** – The ability to articulate speech and use sounds, words, phrases or sentences in meaningful contexts

Parents often overestimate the child's receptive language ability. In the exam situation, as young children tend to spontaneously name objects shown to them, it is usually easier to explore expressive language first.

Expressive language

The available materials may vary, but toys and everyday objects (e.g. spoon, cup, hairbrush, doll and ball) should be to hand. Ideally, real objects should be used for those aged 12 to 24 months. Aim for a choice of 3 items under 16 months, 4 between 16 and 24 months, and above 6 items for more than 24 months. Show the objects one at a time, saying, "what's this?" If the child remains quiet, say, "is it a…?" Offer several alternatives, including the correct answer. Then repeat with another object.

Alternative approaches include sharing a picture book with the child and asking them to describe a scene that depicts everyday childhood experiences (e.g. playing in the park). This is particularly useful to explore higher levels of language in 3 and 4 year olds. Younger children may name or point to items in the picture. Children over 2 can tell simple stories from pictures.

The age ranges within which children obtain expressive language skills are noted in Table 7.41.

Table 7.41	
Expressive language milestones	Normal age range
Consonant babble, e.g. "baba"	By 8 months
Few single words, e.g. "dada", "no", "gone"	12–18 months
Approximately 50 words	18–23 months
2 word phrases, e.g. "Daddy car"	18–24 months
3 elements, e.g. "Boy kick ball"	2 years
4 elements, e.g. "Where Daddy's shoe gone?"	3 years
Complex sentences, multiple clauses	4 years
Names, colours	4 years

Receptive language

Now turn your attention to assessing verbal comprehension. Lay out a number of items and ask:

- "Where's the *spoon*?" (1 key word)
- "Put the *spoon* in the *cup*" or ask for 2 items (2 key words)

If the correct object is chosen, take it, say "thank you" and replace it on the table. If the wrong or no choice is made, request another item. As a last resort, give an item to the child saying, "Give it to Mummy" or encourage them to point to their mouth, eyes, or nose. Make the requests more complex by involving more words that carry key information for older or more able children.

The age ranges within which children obtain receptive language skills are noted in Table 7.42.

Table 7.42	
Receptive language milestones	Normal age range
"Give it to Daddy" 1 key word (mummy/daddy)	12–15 months
"Where is the ball/spoon?" 1 key word	17–23 months
"Put the spoon in the cup" "Give me the brush and the ball" 2 key words	24–30 months
"Put the ball under the table" 3 key words	30–36 months
"Give me the red car and put the fork on the plate" 4 key words	42–52 months

Social communication

Although you are assessing speech and language, consider the quality of the child's social interaction. Do they make good eye contact? Do they share joint attention? For example, when presented with a toy car, is the child clearly delighted and immediately shows his mother, sharing his pleasure? Are they able to tolerate a change in activity without becoming too distressed?

Top tip!
Sometimes, no amount of charm and playfulness will persuade a child that they want to interact with you. Ask the examiners if you are able to take a history from the parent or carer.

Consider the following:

- Do parents have any concerns about *hearing*?
- Establish whether the child is using *single words, phrases or sentences*. Ask for examples.
- Ask about *understanding*, but be wary of contextual clues.
- Ask about *play and interaction* with peers and adults.
- The mother is concerned that Cameron's development is behind that of his cousin; there is a wide range of normal, and both may be developing along normal lines.

Assimilating the signs

Now that you have conducted a thorough assessment of the child's speech and language, you will be expected to assimilate and present your positive clinical findings in order to arrive at a differential diagnosis. Key features from Cameron's assessment include:

Inspection – Cameron has no dysmorphic features or obvious motor problems.
Receptive language – At a 3-key-word level
Expressive language – Single-word level
Social communication – Good eye contact. Shares joint attention. Gestures.

To present...

> "Cameron is a 3 year old boy whose mother is concerned about his speech development. Cameron makes good eye contact and shows a range of facial expressions. He points and shares interest with adults. His understanding is at a 3-word level, but his expressive language is at a single-word level. The mother estimates he has a vocabulary of 40 words.
>
> Cameron's social communication skills and receptive language skills are within the normal range for his age. His expressive language is delayed at an 18-month level. I should like to assess his development more fully to ascertain if this is an isolated expressive language delay, or if there are other developmental issues."

Discussion

■ *What is the differential diagnosis for a child with speech and language delay?*

Disorders that are commonly associated with receptive and expressive communication problems include:

- Hearing loss
- Autism
- Social factors, including neglect
- Global developmental delay
- Physical issues, e.g. cleft lip/palate
- Cerebral palsy
- Specific language impairment
- Oro-motor dyspraxia

■ *How would you manage Cameron?*

- Referral to speech and language therapy
- Referral to audiology
- Referral for health visitor review of development
- Referral to community paediatrician only if delayed in 2 or more developmental domains

■ *What are the types of speech and language impairment? What are the consequences?*

- Speech disorders – Impairment in the articulation of speech sounds, fluency and voice.
- Language disorders – Impairment of the spoken system, involving:
- The form of language (grammar and phonology)
- How language is used in different social contexts (pragmatics)
- The content and meaning of language (semantics)

Language delay is characterised by the late emergence of typically developing language. Speech and language impairments affect 5–8% of preschool children. They can lead to behaviour difficulties, social isolation and literacy problems.

■ Autism can present with delayed and disordered language development. What is autism?

Autism is a lifelong developmental disability that presents with qualitative impairment of reciprocal social communication and interaction, restricted interests, and rigid and repetitive behaviours. Autism spectrum disorders are diagnosed in children, young people and adults if these behaviours meet the criteria defined in the International Statistical Classification of Diseases and Related Health Problems (ICD-10) and the Diagnostic and Statistical Manual of Mental Disorders (DSM-V, fifth edition). Autism is thought to occur in at least 1% of children. Many more children have impairment in their social communication and interaction skills, but do not meet the criteria for a diagnosis.

Children at particular risk of autism include those with:

- A first-degree relative with autism
- Learning disability
- Gestational age less than 35 weeks
- Chromosomal disorders
- Neurofibromatosis
- Tuberous sclerosis

■ How might autism present in children?

Presenting features may include some of the following.

Speech and language:

- Language delay (in babble or words, e.g. less than 10 words by the age of 2 years)
- Regression or loss of speech
- Echolalia

Social interaction:

- Reduced or absent responsive social smiling
- Reduced or absent responsiveness to other people's facial expressions or feelings
- Reduced or absent awareness of personal space
- Reduced or absent social interest in others
- Reduced or absent initiation of social play with others (plays alone)
- Reduced or absent enjoyment of situations that most children enjoy (e.g. parties)
- Reduced eye contact with adequate vision
- Reduced or absent joint attention shown by lack of:
  - Following a point
  - Using pointing at or showing objects to share interest

Play:

- Reduced or absent imagination and variety of pretend play

Behaviours:

- Repetitive 'stereotypical' movements, such as hand flapping, spinning, finger flicking, body rocking while standing
- Repetitive or stereotyped play (e.g. opening and closing doors)
- Unusual interests for their age
- Excessive insistence on following their own agenda
- Difficulty in coping with change
- Overreaction or underreaction to sensory stimuli (e.g. textures)
- Extreme food fads

■ *What is involved in an assessment of a child with significant social communication and interaction difficulties?*

A multidisciplinary team (involving a paediatrician and/or child and adolescent psychiatrist, a speech and language therapist and a clinical and/or educational psychologist, with access to an occupational therapist) carries out the assessment. Not every child will need to see every member of the team. A thorough medical and developmental history is taken and a physical examination is undertaken. It is essential that a direct assessment of the child's social and communication skills and behaviours is undertaken by observation and direct interaction, focusing on features consistent with ICD-10 or DSM-V criteria. Many centres use an autism-specific tool to gather this information. Frequently occurring comorbid conditions (e.g. ADHD, developmental coordination disorder and learning difficulties) need to be considered. The findings of the assessment and the management plan need to be communicated clearly and sensitively to the child and their family. Information on the condition and local and national support groups, as well as advice on welfare benefits and educational support, is important for families.

Syllabus mapping

Neurology and neurodisability

Knowledge

The candidate must:

- Understand the definition and concepts of disability and what this means for the child and family.
- Be familiar with the common causes of disability, disordered development and learning difficulties.
- Be able to take a neurodevelopmental history.
- Know the causes of speech and language delay, and know when to refer to a specialist.
- Be aware of local services/disability allowances.
- Understand the need for multidisciplinary team input in the care of the disabled child, and be aware of the work of the child development team and centre.
- Understand the need to work with other services as required, including education, social services, child protection, and respite care facilities.

- Be aware of how agencies work together to address how children with health and medical needs are managed at school.
- Be able to recognise presenting features of visual or hearing impairment, as well as know when and how to refer for further assessment.

Skills

The candidate must:

- Be able to perform a reliable assessment of the neurodevelopmental status at key stages, including the newborn period, the first year of life, nursery age and school entry.

Further reading and references

1. Hall M, Hill P. *The Child with a Disability*. Blackwell, Oxford, 1996.
2. National Institute for Clinical Excellence. (CG128) – Autism diagnosis in children and young people: Recognition, referral and diagnosis of children and young people on the autism spectrum. 2011. https://www.nice.org.uk/guidance/cg128 (accessed March 2015).
3. Prelock P, Hutchins T, Glascoe F. Speech-Language Impairment: How to identify the most common and least diagnosed disability of childhood. *Medscape J Med* 2008; 10(6): 136
4. Sonksen P. *A developmental approach to the examination of preschool children*. 2015.

SECTION 8:
THE SAFE PRESCRIBING STATION

Chapter 8.1: Introduction
Dr Anna Mathew, Dr Nick Cooper

A challenging task for all practising doctors is to reliably, safely and effectively prescribe. In paediatrics, this is of paramount importance, as some drugs may only be prescribed in specific circumstances, or according to a child's age and weight. Dosages differ between an infant, toddler and adolescent, and some drugs may be 'unlicensed' although accepted in practice as to their use.

During the past decade, there has been increasing awareness about the prevalence of prescribing errors that frequently result in morbidity and, in some cases, mortality of our patients. Possibly as a direct result of these concerns, there is now an established prescribing skills assessment for final year medical students in the UK. For some years, the RCPCH has been reviewing the prescribing of paediatric specialist trainees prior to the completion of specialist training.

Several reports have highlighted the concerns regarding prescribing errors in primary and secondary care, and, therefore, the introduction of a prescribing station in the DCH clinical examination is timely.

The GMC's (general medical council) guidance on good medical practice stipulates that all doctors must recognise and work within the limits of their competence and must keep their knowledge and skills in this area up to date. By maintaining and developing skills in prescribing and medicine management, doctors can develop knowledge and skills in pharmacology and therapeutics. The GMC states that all doctors who prescribe for children must be familiar with the guidance in the BNFC (British National Formulary for Children), which contains essential information to help with prescribing, monitoring, supplying and administering medicines. Doctors should follow the advice in the BNFC on prescription writing, and must ensure that orders are clear, contain all the statutory requirements, and include the author's name (written legibly).

As a candidate for the DCH examination, it is important that you read the section in the BNFC *General guidance* and, in particular, *Prescription writing* and *Prescribing controlled drugs*. It is important to pay special attention to the additional requirements for writing a prescription of a *controlled drug*, as this scenario can appear in the examination.

What to expect

The safe prescribing station assesses your ability to write a comprehensive prescription with the correct dosage according to the child's age and weight, and that is appropriate to the described clinical scenario. An understanding of indication, mode of action and potential adverse reactions will also be assessed.

Scenarios are usually set with the expectation that a GP or a GP trainee would have the competency to prescribe the medication being requested. Therefore, scenarios are set at primary care level, and the setting is either a GP surgery or, at times, the paediatric department in a hospital. In such situations, scenarios are set such that a GP trainee is working in paediatrics as part of their training rotation. Some common scenarios requiring a prescription could include treatment of asthma, infections, or management of epilepsy. It is not possible within the remit of this book to provide an exhaustive list.

Many of you will be familiar with electronic prescribing, which involves either generating a printed FP10 or using the Electronic Prescribing Service (EPS) to send the prescription directly to a pharmacy. In this examination, however, you will be expected to fill out the form provided in the format of a handwritten prescription form (FP10).

The task is to write a prescription on the supplied FP10 (with a copy of the BNFC available), and subsequently discuss with the examiner the implications of your decision with reference to indication, dose calculation, contraindications, potential adverse reactions and specific issues related to taking the medication. Advice on how to complete the FP10 is shown in Figure 8.1.

A copy of the BNFC, a prescription pad and a calculator will be provided at the station.

Once the prescription has been written, **you will not** be allowed to refer to the BNFC during the discussion that follows with the examiner.

Managing time in the safe prescribing station

Timing: This is a 9-minute station. You will be given up to 2 minutes before the start of the station to read the task set (candidate information sheet) outside the room to prepare yourself.

When the bell rings: On entering the room, the examiner will greet you, take your mark sheet, and allow you to proceed with writing the prescription. You may take the candidate instruction sheet into the room, but this must be replaced as you leave the station.

You will be given 6 minutes to write the prescription. A knock at 6 minutes will mark the end of the recommended time to write the prescription. A discussion around the prescription will be undertaken in the final 3 minutes of the station. At this point, **you will not** be allowed to refer back to the BNFC and, therefore, the examiner will be testing your knowledge regarding the prescription you have just filled out.

If you finish early, you will be asked to remain in the room until the session has ended.

How consistency is ensured

RCPCH examiners set questions for the station well before the date of the examination, in groups, and agree the standards of performance required from candidates for the various grades awarded. In addition, on the day of the examination, examiners work in pairs to review and discuss the 'standard setting' that have been agreed by the RCPCH. The pair of examiners can make adjustments at this stage when considering whether the scenario is of an appropriate standard for this examination. This does not happen frequently, but the opportunity still exists should the need arise. Pass/fail criteria and the questions to follow during 'discussion' time are also set by the RCPCH ahead of the examination to help ensure consistency, but these are reviewed again by the pair of examiners on the day as well. This 'standard setting' process is undertaken before each cycle during the clinical examination to ensure consistency.

'Mark sheets', individualised for each station, help to guide examiners in their assessment of candidates. Mark sheets can inform candidates of the different areas examiners consider when awarding marks and, as importantly, areas where marks will be deducted. In the safe prescribing station, mark sheets contain all the necessary details that examiners will look for when scrutinising candidate prescriptions, and can therefore be used as a resource during preparation and training (Appendix 8.11).

The RCPCH has developed 'anchor statements' that examiners refer to when deciding on pass/fail criteria. There are clear, essential and desired criteria for prescribing effectively (assessed through the completion of an appropriate prescription based on the clinical scenario). Candidates should review these documents to familiarise themselves with the scoring categories explained in the anchor statements (Appendix 8.12).

Figure 8.11: FP10 form used in the DCH clinical examination. Follow steps 1-4 highlighted on the mark sheet when completing the prescription

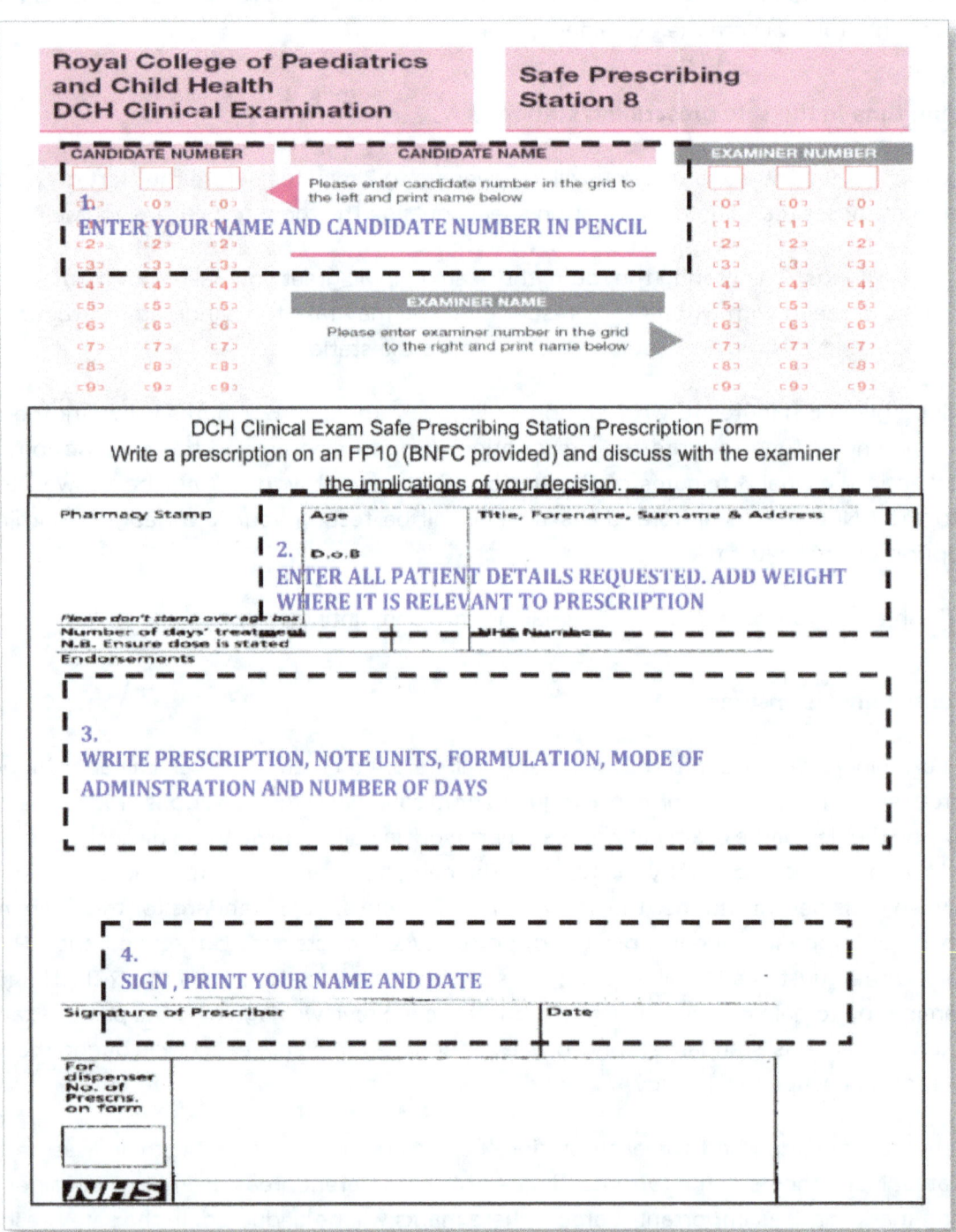

Top tip!
As you will not be able to refer to the BNFC during the 'discussion time' with the examiner, utilise any 'free' time in the first 6 minutes *after* completing the prescription to have a quick look at the side effects of the drug you have prescribed.

Syllabus mapping

Pharmacology, poisoning and accidents

Knowledge

The candidate must:

- Know how to find out information necessary for safe prescribing through the use of paediatric formularies and pharmacy liaison.
- Know the approved indications for prescribing drugs in common paediatric problems.
- Be aware of possible drug interactions and side effects when more than 1 drug is prescribed.
- Know about the licensing of medicines for paediatric patients, unlicensed and off-label use, and the legal aspects of prescribing for children.

Skills

The candidate must:

- Be able to write a legible, clear and complete prescription.
- Be able to make reliable and accurate calculations in order to safely prescribe for babies, children and young people.

Further reading and references

1. Avery AJ, Ghaleb M, Barber N et al. The prevalence and nature of prescribing and monitoring errors in English general practice: A retrospective case note review. *British Journal of General Practice* 2013; 63: 413–414
2. British National Formulary for Children. 2014–2015. http://www.bnf.org/bnf/org_450055.htm (accessed June 2015).
3. DCH clinical syllabus: http://www.rcpch.ac.uk/training-examinations-professional-development/assessment-and-examinations/examinations/syllabus (accessed March 2015).
4. Dornan T, Ashcroft D, Heathfield H et al. An in-depth investigation into causes of prescribing errors by foundation trainees in relation to their medical education. EQUIP study. 2009. General Medical Council. http://www.gmc-uk.org/about/research/25056.asp (accessed July 2015).
5. Good practice in prescribing and managing medicines and devices. 2013. http://www.gmc-uk.org/guidance/ethical_guidance/14316.asp (accessed March 2015).

Clinical Cases in Paediatrics: DCH Clinical Examination

Appendix 8.11: Mark Sheet (Front and Back): Safe Prescribing Station

Royal College of Paediatrics and Child Health
DCH Clinical Examination

Safe Prescribing Station 8

Date: Time: Age of child:

Occasion used (1st, 2nd etc.):

CANDIDATE NUMBER

CANDIDATE NAME — Please enter candidate number in the grid to the left and print name below

EXAMINER NUMBER

Scenario

EXAMINER NAME — Please enter examiner number in the grid to the right and print name below

Do not write in this shaded area

Description of Case

Prescribing Effectively and In Context
(Assessment of the written prescription based on set scenario)

Essential:
Child's name, address, date of birth must be written on the prescription
Prescribes the correct drug
Writes Generic drug name or Trade name if appropriate
Writes legibly
Writes the correct dose (including zero before decimal if appropriate) and the dose strength
Write dose frequency and total number of days of dose indicated
Units are clearly written: g, mg, micrograms, nanograms are acceptable
Completes prescription (signature, name and date of prescription)

Desired:
Checks formulations available and what would be most suitable (capsule or liquid)
Dispensable dose (rounded up)
Writes appropriate route of administration
States weight if relevant

Please record your overall judgement of the candidate's performance

PART A GRADE HERE ▶ Clear Pass | Pass | Bare Fail | Clear Fail | Un-acceptable

Knowledge, Skills and Attitude to Prescribing
(Assessment of the discussion with the examiner)

Explains correct choice (clinical and cost effectiveness) of medication for this scenario (based on clinical reasoning, national guideline or BNFc advice)

Explains relevant patient related factors influencing prescription

Knows contraindications

Knows side effects

Fluent and confident

Please record your overall judgement of the candidate's performance

PART B GRADE HERE ▶ Clear Pass | Pass | Bare Fail | Clear Fail | Un-acceptable

In order that proper feedback is available for the candidate please print your comments on their overall performance on the reverse of this document.

© Speedwell Computing Services +44 (0)1223 815210   enquiries@speedwell.co.uk   www.speedwell.co.uk

☐ Disorganised and unsystematic approach (please add additional comments)

☐ Inappropriate use of tools/assessment aids (please add additional comments)

☐ Poor time management (please add additional comments)

☐ Inaccurate assessment/conclusion (please add additional comments)

Please add any additional comments here:

Appendix 8.12: Anchor Statement: Safe Prescribing Station

Expected Standard	CLEAR PASS	PASS	BARE FAIL	CLEAR FAIL	UNACCEPTABLE
PRESCRIBING EFFECTIVELY AND IN CONTEXT (Assessment of the written prescription based on set scenario)	Achieves both Essential and Desired criteria: **ESSENTIAL:** <ul><li>Child's name, address, date of birth must be written on the prescription</li><li>Prescribes the correct drug</li><li>Writes Generic drug name or Trade name if appropriate</li><li>Writes legibly</li><li>Writes the correct dose (including zero before decimal if appropriate) and the dose strength</li><li>Write dose frequency and total number of days of dose indicated</li><li>Units are clearly written: g, mg, micrograms, nanograms are acceptable</li><li>Completes prescription (signature, name and date of prescription)</li></ul> **DESIRED:** <ul><li>Checks formulations available and what would be most suitable (capsule or liquid)</li><li>Dispensable dose (rounded up)</li><li>Writes appropriate route of administration</li></ul> **Fluent and confident in use of the BNFC (uses BNFC logically, acquires information rapidly, turns to appropriate pages, does not 'browse' or hunt for inspiration)**	Achieves all essential criteria and some desired criteria Prescribes the correct drug OR a clinically appropriate different drug	Misses any essential criteria Prescribes the correct drug OR a clinically appropriate different drug	Misses most essential and desired criteria Prescribes the **wrong drug**	Unsafe prescription:<ul><li>unsafe dose prescribed (correct or the wrong drug)</li><li>unsafe drug prescribed (risk to patient safety)</li></ul>
KNOWLEDGE, SKILLS AND ATTITUDE TO PRESCRIBING (Assessment of the discussion with the examiner)	<ul><li>Explains correct choice (clinical and cost effectiveness) of medication for this scenario (based on clinical reasoning, national guideline or BNFC advice)</li><li>Explains relevant patient related factors influencing prescription</li><li>Knows contraindications</li><li>Knows side effects</li><li>Fluent and confident</li></ul>	<ul><li>Knows indications, important contraindications and side effects of the drug prescribed</li><li>Aware of patient related factors influencing prescription</li><li>Lacks confidence</li></ul>	<ul><li>Limited knowledge of the drug prescribed</li><li>Misses important contraindications, side effects</li><li>Not aware of patient related factors influencing prescription</li><li>Lacks confidence</li></ul>	<ul><li>Limited or poor explanation offered for the choice of the drug prescribed</li><li>Fails to suggest alternative and appropriate drug</li><li>Poor understanding of patient related factors influencing prescription</li><li>Lacks confidence and poor responses</li></ul>	<ul><li>Lack of knowledge or understanding of contraindications, side effects</li><li>Unsafe</li><li>Inappropriate attitude displayed in responses</li></ul>

Chapter 8.2: Case Study 1: Hypoglycaemia in a Newly Diagnosed Diabetic
Dr Duana Cook

This station assesses your ability to write a prescription and then discuss the implications of prescribing this medication with the examiner. An understanding of indication, mode of action, potential adverse reactions and dose calculation will also be assessed during discussion time. Candidates *will not* be allowed to refer to the BNFC for the second part of the assessment.

A copy of the BNFC, a prescription pad and a calculator will be provided at the station.

> **Logistics:**
>
> Timing: This is a 9-minute station. You will have up to 2 minutes before the start of this station to read the candidate sheet and prepare yourself.
>
> *When the bell rings:* On entering the room, the examiner will greet you, take your mark sheet, and allow you to proceed with writing the prescription. You may take the candidate instruction sheet into the room, but this must be replaced as you leave the station.
>
> You will be given 6 minutes to write the prescription. A discussion around the prescription will be undertaken in the final 3 minutes of the station.
>
> If the discussion with the examiner finishes early, you will be asked to remain in the room until the session has ended.

> **Candidate role and task:**
>
> **You are a** GP trainee working on the paediatric day assessment unit.
>
> You have just seen Jessie Thomas (DOB 01/07/2006, 5 Theobalds Road, London WC1X 8SH. Body weight: 24 kg. NHS No: 456 789 1230).
>
> Jessie is a newly diagnosed diabetic on insulin. The diabetic specialist nurse has asked you to prescribe medication to be used in the event of a hypoglycaemic seizure or coma.
>
> **Task: Write a prescription for Jessie based on the information provided, using the BNFC.**
>
> **With the examiner: Discuss issues of safe prescribing.**

Prescription task

Utilise the time given to write a complete prescription, entering all the patient details given in the script. Don't forget to date, sign and print your name at the end of the prescription. Further guidance on filling out a complete prescription can be found in the introductory chapter, as well as on the mark sheets for this station.

> *Top tip!*
> Carefully consider the information you have been given regarding the possible severity of the hypoglycaemic episode being described, and thus the route of administration of the medication you are prescribing (given the clinical condition of the patient).

Figure 8.21: Completed prescription

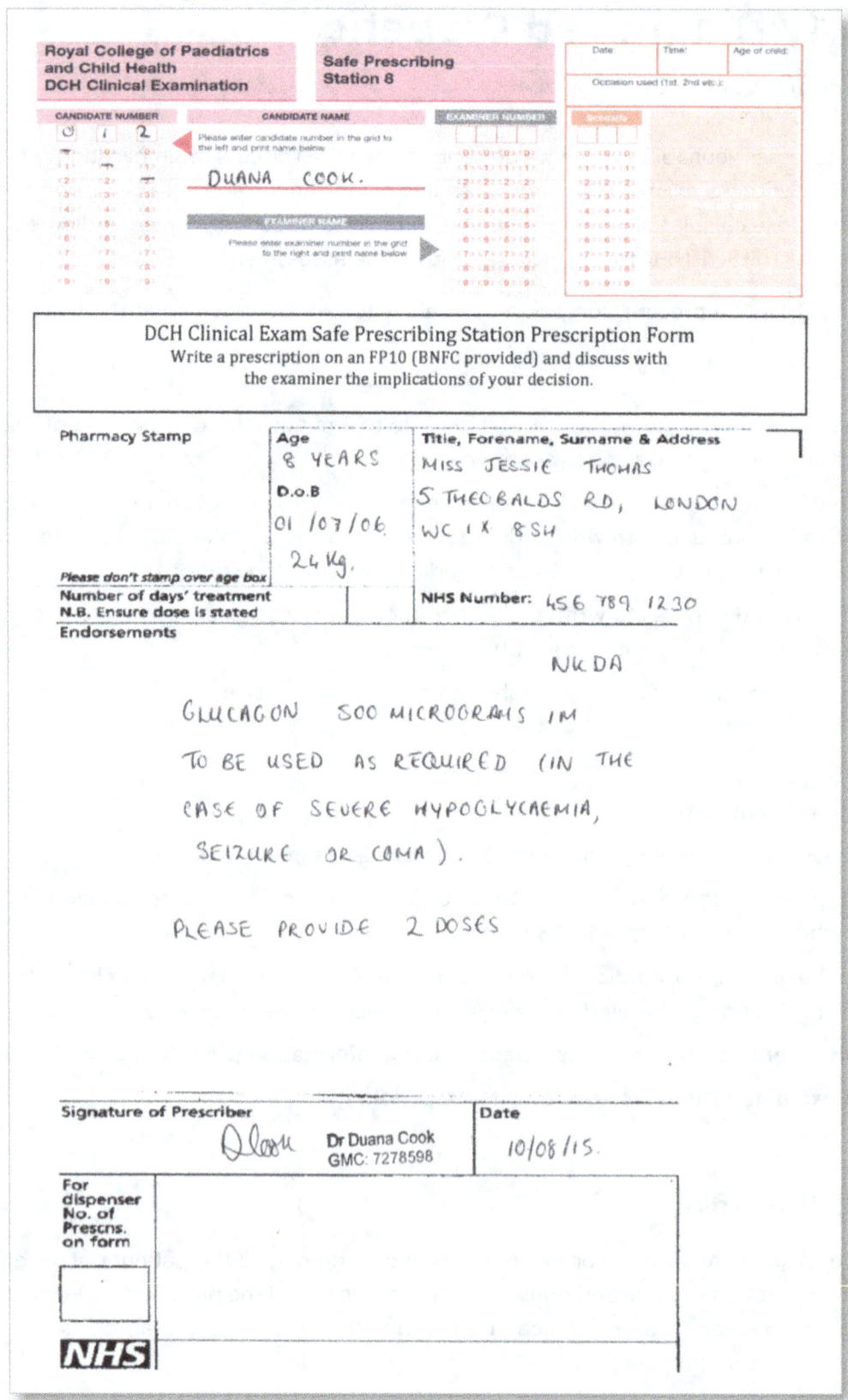

Top tip!
A clear pass candidate will prescribe intramuscular glucagon at an appropriate dose for the child's weight. They must include the child's name, date of birth and address for it to be a safe prescription.

Discussion

In the last 3 minutes of this station, the examiner will discuss with you issues surrounding your prescription. At this point, *you will not* be allowed to refer to the BNFC and, therefore, the examiner will be testing your knowledge regarding the prescription that you have just completed. *Possible* questions from the examiner are highlighted below.

■ *What is the reason for the choice of your medication?*

You have been told that the prescription is for cases of hypoglycaemic seizure or coma. In this situation, it would not be safe to give an oral medication. As the prescription is being written for the parents to take home, it is a 'PRN' prescription to be used in the case of an emergency. The medication prescribed, therefore, should be such that it can be administered quickly and safely by parents or carers, and should act quickly. Glucagon is a polypeptide hormone, produced by the alpha cells of the pancreatic islets of Langerhans. It acts to mobilise the glycogen stored in the liver, converting it into glucose and thereby increasing the blood glucose concentration.

■ *What would you use to treat mild to moderate hypoglycaemia?*

In the case of hypoglycaemia, where the child is still cooperative and able to swallow, they should first be given 10–20 g of glucose orally, which can be either 3 GlucoTabs or 60 ml of Glucojuice or Lucozade, or 100 ml of orange juice or non-diet Coke. In mild hypoglycaemia, the blood glucose should be rechecked 10 minutes after administering the oral glucose, and the treatment can be repeated up to 3 times if the hypoglycaemia persists, before medical help should be sought. In moderate hypoglycaemia, where the patient is conscious but incoherent, if they do not improve after the oral glucose, 1 tube of glucogel should be massaged between the cheek and gum, and medical help sought.

■ *What else do you need to think about when issuing this prescription to Jessie's parents/carers?*

The parents/carers will need to be taught how to recognise hypoglycaemia, and educated on how and when to give the IM glucagon. In most areas, the paediatric diabetes specialist nurses will be involved in teaching parents how to do this. They should be taught about the other oral forms of glucose that are used for milder hypoglycaemic episodes as well.

■ *In the case of a hypoglycaemic seizure or coma, is there anything else you should do in addition to administering the medication you have prescribed?*

A hypoglycaemic episode that causes a seizure or coma is a medical emergency. You need to ensure that parents and carers are aware of this. Ideally, they should check the child's blood glucose level, give the IM glucagon, and then seek medical help immediately by calling an ambulance. If IM glucagon is not effective within 10 minutes, then IV glucose should be given. Once the blood glucose is over 4 mmol/L, and the patient is fully awake and cooperative, they should be given long-acting carbohydrates to eat (e.g. a slice of bread, 2 biscuits, or a meal if one is due). If glucagon was given, then the amount of carbohydrate should be doubled. The usual insulin should still be given, and blood glucose should be monitored regularly for the next 24–48 hours after a severe hypoglycaemic episode. The diabetic team should review the child as a priority.

■ *Are there any situations when the medication you have prescribed will be ineffective?*

The glucagon dose is age and weight dependent. If the glucagon is ineffective, I would ensure that the correct dosage has been prescribed for the age and weight of the child as per the BNFC. Glucagon will be ineffective in treating hypoglycaemia caused by fatty acid oxidation defects and glycogen storage disorders, or in patients with severe liver disease or starved patients. Young people should be informed that, in cases where alcohol consumption has contributed to the hypoglycaemia, glucagon may again be ineffective and IV glucose may be needed.

Additional information

Hypoglycaemia

Hypoglycaemia is one of the acute complications of type 1 diabetes mellitus. It is defined by the World Health Organisation (WHO) as being a blood glucose of <2.5 mmol/L in children, although these children may become symptomatic when the blood glucose is <3.5 mmol/L. All children with type 1 diabetes mellitus will experience an episode of hypoglycaemia at some point, although it occurs more frequently in younger children and in those with more intensive insulin regimens.

Symptoms of hypoglycaemia include:

- Hunger
- Weakness and shakiness/feeling faint and dizzy
- Sweating
- Pallor
- Drowsiness
- Behavioural changes (e.g. irritability, confusion)

Hypoglycaemia is diagnosed based on the presence of 3 criteria, known as Whipple's triad, which consist of low plasma blood glucose, symptoms attributable to this, and the resolution of these symptoms with the correction of the hypoglycaemia.

If hypoglycaemia is not immediately treated with oral glucose, it can rapidly progress to result in seizures or coma. Long-standing hypoglycaemia for several hours can cause brain damage or even death.

Education of parents and children about the signs and symptoms of hypoglycaemia, compliance with insulin regimens, a consistent daily routine, regular BM monitoring, and correct insulin dosages, as well as controlled snacking, are all important factors in helping to prevent hypoglycaemia.

Hypoglycaemia is classified as mild, moderate or severe. Mild hypoglycaemia is self-recognised and the patient responds to it and self-treats. It is therefore rare in children under the age of 6, as they usually are unable to help themselves. In moderate hypoglycaemia, patients are conscious and still able to swallow, but are unable to respond to the hypoglycaemia themselves and, as a result, need someone else to treat them. However, oral treatment should be sufficient. Patients with severe hypoglycaemia will be either semi-conscious or unconscious, and may or may not be having seizures. They will therefore require parenteral therapy with glucagon IM or IV glucose. If IV glucose is needed, then 5 ml/kg of 10% glucose infusion can be given intravenously into a large vein through a large gauge cannula.

When children and young people are diagnosed with type 1 diabetes mellitus, they and their carers need to be educated regarding the importance of always having immediate access to quick acting carbohydrates and blood glucose monitoring equipment, so that they can record and effectively treat any episodes of hypoglycaemia.

Hypoglycaemia unawareness

Children who experience frequent episodes of hypoglycaemia may develop hypoglycaemia unawareness, as their bodies fail to mount the typical adrenergic response to the hypoglycaemia. They are, therefore, asymptomatic during episodes, which can lead to more severe episodes occurring. Good diabetic control and compliance, with careful BM monitoring and correct insulin dosages as previously discussed, should help to avoid hypoglycaemic episodes, leading to a restoration of the warning symptoms.

Nocturnal hypoglycaemia

Up to 50% of those with type 1 diabetes mellitus may experience the phenomenon of nocturnal hypoglycaemia. This may be suspected if the child frequently wakes up with a headache, a clammy neck or damp sheets from sweating overnight, or seems overly tired or complains of interrupted sleep. Children may not complain of these symptoms. Nocturnal hypoglycaemia should be suspected if there are repeatedly high-fasting early morning blood sugars, despite apparently adequate overnight insulin dosing. This is because of the hypoglycaemia counter-regulatory mechanisms. A continuous subcutaneous glucose monitoring system can be used to confirm nocturnal hypoglycaemia and this should be reported to the diabetic team, as adjustments may need to be made to the basal insulin dose or bedtime snacks may be recommended.

Syllabus mapping

Diabetes and endocrinology

Knowledge

The candidate must:

- Know the causes, complications and treatment of hypoglycaemia.
- Be able to discuss blood sugar monitoring.

Pharmacology, poisoning and accidents

Knowledge

The candidate must:

- Know how to find out information necessary for safe prescribing through the use of paediatric formularies and pharmacy liaison.
- Know the approved indications for prescribing drugs in common paediatric problems.

Skills

The candidate must:

- Be able to write a legible, clear and complete prescription.
- Be able to make reliable and accurate calculations in order to safely prescribe for babies, children and young people.

Further reading and references

1. Treatment of Hypoglycaemia. Section 6.1.4. *British National Formulary for Children* (BNFC). London: RCPCH Publications Ltd, 2012-2013.
2. National Institute of Clinical Excellence. (CG15) - Type 1 diabetes: Diagnosis and management of type 1 diabetes in children, young people and adults. 2004. https://www.nice.org.uk/guidance/cg15 (accessed February 2015).
3. Tasker R, McClure R, Acerini C. *Oxford Handbook of Paediatrics*. 2nd edition. Oxford University Press, 2013; 132-133.
4. Western Sussex Hospitals NHS Trust. Paediatric Newly Diagnosed Diabetes Integrated Care Pathway.
5. Willacy H, Rull G. Emergency Management of Hypoglycaemia. 2015. http://www.patient.co.uk/doctor/emergency-management-of-hypoglycaemia (accessed February 2016).

Chapter 8.3: Case Study 2: Anti-Malarial Prophylaxis
Dr Anna Mathew, Dr Nick Cooper

This station assesses your ability to write a prescription and then discuss the implications of prescribing this medication with the examiner. An understanding of indication, mode of action, potential adverse reactions and dose calculation will also be assessed during discussion time. Candidates *will not* be allowed to refer to the BNFC for this part of the assessment.

A copy of the BNFC, a prescription pad and a calculator will be provided at the station.

Logistics:

Timing: This is a 9-minute station. You will have up to 2 minutes before the start of this station to read the candidate sheet and prepare yourself.

When the bell rings: On entering the room, the examiner will greet you, take your mark sheet, and allow you to proceed with writing the prescription. You may take the candidate instruction sheet into the room, but this must be replaced as you leave the station.

You will be given 6 minutes to write the prescription. A discussion around the prescription will be undertaken in the final 3 minutes of the station.

If the discussion with the examiner finishes early, you will be asked to remain in the room until the session has ended.

Candidate role and task:

You are a GP working in a GP surgery.

You have seen the Cameron family, who are going to Tanzania for a 3-week safari. Luke (DOB 12/09/2003) weighs 24 kg. His address is 5 Theobalds Road, London WC1X 8SH and his NHS No: 789 456 0123. He is currently not on any medication.

Task: You wish to prescribe malaria prophylaxis and decide on Malarone (proguanil hydrochloride 25 micrograms, atovaquone 62.5 micrograms).

With the examiner: Discuss issues of safe prescribing.

Top tip!
Consider the issues of safe prescribing. A clear pass candidate will write instructions carefully (see section in the BNFC on prescription writing and anchor statements) and check the regime while remembering that the patient needs to start the tablets before travelling and continue on returning from holiday.

Although this would be a private prescription, for the purpose of the exam, you can use the FP10 form.

Prescription task

Utilise the time given to write a complete prescription, entering all the patient details given in the script. Don't forget to date, sign and print your name at the end of the prescription. Further guidance on filling out a complete prescription can be found in the introductory chapter, as well as on the mark sheets for this station.

**Figure 8.31:
Completed prescription**

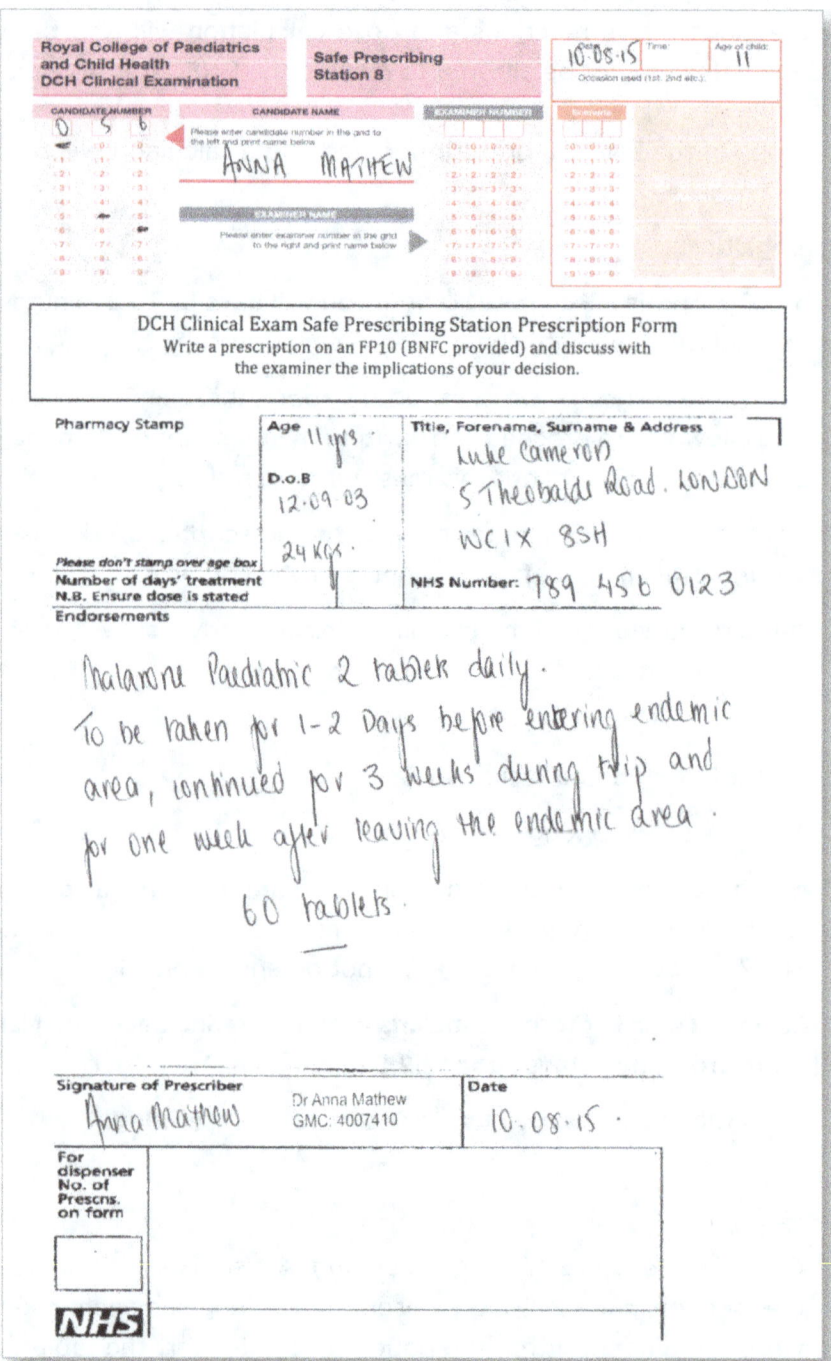

Top tip!
Think of important considerations. A clear pass candidate will have a good understanding of paediatric prescribing practice and additional non-therapeutic precautions, including the importance of raising awareness of any illness after returning from holiday.

Discussion

In the last 3 minutes of this station, the examiner will undertake a discussion around your prescription. At this point, *you will not* be allowed to refer to the BNFC and, therefore, the examiner will be testing your knowledge regarding the prescription you have just completed. *Possible* questions from the examiner are highlighted below.

■ *What specific instructions should be given regarding the prescription?*

Malarone tablets must be started 1–2 days before entering the endemic area, continued for 3 weeks (the duration of holiday), and then for 1 week after leaving the endemic area. Stress the importance of completing the course by continuing on returning from holiday.

■ *What are the possible side effects of this medication?*

These are gastrointestinal disturbances, headache, dizziness, abnormal dreams, rash, and pruritus. There are several other more rare complications. Contraindications include renal impairment.

■ *How is Malarone administered?*

Tablets can be swallowed whole or may be crushed and mixed with food or a milky drink just before administration.

■ *What other pertinent advice could be given to the parents?*

About 300 children annually develop malaria in the UK (imported into the UK), and symptoms can occur several months after the family returns from holiday.

It is important to stress the importance of the ABCD approach towards malaria prevention:

Awareness of risk
Bite prevention
Chemoprophylaxis
Diagnosis

A combination of these preventative measures is more likely to ensure effective protection against malaria, as none of these measures are 100% effective when considered in isolation (see below for further information).

Visit your GP if ill within 12 months and, especially important, if within 3 months of returning from holiday.

> *Top tip!*
> *Be confident when discussing issues of safe prescribing. A clear pass candidate* will have a systematic approach for structuring answers and a good understanding of the evidence base, e.g. available information from websites such as TRAVAX and MASTA (in this scenario) as well as any national guidelines underpinning good paediatric practice.

Additional information

Awareness of risk

Malaria is a disease transmitted by mosquitoes and is caused by the Plasmodium parasite. Five species of the parasite are known to infect humans, the most common being the Falciparum species.

Children can develop generalised non-specific symptoms, such as fever, sweats, rigors, general myalgia and headaches, after visiting an endemic area and should seek medical attention to consider the diagnosis of malaria. Signs of more severe symptoms such as impaired consciousness, seizures and extreme weakness are red flags for immediate assessment and treatment.

Bite prevention

Several factors influence the risk of bites from mosquitoes.

Temperature and season:
Areas of high humidity and temperatures ranging between 20–30°C offer optimal conditions for mosquitoes to breed and, consequently, for visitors to be bitten. Monsoon or rainy seasons also provide optimal conditions for breeding that could result in a higher incidence of new malaria cases.

Type of accommodation:
As transmission of malaria is greater between dusk to dawn due to the activity of the Anopheles mosquito, it is important that preventative measures are addressed when considering the quality of accommodation.

Sleeping in *air-conditioned rooms* where windows and doors can be sealed to prevent entry to mosquitoes, and sleeping under *insecticide-impregnated bed nets* decrease the likelihood of obtaining mosquito bites.

Spraying bedrooms with insecticide to kill any mosquitoes in the room, and the use of a *fine wire mesh over windows and door screens* provide further protection.

Type of clothing:
Wearing loose-fitting long sleeved clothing, with full-length trousers and socks, minimises the exposure of skin to potential mosquito bites.

Application of topical insect repellent:
DEET-based insect repellents at concentrations of over 20% give a longer duration of protection than other formulations.

Chemoprophylaxis

All travellers from the UK should obtain the medication required for chemoprophylaxis before travelling overseas for quality standard purposes. It is important that all travellers comply with the duration of their prescription, and continue with their medication after returning to the UK. Weight is a better guide than age when prescribing for children and should be used when deciding on dosage calculations. The chosen prophylaxis will be dependent on the area of travel and the endemicity of the different strains of the Falciparum parasite in that particular area.

Diagnosis

Suspected malaria is a medical emergency, and should be considered in every patient who has returned from an endemic area (particularly in the last 3 months, but can be within the last year inclusive). Malaria cannot be diagnosed on clinical grounds alone, and all susceptible patients should have a thick blood film diagnosis as a matter of urgency. This should be repeated in a couple of hours if initially negative, due to the cyclical nature of the parasitaemia.

Malaria is a notifiable disease in the UK, and all clinicians treating such patients should ensure they complete a notification form.

Syllabus mapping

Infection, immunity and allergy

Knowledge

The candidate must:

- Be aware of common infections of the foetus, newborn, and children in Britain and important worldwide infections (e.g. TB, HIV, hepatitis B, malaria, polio).

Pharmacology, poisoning and accidents

Knowledge

The candidate must:

- Know how to find out information necessary for safe prescribing through the use of paediatric formularies and pharmacy liaison.
- Know the approved indications for prescribing drugs in common paediatric problems.
- Be aware of possible drug interactions and side effects when more than 1 drug is prescribed.

Skills

The candidate must:

- Be able to write a legible, clear and complete prescription.
- Be able to make reliable and accurate calculations in order to safely prescribe for babies, children and young people.

Further reading and references

1. *British National Formulary for Children* (BNFC). London: RCPCH Publications Ltd, 2014. ISBN 978 0 85711 136 4
2. Public Health England. Guidelines for malaria prevention in travellers from the UK. 2014. https://www.gov.uk/government/publications/malaria-prevention-guidelines-for-travellers-from-the-uk (accessed February 2015).
3. TRAVAX (Health Protection Scotland). www.travax.nhs.uk (accessed February 2015).

Chapter 8.4: Case Study 3: Pain Management in Knee Injury
Dr Duana Cook

This station assesses your ability to write a prescription and then discuss the implications of prescribing this medication with the examiner. An understanding of indication, mode of action, potential adverse reactions and dose calculation will also be assessed. Candidates *will not* be allowed to refer to the BNFC for this part of the assessment.

A copy of the BNFC, a prescription pad and a calculator will be provided at the station.

> **Logistics:**
>
> *Timing:* This is a 9-minute station. You will have up to 2 minutes before the start of this station to read the candidate sheet and prepare yourself.
>
> *When the bell rings:* On entering the room, the examiner will greet you, take your mark sheet, and allow you to proceed with writing the prescription. You may take the candidate instruction sheet into the room, but this must be replaced as you leave the station.
>
> You will be given 6 minutes to write the prescription. A discussion around the prescription will be undertaken in the final 3 minutes of the station.
>
> If the discussion with the examiner finishes early, you will be asked to remain in the room until the session has ended.

> **Candidate role and task:**
>
> **You are a** GP working in a GP practice.
>
> You have just seen Ross Valentine (DOB 22/05/2005, 5 Theobalds Road, London, WC1X 8SH, NHS No: 999 1234 8765) with his mother.
>
> Ross came to your Monday morning surgery having injured his right knee playing football at the weekend. He is able to weight-bear, but the knee remains swollen and painful despite a maximum dose of paracetamol over the previous 2 days. His weight is 24 kg and his height is 125 cm.
>
> **Task: Write a prescription for Ross based on the information provided using the BNFC.**
>
> **With the examiner: Discuss issues of safe prescribing.**

Prescription task

Utilise the time given to write a complete prescription, entering all the patient details given in the script. Don't forget to date, sign and print your name at the end of the prescription. Further guidance on filling out a complete prescription can be found in the introductory chapter, as well as on the mark sheets for this station.

> *Top tip!*
> It is important to consider the WHO pain ladder when completing the prescription, which promotes a step-wise approach to pain management. You also need to consider the type of pain that you are treating, and select a drug with an appropriate mechanism of action.

Figure 8.41: Completed prescription

DCH Clinical Exam Safe Prescribing Station Prescription Form
Write a prescription on an FP10 (BNFC provided) and discuss with the examiner the implications of your decision.

Pharmacy Stamp

Age: 10 YEARS
D.o.B: 22/05/05
24 kg

Please don't stamp over age box

Title, Forename, Surname & Address:
MASTER ROSS VALENTINE
5 THEOBALDS RD, LONDON
WC1X 8SH

Number of days' treatment
N.B. Ensure dose is stated: 7

NHS Number: 999 1234 8765

Endorsements

NKDA.

IBUPROFEN ORAL SUSPENSION

200 mg PO TDS

FOR 7 DAYS

Signature of Prescriber: Dr Duana Cook GMC: 7278598

Date: 23/06/15

For dispenser No. of Prescns. on form

NHS

Top tip!
A clear pass candidate will prescribe a non-steroidal anti-inflammatory drug (NSAID) in an appropriate formulation, according to its generic name, and dosed for the child's weight. The candidate must include the child's name, date of birth and address for it to be a safe prescription.

Discussion

In the last 3 minutes of this station, the examiner will discuss with you issues surrounding your prescription. At this point, you *will not be* allowed to refer to the BNFC and, therefore, the examiner will be testing your knowledge regarding the prescription that you have just completed. *Possible* questions from the examiner are highlighted below.

■ *What is the reason for the choice of your medication?*

As paracetamol alone has been ineffective in this scenario, the WHO pain ladder for children suggests another non-opioid adjuvant in the form of an NSAID, which is particularly useful for pain caused by muscle sprains and strains.

NSAIDs are anti-inflammatory when used regularly and in higher doses. They work via the inhibition of cyclooxygenase (COX) 1 and 2, thus reducing the production of inflammatory molecules such as prostaglandins and thromboxane. This, in turn, reduces inflammation and pain.

■ *Are there any adverse effects of the medication that you have prescribed?*

COX-1 produces prostaglandins, which support platelets and help to protect the stomach. NSAIDs impair the synthesis of these gastroprotective prostaglandins, which can lead to gastrointestinal disturbances, including discomfort, nausea, diarrhoea and (more occasionally) ulcers and gastrointestinal bleeds. Children tend to tolerate NSAIDs more than adults and gastrointestinal side effects are less commonly seen. However, they do still occur. Other side effects can include hypersensitivity reactions, particularly rashes, angioedema and bronchospasm.

■ *Given these adverse effects, is there anything else to consider when prescribing this medication?*

Given the risks of gastrointestinal irritation, you may want to consider also prescribing a gastroprotective drug such as an H2-receptor antagonist or a proton pump inhibitor (PPI) – e.g. ranitidine or omeprazole – particularly if the patient is likely to be taking the NSAID long term.

■ *When should you exercise caution in prescribing these medications?*

All NSAIDs can potentially worsen asthma, causing bronchoconstriction and induction of rhinitis-type symptoms. Therefore, they should be used with caution in any child with asthma, a history of allergic disorders, or a previous hypersensitivity reaction to an NSAID.

NSAIDs can result in a bleeding tendency through the impairment of thromboxane A2, which is required for platelet aggregation. Without it, the bleeding time is prolonged. Caution should therefore be exercised in a child with thrombocytopenia or pre-existing platelet disorders.

■ *Are there any absolute contraindications for these medications?*

All NSAIDs are contraindicated in children with active gastrointestinal bleeding or ulceration, or if they have a history of recurrent gastrointestinal ulceration or haemorrhage. In addition, NSAIDs can exacerbate Crohn's disease and ulcerative colitis, and should be avoided in these conditions if possible.

In children with renal impairment, NSAIDs should be avoided whenever possible and only used with extreme caution. When being used, the lowest effective dose should be prescribed and for the shortest possible duration. Renal function should always be monitored when using NSAIDs in a patient with renal impairment. The renal system is dependent on prostaglandins synthesised primarily by COX-2 for their vasodilatory actions. By inhibiting the production of these prostaglandins, NSAIDs can cause volume-dependent renal failure, as well as provoke renal failure through papillary necrosis and interstitial nephritis. As they can cause fluid retention and impair renal function, they are also contraindicated in children with heart failure. In children with severe liver impairment, there is an increased risk of gastrointestinal bleeding and fluid retention; hence, NSAIDs should be avoided in such patients.

■ *What should be your next course of action if swelling and pain persist after a course of ibuprofen?*

Undertake an urgent referral to the orthopaedic surgeons, asking them to explore any underlying ligament or menisci injuries rather than attributing this to simple soft tissue injury.

Additional information

Management of musculoskeletal pain

Soft tissue trauma can cause injuries such as sprains and strains, which are relatively common in children and may require analgesia.

A sprain refers to the stretching of a ligament, or a strain or stretch of a muscle or tendon. Severe sprains are associated with complete disruption of the ligament, which leads to joint instability. Milder sprains result in localised pain and swelling, but the joint is stable and intact, as the ligament is not completely torn.

Initial management of a mild to moderate soft tissue injury is rest, ice, compression and elevation (RICE). In addition to this, analgesia is often required.

Regular paracetamol is usually advocated as first-line treatment. When used regularly, and at an appropriate dose for the weight of the child, paracetamol has been shown to be very effective. It has an excellent safety profile, with very few reported cases of toxicity at therapeutic levels. It is also cost-effective when compared to other analgesics.

The WHO pain ladder is a step-wise approach to pain management, which can be applied when paracetamol alone is insufficient. The ladder starts with a non-opioid analgesic, and progresses through to potent opioids. Whenever you are climbing a step up the ladder, the non-opioid analgesic should always be continued.

For musculoskeletal pain, NSAIDs can be used as an adjunct to paracetamol on the pain ladder, although they are sometimes used as first-line treatment for inflammatory pain if the cautions and side effects discussed above have been taken into consideration. The NSAID of choice in children is usually ibuprofen, as none of the other NSAIDs have been adequately studied for their safety and efficacy in the paediatric population.

The combination of paracetamol with an NSAID may enable lower doses of the NSAID to be therapeutic, hence reducing the likelihood of adverse effects such as gastrointestinal bleeding. Whether using only a paracetamol or both a paracetamol and an NSAID for persisting musculoskeletal pain, they should be given at regular intervals and not on an 'as required' basis.

In children, the WHO now recommends a 2-step ladder for pain management, which involves the prescription of a strong opioid (namely morphine) for pain assessed as being moderate to severe in nature (Figure 8.41). Milder opioids such as codeine and tramadol, which feature in the second step of the adult pain ladder, are no longer recommended in children, as the response is unpredictable and the safety and efficacy records for these medications in children are currently inadequate.

Figure 8.42: The WHO 2-step pain ladder for children (Illustrated by Dr D Cook)

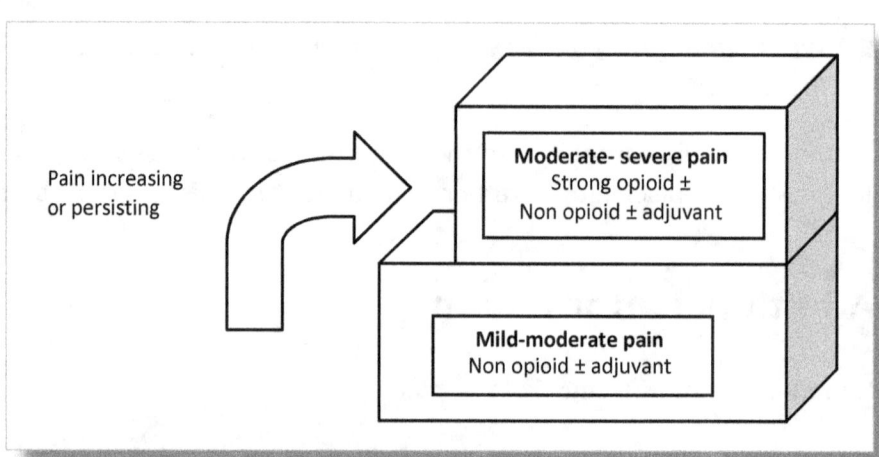

If prescribing opioid medication for a child, the dose should be increased gradually until adequate pain relief is achieved without unacceptable side effects. The lowest effective dose will vary between patients, and is unrelated to weight. There is no maximum dose limit, as there is for paracetamol and NSAIDs. If the patient is experiencing side effects such as nausea, vomiting, sedation or confusion, an alternative opioid should be used. If a child requires high doses of opioid medication, then further escalation should probably be done in a hospital to enable better monitoring and observation.

When to undertake investigations and seek specialist opinion

When a child presents with a musculoskeletal injury, the history regarding the nature of the pain and mechanism of injury are important, as is direct physical examination (which may reveal swelling, tenderness, deformity or instability).

A mild strain will usually cause only tenderness, whereas a mild to moderate sprain may result in localised swelling as well as pain. Such injuries can generally be managed, as discussed above, with RICE and regular Step 1 analgesics such as paracetamol and ibuprofen. No further investigations are usually required in such cases.

If examination reveals joint deformity or instability, or the history is of more severe trauma, then a radiographic investigation of the joint is warranted. Joint instability may mean that surgical repair is required, and hence an orthopaedic opinion should be sought.

The finding of an effusion around the knee after trauma also necessitates orthopaedic referral, as this may result from a torn ligament, torn meniscus or an osteochondral fracture. Locking of the knee may also indicate a meniscal injury and, again, is a cause for referral. In addition, if, after injury, you find tenderness present on both sides of the metaphysis of the femur on examination, then epiphyseal injury needs to be eliminated and an x-ray investigation and referral is again required.

With regard to the foot, the Ottawa rules are used to predict the likelihood of midfoot fractures. X-rays are required if any of the following are present:

- Point tenderness over the base of the fifth metatarsal
- Point tenderness over the navicular bone
- Inability to take 4 steps, both immediately after injury and when seen for assessment

In addition to these specific examination findings, the degree of pain and the analgesia requirement should also be taken into account. Most soft tissue injuries are generally responsive to simple analgesia with paracetamol and NSAIDs. If you need to progress up the pain ladder because these are inadequate, then further investigation may be indicated.

Syllabus mapping

Musculoskeletal

Knowledge

The candidate must:

- Be able to discuss the causes of joint swelling and their initial management.

Pharmacology, poisoning and accidents

Knowledge

The candidate must:

- Know how to find out information necessary for safe prescribing through the use of paediatric formularies and pharmacy liaison.
- Know the approved indications for prescribing drugs in common paediatric problems.

Skills

The candidate must:

- Be able to write a legible, clear and complete prescription.
- Be able to make reliable and accurate calculations in order to safely prescribe for babies, children and young people.

Further reading and references

1. *British National Formulary for Children* (BNFC). Section 1.3; 10.1.1. London: RCPCH Publications Ltd, 2012-2013.
2. Hauer J, Jones BL, Poplack DG. Evaluation and management of pain in children. 2014. http://www.uptodate.com/contents/evaluation-and-management-of-pain-in-children (accessed February 2015).
3. Hay W, Levin M, Sondheimer J, Deterding R. *Current Diagnosis and Treatment Pediatrics*. 19th edition. McGraw Hill Medical, 2009.
4. NPS Prescribing Practice Review 22: Analgesics in musculoskeletal pain. 2006. http://www.nps.org.au/publications/health-professional/prescribing-practice-review/2006/prescribing-practice-review-22 (accessed February 2015).
5. Risser A, Donovan D, Heintzmann J, Page T. NSAID Prescribing Precautions. *Am Fam Physician* 2009; 15; 80(12): 1371-1378
6. Schafer AI. Effects of nonsteroidal anti-inflammatory drugs on platelet function and systemic hemostasis. *J Clin Pharmacol* 1995; 35(3): 209-1
7. World Health Organization (WHO) Geneva. *Cancer pain relief and palliative care in children*. Geneva: WHO, 1998.
8. World Health Organisation (WHO). WHO guidelines on the pharmacological treatment of persisting pain in children with medical illnesses. 2012. http://whqlibdoc.who.int/publications/2012/9789241548120_Guidelines.pdf? ua=1 (accessed February 2015).

Chapter 8.5: Case Study 4: Eczema Treatment and Management

Dr Ciara Holden

This station assesses your ability to write a prescription and then discuss the implications of prescribing this medication with the examiner. An understanding of indication, mode of action, potential adverse reactions and dose calculation will also be assessed. Candidates *will not* be allowed to refer to the BNFC for this part of the assessment.

A copy of the BNFC, a prescription pad and a calculator will be provided at the station.

Logistics:

Timing: This is a 9-minute station. You will have up to 2 minutes before the start of this station to read the candidate sheet and prepare yourself.

When the bell rings: On entering the room, the examiner will greet you, take your mark sheet, and allow you to proceed with writing the prescription. You may take the candidate instruction sheet into the room, but this must be replaced as you leave the station.

You will be given 6 minutes to write the prescription. A discussion around the prescription will be undertaken in the final 3 minutes of the station.

If the discussion with the examiner finishes early, you will be asked to remain in the room until the session has ended.

Candidate role and task:

You are a GP working in a GP surgery.

You have just seen Sally Hope (DOB 04/07/2008, 5 Theobalds Road, London, WC1X 8SH, NHS No: 123 456 789) with her mother.

Sally has atopic eczema. Her mother has been applying topical emollients but the flexures of her elbows remain itchy, red and inflamed. They do not appear to be infected.

Her weight is 16 kg and her height is 100 cm. You decide to treat the eczema.

Task: Write a prescription for Sally based on the information provided using the BNFC.

With the examiner: Discuss issues of safe prescribing.

Prescription task

Utilise the time given to write a complete prescription, entering all the patient details given in the script. Don't forget to date, sign and print your name at the end of the prescription. Further guidance on filling out a complete prescription can be found in the introductory chapter, as well as on the mark sheets for this station.

Figure 8.51: Completed prescription

DCH Clinical Exam Safe Prescribing Station Prescription Form

Write a prescription on an FP10 (BNFC provided) and discuss with the examiner the implications of your decision.

Pharmacy Stamp

Please don't stamp over age box

Age 6 years

D.o.B 04/07/08

Title, Forename, Surname & Address
Miss Sally Hope
5 Theobalds Road
London
WC1X 8SH

Number of days' treatment
N.B. Ensure dose is stated: 28

NHS Number: 123456789

Endorsements

Hydrocortisone cream 1%
Apply thinly over area of dry skin
2 times per day
Total of 28 days

Signature of Prescriber: J. Smith GMC 7166732

Date: 1/8/2014

For dispenser
No. of
Prescns.
on form

NHS

Top tip!

Consider the issues of safe prescribing. A clear pass candidate will write instructions carefully (see section in the BNFC on prescription writing and anchor statements) and carefully consider national guidelines for the management of eczema, which utilise a step-wise approach with regard to treatment.

Discussion

Top tip!
A clear pass candidate will prescribe a low-potency topical steroid and must include the child's name, date of birth and address for it to be a safe prescription.

In the last 3 minutes of this station, the examiner will discuss with you issues surrounding your prescription. At this point, *you will not* be allowed to refer to the BNFC and, therefore, the examiner will be testing your knowledge regarding the prescription you have just filled out. *Possible* questions from the examiner are highlighted below.

■ **What is the reason for the choice of your medication?**

As topical emollients have been insufficient in controlling Sally's eczema, it is important to progress according to the recommendations made by the NICE atopic eczema in children guidelines, which provide a stepped approach according to the severity and location of the eczema. In this instance, these guidelines would recommend the addition of topical steroids.

■ **Are there any adverse effects of the medication that you have prescribed?**

Mild and moderate potency corticosteroids are reported to have few side effects.

Steroid phobia is a major cause for steroids not being administered by parents. The risks of skin thinning and systemic effects are very low when topical corticosteroids are used appropriately. The importance of compliance needs to be discussed.

Application of 1 to 2 times daily is usually prescribed. The amount will vary according to the site of the body that requires treatment, and should be spread thinly over the skin.

Top tip!
A clear pass candidate will explain the correct choice of medication and the patient-related factors influencing the prescription (discussed above).

■ **What further advice could you give the parents?**

- To consider environmental factors that could be contributing to the flare-up of the eczema. Common trigger factors that must be explained to parents are noted in the general measures below.
- To be aware of the social and psychological effects of eczema on the child and carers. This should include sleep disturbance and possible effects on school attendance.
- To plan a review of the child should there be no improvement after a month of appropriate treatment.
- To consider referral to a paediatrician or dermatologist if the eczema is not improving to a satisfactory level with appropriate first-line management.

Additional information

Atopic eczema

Atopic eczema is a chronic, inflammatory skin condition. It is characterised by areas of dry, erythematous and itchy skin.

It is a multifactorial condition with a strong genetic component. An important factor in the development of eczema is the defects in skin barrier function, particularly in the filaggrin protein.

Atopic eczema is part of the group of atopic conditions, including asthma and allergic rhinitis. Atopic individuals are more likely to become sensitised to common aeroallergens and food components. Children with atopic eczema will often develop allergic rhinitis and/or asthma in later life.

Epidemiology

Atopic eczema affects approximately 1 in 5 children in the UK. In primary care, it is the reason for up to 1 in 30 consultations. Most children with atopic eczema develop it before 1 year of age.

Presentation

Diagnostic criteria: UK NICE guidelines state that atopic eczema can be diagnosed when a child has an itchy rash, plus 3 of the following criteria:

- Current dermatitis affecting the flexures (or the extensor areas and/or cheeks in a child under 18 months)
- A history of dermatitis affecting the flexures (or the extensor areas and/or cheeks in a child under 18 months)
- A history in the last 12 months of dry skin
- Onset of signs and symptoms under the age of 2 years. However, if the child is under 4 years, this criterion should not be applied yet
- History of allergic rhinitis or asthma. If the child is under 4 years, then a history of atopic disease in a first-degree relative

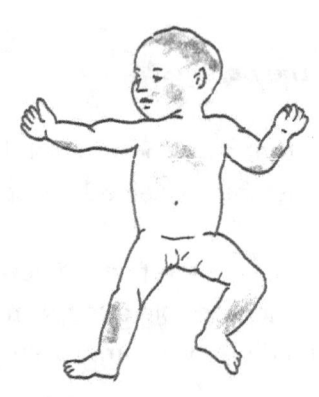
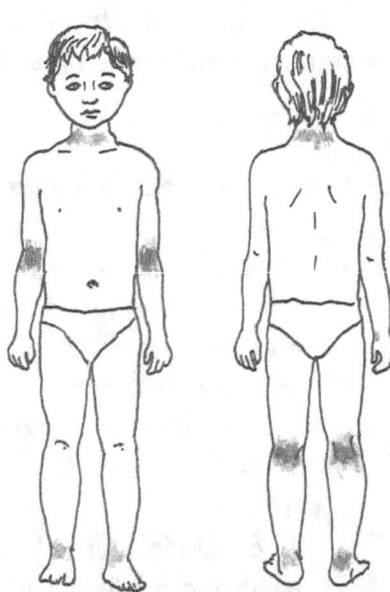

Figure 8.52: Distribution of eczema. The infant on the left shows the distribution mainly on the face, scalp, trunk and extensor areas. The child on the right shows the distribution mainly on the flexor areas. (Illustration by Dr G Bandaranayake)

Investigations

Atopic eczema is mainly made as a clinical diagnosis. A child with a suspected food allergy should be referred for review and possible investigations (depending on the food allergy).

Management

Management of atopic eczema can be divided into general measures and specific measures.

General measures

Factors that exacerbate the child's eczema should be identified and avoided. The possible trigger factors include irritant products, food allergens, inhalant allergens and contact allergens. Irritant washing detergents and soaps should be avoided. Emollients can be used as soap substitutes and should be reapplied after washing. Non-irritant clothing such as cotton is helpful. Nails should be kept short.

Specific measures

A stepped approach to treatment, with education on management for the parents and child, is important.

Emollients should be used regularly throughout the day for moisturising and washing. The use of emollients is continuous, even when a flare of eczema has resolved. The family should be given a choice of emollients so that they may choose which product/products are most suitable for them.

Topical corticosteroids are prescribed according to the severity of the eczema and the area of the body affected (Table 8.51).

Table 8.51		
Severity of eczema	Topical corticosteroid	Example of brand names
Mild atopic eczema	Mild potency	Hydrocortisone 0.1–2.5%, Dioderm, Efcortelan, Mildison
Moderate atopic eczema	Moderate potency	Betnovate-RD, Eumovate, Haelan Modrasone
Severe atopic eczema	High potency	Betamethasone valerate 0.1%, Betnovate-C, Diprosone, Elocon, Hydrocortisone butyrate

For the face and neck, corticosteroids of mild potency are recommended. A severe flare may require moderate potency corticosteroids for a 3-to-5-day course only.

For vulnerable sites, including the axilla and groin, only short courses (7–14 days) of moderate and potent corticosteroids are recommended.

Very potent corticosteroids (such as Clobetasol propionate – Dermovate) should only be prescribed after dermatology specialist advice.

Treatment of infection

Parents and children should be educated about the signs and symptoms of bacterial infection. The common bacterial infections are caused by Staphylococcus and Streptococcus. A swab should be taken first, and then topical or systemic antibiotics prescribed according to the severity of the infection.

Parents need to be aware of the signs and symptoms of eczema herpeticum. Prompt antiviral treatment is needed with specialist supervision.

Other treatment options

- Bandages with zinc impregnation or ichthammol. These are helpful for itching and particularly for areas of chronic limb eczema.
- Wet wraps can be worn overnight and increase the efficacy of treatment.
- Topical calcineurin inhibitors (e.g. Tacrolimus), systemic therapy and phototherapy are management options that would require dermatology supervision.

Syllabus mapping

Dermatology

Knowledge

The candidate must:

- Be able to diagnose, investigate and manage common skin rashes – eczema, acne, impetigo, ammoniacal dermatitis (Staphylococcal scalded syndrome, seborrheic dermatitis, cradle cap, and nappy rash).
- Be aware of the different potencies of topical steroids and of their side effects.
- Be able to understand the impact of severe dermatological problems on children.
- Recognise when to consult a dermatologist.

Pharmacology, poisoning and accidents

Knowledge

The candidate must:

- Know how to find out information necessary for safe prescribing through the use of paediatric formularies and pharmacy liaison.
- Know the approved indications for prescribing drugs in common paediatric problems.

Skills

The candidate must:

- Be able to write a legible, clear and complete prescription.
- Be able to make reliable and accurate calculations in order to safely prescribe for babies, children and young people.

Further reading and references

1. British Association of Dermatologists. http://www.bad.org.uk/ (accessed September 2014).
2. British National Formulary for Children. http://www.bnf.org/bnf/org_450055.htm (accessed February 2015).
3. Lewis-Jones S, Mugglestone M. Management of atopic eczema in children aged up to 12 years: Summary of NICE guidance. *BMJ* 2007; 335: 1263.
4. National Institute of Clinical Excellence. (CG57) – Atopic eczema in children: Management of atopic eczema in children from birth up to the age of 12 years. 2007.
5. van Den Oord RA, Sheikh A. Filaggrin gene defects and risk of developing allergic sensitisation and allergic disorders: Systematic review and meta-analysis. *BMJ* 2009; 339: b2433
6. Williams H, Bigby M, Diepgen T et al. *Evidence-Based Dermatology*, 2nd edition. John, 2009.

Chapter 8.6: Case Study 5: Treatment and Management in Asthma
Dr Thomas Ruffles

This station assesses your ability to write a prescription and then discuss the implications of prescribing this medication with the examiner. An understanding of indication, mode of action, potential adverse reactions and dose calculation will also be assessed. Candidates *will not* be allowed to refer to the BNFC for this part of the assessment.

A copy of the BNFC, a prescription pad and a calculator will be provided at the station.

Logistics:

Timing: This is a 9-minute station. You will have up to 2 minutes before the start of this station to read this sheet and prepare yourself.

When the bell rings: On entering the room, the examiner will greet you, take your mark sheet, and allow you to proceed with writing the prescription. You may take the candidate instruction sheet into the room, but this must be replaced as you leave the station.

You will be given 6 minutes to write the prescription. A discussion around the prescription will be undertaken in the final 3 minutes of the station.

If the discussion with the examiner finishes early, you will be asked to remain in the room until the session has ended.

Candidate role and task:

You are a GP working in a GP surgery.

You have seen Christine Hope (DOB 10/05/2009, 5 Theobalds Road, London, WC1X 8SH, NHS No: 919 743 8266) with her mother.

Christine has a history of several attendances at the accident and emergency department with recurrent wheeze requiring oral prednisolone and nebulisers. There is a strong family history of atopy.

Christine already has a 'blue' inhaler (salbutamol) and a spacer. Her mother has been told that Christine needs preventative medication.

Task: Write a prescription for Christine based on the information provided using the BNFC. With the examiner: Discuss issues of safe prescribing.

Prescription task

Utilise the time given to write a complete prescription, entering all the patient details given in the script. Don't forget to date, sign and print your name at the end of the prescription. Further guidance on filling out a complete prescription can be found in the introductory chapter, as well as on the mark sheets for this station.

Figure 8.61: Completed prescription

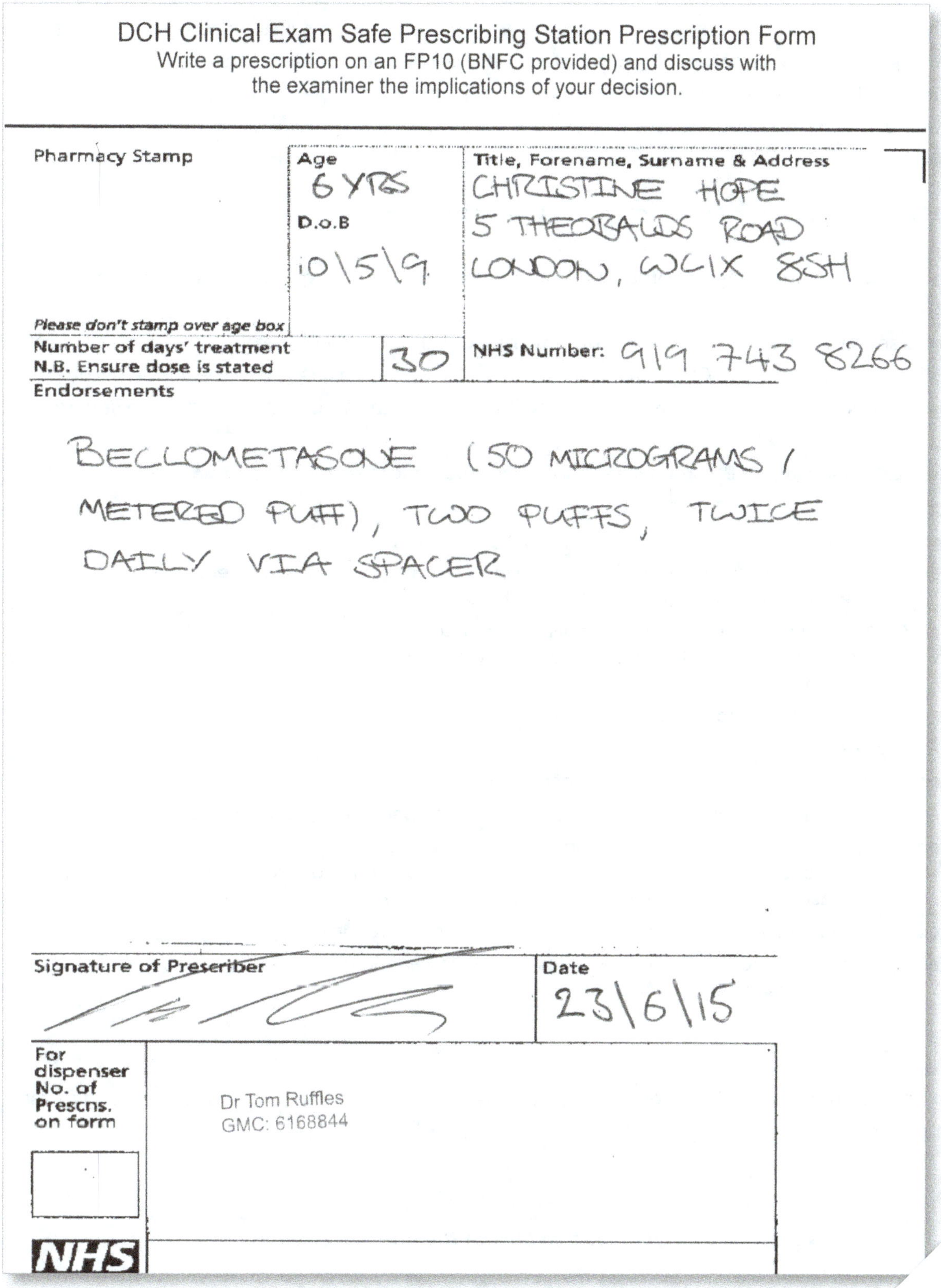

DCH Clinical Exam Safe Prescribing Station Prescription Form

Write a prescription on an FP10 (BNFC provided) and discuss with the examiner the implications of your decision.

Pharmacy Stamp

Please don't stamp over age box

Age: 6 YRS

D.o.B: 10\5\9

Title, Forename, Surname & Address: CHRISTINE HOPE, 5 THEOBALDS ROAD, LONDON, WC1X 8SH

Number of days' treatment N.B. Ensure dose is stated: 30

NHS Number: 919 743 8266

Endorsements

BECLOMETASONE (50 MICROGRAMS / METERED PUFF), TWO PUFFS, TWICE DAILY VIA SPACER

Signature of Prescriber

Date: 23\6\15

For dispenser No. of Prescns. on form

Dr Tom Ruffles
GMC: 6168844

NHS

Top tip!

It is important to carefully consider national guidelines for the management of a
utilise a step-wise approach with regard to treatment and are age-specific
medications should specify the inhaler device to be used!

Discussion

In the last 3 minutes of this station, the examiner will undertake a discussion around your prescription. At this point, *you will not* be allowed to refer to the BNFC and, therefore, the examiner will be testing your knowledge regarding the prescription you have just completed. *Possible* questions from the examiner are highlighted below.

■ *What is the reason for the choice of your medication?*

The BTS guidelines provide comprehensive advice on the management of paediatric asthma.

In this scenario, it would be appropriate to prescribe an inhaled steroid such as beclometasone. This is usually initiated at 100 micrograms twice a day, although it is within the scope of the guideline to commence 200 micrograms twice a day if the presentation is considered more severe.

Table 8.61: Summary of BTS guidelines for the management of paediatric asthma	
Age <5 years	
Step 1	Use inhaled short-acting beta-agonist, e.g. salbutamol.
Step 2	Add inhaled corticosteroid 200–400 micrograms per day, e.g. beclometasone. Alternately, add leukotriene receptor antagonist, e.g. montelukast.
Step 3	Add leukotriene receptor antagonist, e.g. montelukast. Alternately, add inhaled corticosteroid 200–400 micrograms per day, if already on a leukotriene receptor antagonist.
Step 4	Refer to respiratory paediatrician.
Age 5–12 years	
Step 1	Use inhaled short-acting beta-agonist, e.g. salbutamol.
Step 2	Add inhaled corticosteroid 200–400 micrograms per day, e.g. beclometasone.
Step 3	Add inhaled long-acting beta-agonist, e.g. salmeterol. If nil response to long-acting beta-agonists, consider a trial of a leukotriene receptor antagonist. Increase inhaled steroid to 400 micrograms per day if not already done.
Step 4	Increase inhaled corticosteroids to 800 micrograms per day.
Step 5	Use daily steroid tablet in lowest dose, providing adequate control. Refer to respiratory paediatrician.

Top tip!
In patients not responding to escalating management, it is important to consider other differential diagnoses at every step.

■ *What side effects would you need to inform the parents about?*

Inhaled corticosteroids

These have been shown to improve lung function, reduce asthma symptoms and the use of reliever medications, as well decreasing GP appointments and hospital admissions by up to 50%.

Side effects

- Oral candidiasis
- Hoarse voice

These side effects are dose dependent and can be minimised by the use of a spacer and mouth rinsing after each administration.

- Growth suppression

These effects are also dose dependent, with some studies showing a decreased growth velocity in the short to medium term. However, long-term follow-up studies are reassuring, showing no significant decrease in estimated mid-parental height between children treated with inhaled corticosteroids and controls. This suggests that suppressing asthma disease activity in children usually outweighs any potential systemic side effects of inhaled corticosteroids.

■ *What additional steps do you need to undertake to ensure appropriate administration of this medication?*

Knowledge of the correct inhaler technique is essential for all health professionals, who should routinely check that children and their guardians are aware and can demonstrate this.

Inhaler technique

1. Insert metered dose inhaler (MDI) into spacer.
2. Shake the canister for 5 seconds.
3. Breathe out through your mouth. *This step can be omitted for children using a spacer and mask.*
4. Put your mouthpiece between your teeth and close your lips tightly around the mouthpiece. *For younger children using a spacer with a mask, apply the mask securely, covering the mouth and nose.*
5. Press down on the top of the canister with the index finger to release the medicine.
6. At the same time, breathe in and out slowly through the mouth for 5–10 breaths.
7. If you need more than 1 puff, repeat steps 1–6 for each puff required.
8. If your inhaler contains a steroid medication, rinse your mouth and gargle with water before spitting out. *For younger children using a spacer and mask, wash the face as well after each administration.*

Top tip!
An important part of the process of prescribing is to look at inhaler technique and to give advice on "spacer care".

Spacer devices

In children under 5 years and those using inhaled corticosteroids, MDIs and a spacer device (e.g. Volumatic or Aerochamber) are the recommended delivery methods. Spacers hold the medicine in a chamber after its release, allowing the child to inhale slowly and decreasing the amount of medication deposited in the mouth.

When a spacer is cleaned, it should be rinsed in soapy water and left to drip dry. It should not be rinsed in running water or dried with a cloth, as the static reduces effective particle delivery to the lungs. This should be done when new, and every month. Spacers should be replaced if they become scratched.

The asthma.org.uk website contains useful videos instructing one on the use of the varying types of inhalers and spacers available.

Top tip!
A spacer device is recommended in all children under 5 years and those using inhaled corticosteroids.

Additional information

Asthma is a chronic inflammatory condition, resulting in episodic reversible airflow obstruction. This chronic inflammatory process increases the airway's responsiveness to specific triggers.

Prevalence

Asthma has increased in prevalence in recent years, and affects 10–20% of children in the UK. Acute exacerbations account for 10–15% of paediatric hospital admissions and there are approximately 30 deaths under the age of 19 per year in the UK.

Clinical features

Features suggestive of asthma include recurrent:

- Wheeze
- Cough
- Shortness of breath
- Chest tightness

This is classically worse at night or in the early morning, and can occur in response to specific triggers:

- Exercise
- Pets
- Cold or damp weather
- Emotion

Other factors supportive of a diagnosis are:

- Personal history of atopic disorder.
- Family history of atopic disorder and/or asthma.
- History of improvement in symptoms in response to adequate therapy.

Long-term management

Assessment and monitoring – Successful asthma treatment relies on an ability to monitor the condition over time. This can be achieved by recording the frequency and severity of symptoms, and by measuring lung function with a peak flow meter.

Asthma diary – A diary is a useful adjunct to reviewing the severity of asthma symptoms and peak flow readings, and is particularly useful in assessing response to instigation of new treatments.

Peak expiratory flow (PEF) meter – PEF meters measure airflow obstruction during exhalation. PEF monitoring is started by measuring morning and evening PEFs to determine a baseline, and correlating values with symptoms to determine the efficacy of trialled treatments. PEF meters are inexpensive and easy to use, and children as young as 4 are able to master the technique required.

Spirometry – In asthma, constriction of the airways results in diminished airflow during forced expiration. A ratio of forced expiratory volume in 1 second (FEV1) to forced vital capacity = total volume exhaled (FVC) that is <0.8 indicates significant airflow obstruction.

These measures are not diagnostic of asthma, as there are several disorders that obstruct airflow. However, an increase in FEV_1 >15% following the administration of an inhaled β2 agonist (e.g. salbutamol) is strongly supportive of asthma.

> *Top tip!*
> Reproducible spirometry readings are usually possible in children aged 6 and above.

Patient education

Patient and family education is particularly important in checking inhaler technique, as well as maintaining treatment adherence and thus symptom control. The role of respiratory specialist nurses in supporting children and their families has become particularly important.

Patients with asthma benefit from a written asthma action plan that describes their regular asthma medication use, as well as a step-wise approach to managing worsening asthma (including what medications to take and when to seek medical care).

(See sections on inhaler technique and spacer care.)

Pharmacotherapy

Knowledge of the BTS guidelines for the management of paediatric asthma is essential for all GP trainees.

(See sections on medication choice and side effects.)

Pharmacology, poisoning and accidents

Knowledge

The candidate must:

- Know how to find out information necessary for safe prescribing through the use of paediatric formularies and pharmacy liaison.
- Know the approved indications for prescribing drugs in common paediatric problems.
- Be aware of possible drug interactions and side effects when more than 1 drug is prescribed.

Skills

The candidate must:

- Be able to write a legible, clear and complete prescription.
- Be able to make reliable and accurate calculations in order to safely prescribe for babies, children and young people.

Respiratory medicine with ENT

Knowledge

The candidate must:

- Be able to discuss the assessment and management of children with acute asthma and plan long-term management (BTS guidelines for management of asthma).
- Be aware of the long-term complications of medications used for asthma.

Further reading and references

1. Asthma UK Inhaler Demos: www.asthma.org.uk/inhaler-demos (accessed March 2015).
2. British National Formulary for Children. http://www.bnf.org/bnf/org_450055.htm (accessed February 2015).
3. British Thoracic Society/Scottish Intercollegiate Guidelines Network. British Guideline on the Management of Asthma. 2014. https://www.brit-thoracic.org.uk/guidelines-and.../asthma-guideline (accessed March 2015).
4. Pedersen S. Clinical Safety of Inhaled Corticosteroids for Asthma in Children: An Update of Long-Term Trials Drug Safety 2006; 29(7): 599–612

SECTION 9:
PROBLEM BASED LEARNING

Chapter 9.1: Introduction

Dr Anna Mathew, Dr P Venugopalan, Dr Nick Cooper, Dr Geethika Bandaranayake, Dr Usha Natarajan, Dr Asya Al-Kharusi

This section of the book is intended to help in the revision of certain key areas of the curriculum. When preparing for a clinical examination, it is important to have a strong foundation in both theoretical knowledge and clinical skills. Both these areas are tested in the DCH clinical examination, and both the candidate and the examiner feel a great sense of satisfaction when candidates are able to perform well. Candidates may not realise this, but examiners remember the 'good' candidates and these candidates are often the focus of discussion at examiner meetings when comments are made about the uplifting experience of a good performance! Sadly, the converse is also true.

Several problem-based scenarios have been generated around key clinical areas; to get the most out of these short scenarios, we would advise that each candidate should make an attempt to answer the questions in their own time and by themselves initially, making notes as they go along. By undertaking self-directed learning, each candidate determines the time, pace and depth to which they would like to work.

We would then advise a small group session, where each of these scenarios can be discussed. This forum encourages participation, discussion, feedback and reflection, and encourages a more collaborative way of learning. A local tutor or supervisor could facilitate each session to help provide direction, expertise and generate self-reflection among those present. Recommended textbooks provide useful additional reading material to facilitate learning. Ideally, each session would last about 60–90 minutes.

We would recommend that all candidates follow 'discussion time' by revising around these topics, ideally after each session, to maximise the benefits of the session and help consolidate knowledge.

We would like to point out that we have covered only selected portions of the curriculum in this section. We hope these exercises will give candidates and supervisors/tutors a flavour of the type of self-learning material they can independently generate to aid preparation for the DCH examination.

The DCH question-writing group of the RCPCH created this section of the book. Hopefully, this will prove to be a useful educational resource.

Recommended textbooks

1. *British National Formulary for Children* (BNFC). London: RCPCH Publications Ltd, 2014. ISBN 978 0 85711 136 4 (and subsequent updates)
2. Kliegman RM, Stanton BF, St Geme JW et al. *Nelson Textbook of Pediatrics*, 20th edition. Philadelphia: Elsevier, 2015. ISBN 978-1-4557-7566-8
3. Lissauer T, Clayden G. *Illustrated Textbook of Paediatrics*, 4th edition. Edinburgh: Mosby, 2012. ISBN 978-0-7234-3565-5
4. McIntosh N, Helms P, Smyth R et al. *Forfar and Arneil's Textbook of Pediatrics*, 7th edition. Edinburgh: Churchill Livingstone, 2008. ISBN 978-0-443-10396-4
5. Rudolf M, Lee T, Levene M. *Paediatrics and Child Health*, 3rd edition. Chichester: Wiley-Blackwell, 2011. ISBN 978-1-4051-9474-7

Chapter 9.2: The Child with a Respiratory/ENT Problem

Resp 1 A 4 year old boy presents to you with delayed speech development and difficulty in pronouncing certain sounds. His mother says he always has a 'cold' and has been treated several times with antibiotics. *What is the differential diagnosis? Discuss management options.*	*Tip:* Ensure you are able to discuss common causes and the management of earache, ear discharge, otitis media and glue ear. *(DCH2013 Curriculum-Resp1)*
Resp 2 An 8 year old girl complains of severe pain when touching her ear. She swims in the local pool. Her external ear canal looks red and has purulent discharge. *What is the diagnosis? Discuss your management plan.*	*Tip:* Ensure you are able to discuss common causes and the management of earache, ear discharge, otitis media and glue ear. *(DCH2013 Curriculum-Resp1)*
Resp 3 A 3 year old has had several episodes of otitis media that you have treated with antibiotics in the last year. He presents again with another infection. *What management options should you consider?*	*Tip:* Ensure you are able to discuss common causes and the management of earache, ear discharge, otitis media and glue ear. *(DCH2013 Curriculum-Resp1)*
Resp 4 A 3 year old girl presents with recurrent tonsillitis associated with high temperatures. She has had 3 febrile convulsions associated with these episodes. The parents approach you for further management. *How would you take this forward?*	*Tip:* Know the common causes and the management of nosebleeds, allergic rhinitis, and sore throat, including tonsillitis. *(DCH2013 Curriculum-Resp2)*
Resp 5 A 6 year old boy presents with enlarged cervical lymph nodes for 2 weeks; these haven't responded to antibiotics. These nodes are non-tender and he looks pale and lethargic. *What differentials should you consider and how would you approach his management?*	*Tip:* Be aware of the differential diagnosis of neck swellings (including malignancies). *(DCH2013 Curriculum-Resp4)*
Resp 6 A 2 year old unimmunised child presents with a diffused and painless swelling on the cheek that extends to the mandible. *What differentials should you consider and how would you manage this child?*	*Tip:* Be aware of the differential diagnosis of neck swellings, including parotitis (due to infection (mumps), immunocompromised state (e.g. HIV), and malignancy). *(DCH2013 Curriculum-Resp4)*
Resp 7 A 3 year old asthmatic child presents with a cough, wheeze and difficulty in breathing. Salbutamol has not been effective in relieving the symptoms. *How would you manage this child?*	*Tip:* Ensure you are able to discuss the assessment and the management of children with acute asthma, and plan long-term management (BTS/SIGN guidelines). *(DCH2013 Curriculum-Resp5)*
Resp 8 A 7 year old girl presents with a cough and wheeze, which are worse at night. She has a background history of troublesome asthma and is on regular inhaled steroids and long-acting beta-agonists. *How would you assess and manage her?*	*Tip:* Be aware of the long-term management of asthma (BTS/SIGN guidelines). *(DCH2013 Curriculum-Resp5)*

Resp 9 An 8 year old child presents with a 3-day history of wet cough, high fever of 39°C and right sided chest pain. The chest x-ray shows patchy opacities over both lung fields. *What other investigations would you like to do, and what would be your approach to management?*	*Tip:* Know the causes and the management of respiratory tract infections, including the association of pneumonia with pleurisy. *(DCH2013 Curriculum-Resp9)*
Resp 10 A 2 year old presents as very unwell with a cough and stridor. *What important aspects of the clinical history would you obtain? What would be your approach and management?*	*Tip:* Ensure you are able to discuss the causes of infective and allergic stridor, and the management of acute or recurrent stridor. *(DCH2013 Curriculum-Resp9)*
Resp 11 A 6 month old baby develops a cough and difficulty in breathing and struggles to complete her feeds. She sounds audibly wheezy and crackles are heard on auscultation. *What further steps would you take in her evaluation and how would you manage this baby?*	*Tip:* Know the causes and management of respiratory tract infections, including bronchiolitis. *(DCH2013 Curriculum-Resp9)*
Resp 12 A 6 year old child presents with a 3-month history of intermittent fever, night sweats and weight loss associated with a cough. A chest x-ray shows patchy infiltrates in both lungs. *What further steps would you take to make a diagnosis and how would you manage this child?*	*Tip:* Know the causes and management of chronic respiratory tract infections, including tuberculosis. *(DCH2013 Curriculum-Resp9)*
Resp 13 A 2 year old unimmunised boy presents as an emergency with a harsh barking cough and audible stridor. He looks very ill, has a temperature of 39°C and is drooling saliva. *What is your differential diagnosis and how would you approach the management of this child?*	*Tip:* Know the causes and the management of respiratory tract infections, including epiglottitis. *(DCH2013 Curriculum-Resp9)*
Resp 14 A 2 year old boy presents with a cough and difficulty in breathing. On auscultation, you hear a wheeze on the right side of the chest. *What further history would you seek and how would you approach his management?*	*Tip:* Ensure you are able to examine the respiratory system, interpret and discuss physical findings, and include consideration of an inhaled foreign body. *(DCH2013 Curriculum-Resp10)*

Chapter 9.3: The Child with a Cardiovascular Problem

Cardio 1: A 2 year old presents with bluish discolouration of hands and feet when exposed to the cold. He is otherwise well and a clinical examination of the heart is normal. *What is the probable cause of the symptom and how would we counsel the parents?*	*Tip:* Know the differences between central and peripheral cyanosis, and read about acrocyanosis. *(DCH2013 Curriculum-Card1)*
Cardio 2 You are performing blood pressure screening for children in a nursery school. You find that a 4 year old boy has a blood pressure of 140/80 mmHg. *Outline a plan of management.*	*Tip:* Understand the measurement and interpretation of blood pressure in different age groups (including referral indications). *(DCH2013 Curriculum-Card2)*
Cardio 3 A 2 year old child brought to your clinic with a cold and cough suddenly becomes unresponsive and blue. You do not have any equipment for advanced life support in your clinic. *Discuss the steps in the initial assessment and resuscitation of this child, in the context of current resuscitation guidelines followed in your country.*	*Tip:* Be well versed with the theory and practice of basic life support in the primary care setting. *(DCH2013 Curriculum-Card3)*
Cardio 4 A 12 year old boy complains of chest pain and palpitations first noted while he was playing football. He has continued to experience this pain while watching television. *Discuss the differential diagnosis.*	*Tip:* Know the common causes of palpitations, syncope and chest pain, and know when to refer. *(DCH2013 Curriculum-Card4)*
Cardio 5 A 6 month old girl is brought to you with a history of poor feeding and fast breathing. You note that she has a heart murmur and the femoral pulses are difficult to feel. *Discuss the differential diagnosis and outline initial steps in the management.*	*Tip:* Be aware of the causes of heart failure, its clinical features, initial management, and when to refer for further assessment. *(DCH2013 Curriculum-Card5)*
Cardio 6 You receive a phone call from the dentist. He has a 10 year old boy whose mother tells him he has a hole in the heart. The dentist wants to know whether he needs to give him an antibiotic prior to a dental extraction. *In this context, discuss the current recommendations on antibiotic prophylaxis for children with heart diseases.*	*Tip:* Be aware of the current recommendations for endocarditis prophylaxis in children with heart disease. *(DCH2013 Curriculum-Card6)*
Cardio 7 A 2 year old boy is brought to you with a heart murmur. The murmur is systolic, grade 4/6, and best heard over the pulmonary area. *Discuss the differential diagnosis, initial investigations, and management.*	*Tip:* Be aware of the clinical features, investigations and the management of common congenital heart diseases. *(DCH2013 Curriculum-Card7)*
Cardio 8 A 2 month old baby with trisomy 21 (Down's syndrome) is referred to you for a full assessment. Parents have read on the internet about the association of heart disease with Down's syndrome. *Discuss the common syndromes associated with heart defects and, in general, discuss the aetiology of congenital heart diseases.*	*Tip:* Know the common congenital heart diseases, including their aetiological factors. *(DCH2013 Curriculum-Card8)*

Chapter 9.4: The Neonate

Neo 1 A term baby weighed 1.8 kg at birth. There were antenatal concerns related to maternal alcohol use and intrauterine growth retardation. *Discuss the possible complications to the baby associated with this history.*	*Tip:* Know and understand the effects of antenatal and perinatal events on short-term and long-term outcomes. *(DCH2013 Curriculum-Neo1)*
Neo 2 A 3 day old full-term baby is seen with jaundice. On examination, she has a unilateral swelling on her scalp, to 1 side of the midline. *Outline the causes and differential diagnosis of scalp swellings in a neonate. What are the causes of jaundice in this baby?*	*Tip:* Be able to recognise and outline the management of common disorders in the newborn, including scalp swellings and jaundice. *(DCH2013 Curriculum-Neo3)*
Neo 3 A term baby on its day 1 check is noted to have 'clicky' hips. There is also a family history of hip problems. *Discuss the causes of a 'clicky' hip and outline the management.*	*Tip:* Know about developmental dysplasia of the hip, its diagnosis and management. *(DCH2013 Curriculum-Neo7)*
Neo 4 An otherwise normal term baby is noted to have a haemangioma on the upper eyelid. The mother is concerned that this might bleed and cause problems. *Discuss the natural history and possible complications of a haemangioma.*	*Tip:* Know about common minor congenital abnormalities. *(DCH2013 Curriculum-Neo8)*
Neo 5 A newborn is jaundiced at 36 hours of age. She is slightly lethargic and slow to feed. She weighed 3.5 kg at birth and had a normal APGAR. She is solely breastfed. *What are the causes of jaundice in the newborn period? Outline differential diagnosis and management.*	*Tip:* Understand physiological jaundice and breast milk jaundice, and recognise the early presentation of neonatal hepatitis and biliary atresia. *(DCH2013 Curriculum-Neo9)*
Neo 6 A term baby is noted to be cold and lethargic at 3 hours of age. There is a history of maternal fever; the mother's membranes had ruptured 48 hours prior to delivery. The baby did not require any resuscitation at the time of birth. *What is the most likely diagnosis? Discuss management. What are the risk factors in the history that would alert you?*	*Tip:* Demonstrate early recognition, and understand the importance of the timely treatment of sepsis in the neonate. *(DCH2013 Curriculum-Neo10)*
Neo 7 A preterm baby born at 28 weeks gestation is noted to be grunting and tachypnoeic soon after birth. The baby is saturating 85% on 2 litres per minute nasal oxygen. *Discuss the causes, investigations and the management of respiratory distress in this baby.*	*Tip:* Be aware of problems associated with prematurity. *(DCH2013 Curriculum-Neo13)*

Chapter 9.5: The Child with a Neurological Problem

Neuro 1 An 8 month old baby is being routinely followed-up as he was born prematurely at 28 weeks gestation and had an intraventricular haemorrhage. On examination, he is noticed to have increased muscle tone and scissoring of his lower limbs. Upper limbs appear normal. *What is the likely problem? What other comorbidities are likely to be associated with such a problem? How will you manage this child?*	*Tip:* Ensure you are able to discuss the different types of cerebral palsy. Understand the possible comorbidities, such as epilepsy, gastro-oesophageal reflux, feeding difficulty, visual and hearing impairment, learning difficulties, neurodevelopmental delay, etc. Appreciate the importance of the multidisciplinary team in helping evaluate independent skills, mobility, comorbidities, quality of life, etc. *(DCH2013 Curriculum-Neuro1)*
Neuro 2 A 10 year old boy with learning difficulties and epilepsy is noticed to have acne-like spots and hypopigmented patches on his trunk. *What is the likely diagnosis? Discuss inheritance, and clinical features. Name 2 other neurocutaneous syndromes.*	*Tip:* Ensure you are able to discuss neurocutaneous syndromes (NF1, tuberous sclerosis, Sturge-Weber syndrome) *(DCH2013 Curriculum-Neuro2)*
Neuro 3 An 18 month old boy has been vomiting daily for the last 3 weeks. He appears miserable and has stopped walking. His mother has noticed a new squint. *What is the most likely diagnosis? Discuss differential diagnosis. What are the features in the history and clinical examination that would help to make a diagnosis?*	*Tip:* Ensure you are able to discuss the symptoms and signs of raised intracranial pressure and a space occupying lesion. Be able to discuss differential diagnosis – neoplastic, infective, etc. *(DCH2013 Curriculum-Neuro3)*
Neuro 4 A 5 year old boy has difficulty in mounting stairs. He walked at the age of 2 and half years. He is clumsy and slower than his peers. *Name 2 clinical features that may help in diagnosis.* *Discuss your management.*	*Tip:* Ensure you are able to discuss causes of delayed walking. Be able to discuss genetic inheritance, investigations and multidisciplinary management of muscular dystrophy. *(DCH2013 Curriculum-Neuro4)*
Neuro 5 A 4 month old baby has a frog-like posture, and poor anti-gravity movements. When picked up, he tends to slip through the fingers. *Discuss differential diagnosis. How will you manage this child?*	*Tip:* Be aware of the differential diagnoses of hypotonia, including neuromuscular disorders such as spinal muscular atrophy, myopathies, and central hypotonia. Be aware of the management options, including common investigations, counselling, prognosis and supportive measures. *(DCH2013 Curriculum-Neuro5)*

Neuro 6 A 7 year old is referred by his class teacher as he is noted to have brief vacant spells several times a day. His schoolwork has deteriorated. *What are the management options?*	*Tip:* Be aware of fits, faints and funny turns, and understand the principles of the management of common epileptic disorders, including side effects of commonly used drugs (in this case, absence seizures). *(DCH2013 Curriculum-Neuro10, 13)*
Neuro 7 A 4 week old baby is brought to the hospital with rapid jerking episodes that happen every time the baby goes to sleep. They are not distressing to the baby and the baby sleeps through each episode. The baby is otherwise well and thriving. *What advice would you give the mother?*	*Tip:* Be aware of fits, faints and funny turns, including benign sleep myoclonus. *(DCH2013 Curriculum-Neuro10, 13)*
Neuro 8 A 13 year old girl is seen in the clinic for unexplained clumsiness. This seems worse shortly after waking up in the morning. She often smears her eyeliner when applying it, and finds it difficult to brush her hair. At breakfast, she often spills her cereal as she notices her arms suddenly jerk. *What would be your investigation and management plan?*	*Tip:* Be aware of fits, faints and funny turns, and understand the principles of the management of common epileptic disorders, including side effects of commonly used drugs (in this case, juvenile myoclonic epilepsy). *(DCH2013 Curriculum-Neuro10, 13)*
Neuro 9 A 4 year old boy wakes up at night a couple of hours after going to sleep screaming and looking very scared. He is inconsolable for a few minutes and then goes back to sleep. He has no recollection of these events the following day. He is otherwise well and doing well at school. *What advice would you give the mother?*	*Tip:* Be aware of fits, faints and funny turns, including night terrors. *(DCH2013 Curriculum-Neuro10, 13)*

Chapter 9.6: The Child with a Genetic Disorder

Gene 1 A 14 year old girl has not yet attained menarche. On examination, she is noticed to be small for mid-parental height, has slightly protruding ears, pectus excavatum, and widely spaced nipples. *What is the likely diagnosis and how would you confirm this? What other features are likely to be present in this condition?*	*Tip:* Be able to discuss syndromic diagnosis and associated features, including Turner syndrome. *(DCH2013 Curriculum-Gene1)*
Gene 2 A newborn baby has been noticed to have several characteristic facial features, hypertelorism, upward slanting palpebral fissures, a depressed nasal bridge, and a small mouth. *How will you confirm your diagnosis?* *Discuss genetic counselling. What other features are likely to be seen in this condition? Discuss complications and management.*	*Tip:* Be able to discuss clinical features, complications, genetic counselling and the management of syndromes, including Down's syndrome. *(DCH2013 Curriculum-Gene2)*
Gene 3 A 4 year old boy and his older brother have learning difficulties and autism. On examination, he has a long face with coarse features, and large everted ears. His mother also has mild learning difficulties. *What syndrome do the features suggest?* *How will you confirm the diagnosis?* *Discuss the mode of inheritance.*	*Tip:* Be able to discuss syndromic diagnosis and unusual genetic inheritance (repeat expansion mutations), including fragile X syndrome. *(DCH2013 Curriculum-Gene3)*
Gene 4 A 6 year old child presents with obesity, learning difficulties, hypogonadism and almond-shaped palpebral fissures. He had neonatal feeding difficulties, hypotonia and failure to thrive during infancy. *What is the diagnosis? Discuss the mode of inheritance and genetics of this condition.*	*Tip:* Be able to discuss the clinical features of this syndrome. Be aware of the unusual genetics of imprinting and uniparental disomy in the Prader-Willi syndrome. *(DCH2013 Curriculum-Gene4)*
Gene 5 A 9 year old boy has multiple café-au-lait spots. His mother and maternal aunt have a few superficial lumps on their bodies. His 6 year old sister has similar skin lesions, but also has epilepsy. The father and brothers have no clinical features. *What is the diagnosis? How is this condition inherited? Name 5 other conditions with a similar mode of inheritance. Draw a pedigree chart for the family.*	*Tip:* Be able to discuss clinical features and complications of the condition. Be able to discuss autosomal dominant inheritance with examples, including neurofibromatosis type 1. Be able to draw a typical pedigree chart. *(DCH2013 Curriculum-Gene5)*

Chapter 9.7: The Child with a Gastroenterology or Hepatology Problem

Gastro 1 A 6 week old infant presents with vomiting after feeding. He is irritable and difficult to console. He frequently cries, draws up his legs and arches his back after feeds. Weight gain is slow. *What would be your approach and management?*	*Tip:* Know the causes of vomiting at different ages (including gastro-oesophageal reflux) and be able to assess and manage this problem. *(DCH2013 Curriculum-Gastro2)*
Gastro 2 A 3 year old girl presents with poor weight gain. She complains of intermittent abdominal pain and has been "off-colour" for the last few months. Her weight has dropped across 2 centiles from the 50th to below the 9th centile. Both her parents are above the 90th centile for height and weight. *What investigations would you like to perform and how do you manage this case?*	*Tip:* Ensure you are able to discuss causes, assessment and management of the failure to thrive, including coeliac disease. *(DCH2013 Curriculum-Growth and Dev2)*
Gastro 3 A 12 year old girl presents with a 6-month history of abdominal pain and intermittent diarrhoea. She is constantly tired and finds it difficult to concentrate at school. Her parents feel she has lost weight in the last few months. The full blood count performed by the GP 2 months ago was normal. *What further information would you like to obtain and how do you manage her?*	*Tip:* Know the causes of acute and chronic diarrhoea and vomiting, and be able to assess and manage Crohn's Disease, inflammatory bowel disease, and/or chronic malabsorption. *(DCH2013 Curriculum-Gastro3)*
Gastro 4 A 5 year old presents with abdominal pain. His bowel habit is irregular and has recently started having 'accidents' in his pants. On examination, a few hard masses are felt on the left side of the abdomen. *What management options do you have?*	*Tip:* Be familiar with the diagnosis and management of constipation. *(DCH2013 Curriculum-Gastro4)*
Gastro 5 A 2 week old baby is referred for further assessment and the management of jaundice. He was born at term in good condition and had an uneventful postnatal period. He has regained his birth weight and is exclusively breastfed. His stool and urine colour are normal. *What would be your approach and management?*	*Tip:* Know the causes of neonatal and childhood jaundice, including breast milk jaundice, and when to refer. *(DCH2013 Curriculum-Gastro5)*
Gastro 6 A 9 month old infant presents to the emergency department with bleeding per rectum. The parents report he has had a few episodes of vomiting and intermittent excessive crying associated with the drawing up of legs. In between these episodes, he is settled and appears well. On examination, he looks irritable and dehydrated. *How would you approach and manage this baby?*	*Tip:* Know the common causes of upper and lower gastrointestinal bleeding, including intussusception. *(DCH2013 Curriculum-Gastro6)*
Gastro 7 You receive an emergency call from the labour room to assess a term baby born in poor condition. On arrival, the baby is cyanosed, tachypnoeic and has increased work of breathing. The baby fails to respond to conventional resuscitation and needs to be intubated. The baby also has a significant scaphoid abdomen and poor chest expansion on the left. *Consider the differential diagnosis and the basic approach in management.*	*Tip:* Know the presenting features of congenital abnormalities, including tracheoesophageal fistula, malrotation, bowel atresias, Hirschsprung's disease, abdominal wall defect, and diaphragmatic hernia. *(DCH2013 Curriculum-Gastro8)*

Chapter 9.8: The Child with a Musculoskeletal Problem

MSK 1 A 7 year old boy presents with intermittent right sided thigh pain and a limp over the last 3 weeks. On examination, he has a reduced range of movement in the right hip. *Consider the differential diagnosis and outline a management approach.*	*Tip:* Know the differential diagnosis of a limp, including Perthes disease. *(DCH2013 Curriculum-Msk2)*
MSK 2 A 9 year old boy presents with intermittent back pain over the last 2 weeks. He has had a low-grade temperature and 2 episodes of bleeding gums during this period. Other than pallor, his systemic examination is unremarkable. Blood tests show a low haemoglobin, neutropaenia and atypical lymphocytes. *Consider the differential diagnosis and the approach to the management of this child.*	*Tip:* Be aware of serious causes of back pain, including haematological malignancy. *(DCH2013 Curriculum-Msk3)*
MSK 3 An 11 year old girl presents with excessive tiredness and poor concentration in school for the last 4 months. Despite adequate rest, her tiredness does not improve. She has had difficulty in sleeping, muscular pains and 2 episodes of a sore throat during this period. She has a supportive family and normally enjoys school. *What would be your approach and management in this case?*	*Tip:* Be aware of the presentation of chronic fatigue syndrome, and refer to NICE guidance for a diagnostic workup and management strategies. *(DCH2013 Curriculum-Msk5)*
MSK 4 A 6 year old boy presents to the emergency department with a 24-hour history of a high fever and a swollen right elbow joint. *Discuss the differential diagnosis and management.*	*Tip:* Be able to discuss the causes of joint swelling and the initial management. Be able to discuss the causes of acute and chronic arthritis. *(DCH2013 Curriculum-Msk1, Msk6)*
MSK 5 A 6 year old girl presents with a 7-week history of joint swelling, intermittent fever and being generally unwell. On examination, she has hepatosplenomegaly and both knee joints are swollen with reduced movement. Her full blood count shows normal white blood cells with neutrophilia and raised platelets. *Consider the differential diagnosis and approach to management.*	*Tip:* Be able to discuss causes of acute and chronic arthritis, including juvenile inflammatory arthritis (JIA). *(DCH2013 Curriculum-Msk6)*
MSK 6 A 9 year old girl presents with red and mildly painful eyes over the last 48 hours. She was diagnosed with oligoarticular juvenile arthritis 4 years ago, and her antinuclear antibody (ANA) was positive. *What would be your approach and management in this case?*	*Tip:* Understand the disease associations of rheumatological conditions, particularly juvenile idiopathic arthritis and eye disease (in this case, uveitis). *(DCH2013 Curriculum-Msk7)*
MSK 7 A 9 month old infant who has been exclusively breastfed presents with poor growth and lethargy. On examination, he has broad wrists and ankles, widely opened fontanelle and prominent costochondral junctions. *What further steps/investigations should you perform to make a diagnosis and how do you manage this child?*	*Tip:* Understand the clinical presentation, and the management of nutritional rickets. *DCH2013 Curriculum-Msk10)*

Chapter 9.9: The Child with Diabetes or an Endocrine Problem

Endo 1 A 5 year old previously well boy presents with a 5-day history of polyuria and polydipsia. On examination, he is well hydrated and well perfused. His baseline observations, including blood pressure, are within normal limits. His urine shows glycosuria. *What would be your approach to management in this case?*	*Tip:* Be able to recognise the early features of a child or young person presenting with diabetes and know the principles of management. *(DCH2013 Curriculum-Endo1)*
Endo 2 A 13 year old, under treatment for type 1 diabetes, presents with abdominal pain and vomiting of 24-hour duration. She missed her last insulin dose and has only had a small meal. On examination, she looks ill and dehydrated with rapid breathing. *Outline your plan of emergency management and the principles of subsequent care?*	*Tip:* Be aware of the potential complications relating to diabetic ketoacidosis and understand the principles of treatment. *(DCH2013 Curriculum-Endo2)*
Endo 3 You are called to assess a 3 hour old newborn in the postnatal ward. The baby was born at term with a birth weight of 1.96 kg. On examination, the baby is irritable, with poor tone and jitteriness. Since birth, the baby has had only a small amount of breast milk. *What is the urgent investigation you would like to perform and how would you plan further management of this baby?*	*Tip:* Know the causes, complications and treatment of hypoglycaemia. *(DCH2013 Curriculum-Endo3)*
Endo 4 A 7 year old boy presents with excessive tiredness and increased thirst over the last few weeks. His mother reports he also passes large volumes of colourless urine and has wet his bed unusually in this period. *What investigations would you like to perform and how do you manage this boy?*	*Tip:* Know the causes of polyuria and polydipsia, and be able to identify children who require referral. *(DCH2013 Curriculum-Endo5)*
Endo 5 A 13 year old girl presents with deteriorating school performance and intermittent palpitations. On examination, she has prominent eyes, increased heart rate and a lump in her neck. *What would be your approach to the management of this child?*	*Tip:* Know the causes and management of hypo/hyperthyroidism. *(DCH2013 Curriculum-Endo6)*
Endo 6 A 3 week old neonate presents with poor feeding, lethargy and constipation since birth. On examination, the baby is jaundiced with a prominent tongue and poor muscle tone. The family moved to the UK only a week ago. *What would be your approach to management?*	*Tip:* Know about the national screening programme for hypothyroidism. *(DCH2013 Curriculum-Endo7)*
Endo 7 A 6 day old neonate presents to the emergency department with poor feeding, vomiting and lethargy. On examination, the baby looks dehydrated and has scrotal hyperpigmentation. *What further investigations would you like to perform and how do you manage this case?*	*Tip:* Be aware of the causes and presentation of ambiguous genitalia, including congenital adrenal hyperplasia. *(DCH2013 Curriculum-Endo8)*

Chapter 9.10: The Child with a Safeguarding Problem

Safe 1 A 3 month old baby was noted to have a nosebleed. His primary care health worker noted a recent significant increase in his head circumference, crossing more than 2 centile lines. *What should be her next action? If you are the receiving paediatrician, how will you manage this? What would be your differential diagnosis?*	*Tip:* Be aware of the different categories of non-accidental injury – physical, emotional, sexual, neglect, and fabricated illness. Know what steps need to be taken when a non-accidental injury is suspected. Understand the local referral pathway and key professionals who can help. *(DCH2013 Curriculum-Safe1, Safe 3)*
Safe 2 A 6 year boy has been seen repeatedly in the accident and emergency department regarding his mother's concerns around fits. He has also been investigated in a neighbouring hospital for the same concerns, with no abnormality identified. His mother has also sought advice from other paediatricians privately for the same concerns. *What issues will you consider in this situation?*	*Tip:* Be aware of the different categories of non-accidental injury – physical, emotional, sexual, neglect, and fabricated illness. Know what steps need to be taken when non-accidental injury is suspected. Understand the local referral pathway and key professionals who can help. *(DCH2013 Curriculum-Safe1, Safe3)*
Safe 3 A 13 year old boy is often late to school. He is also frequently noted to be unkempt, wearing the same clothes for a week. He asks other children to share their food with him. He lives with his mother who is unemployed and an alcoholic. *Discuss the reasons for this boy's behaviour. How will you manage this situation?*	*Tip:* Be aware of the different categories of non-accidental injury – physical, emotional, sexual, neglect, and fabricated illness. Be able to discuss the socio-economic factors that predispose one to non-accidental injury. *(DCH2013 Curriculum-Safe1, Safe2)*
Safe 4 An 8 month old infant with Down's syndrome is referred for poor weight gain (weight plotted on the Down's syndrome growth chart). The father works in a local shop and the mother is unemployed and has learning difficulties. Clinical examination and investigations do not reveal any specific cause for the failure to thrive. *What will be your next step?* *How will you manage this child?*	*Tip:* Be aware of the different categories of non-accidental injury – physical, emotional, sexual, neglect, and fabricated illness. Know what steps need to be taken when non-accidental injury is suspected. Understand the local referral pathway and key professionals who can help. *(DCH2013 Curriculum-Safe1, Safe3)*
Safe 5 A teacher observed a 6 year old child being pulled around by his father, who was noted to be very emotional and angry. *What should be the teacher's next steps?*	*Tip:* Know what steps need to be taken when non-accidental injury is suspected. Understand the local referral pathway and key professionals who can help. *(DCH2013 Curriculum-Safe3)*
Safe 6 A 12 year old girl has recently been noticed to be subdued and reluctant to go home after school. When approached by her class teacher to discuss her schoolwork, she discloses that her uncle, who has recently been visiting the family, has sexually abused her. *What should be the next step?*	*Tip:* Know what steps need to be taken when non-accidental injury is suspected. Understand the local referral pathway and key professionals who can help. *(DCH2013 Curriculum-Safe3)*

Chapter 9.11: The Child with an Infection/Immunology/Allergy-Related Problem

IIA 1 A 2 month old baby presents with a failure to thrive. He was born at full term, but had a low birth weight of 1.7 kg. The mother was noted to have a positive screen for cytomegalovirus (CMV) during the third trimester, but she did not receive any treatment. *Discuss the assessment and management of this baby.*	*Tip:* Appreciate the occurrence of maternal to foetal transmission of infection and the clinical manifestations of these infections. Be able to recognise clinical features that suggest congenital infections. *(DCH2013 Curriculum-IIA1, IIA11)*
IIA 2 A 10 year old boy presents with high-grade intermittent fever and rigors. He has recently returned to the UK after a holiday in Africa. *What is your differential diagnosis? Outline an approach to diagnosis and management.*	*Tip:* Be aware of the common infections of the foetus, newborn, and children, including important worldwide infections, e.g. TB, HIV, hepatitis B, malaria, polio. *(DCH2013 Curriculum-IIA2)*
IIA 3 A 2 month old baby presents with a fever of 40°C over the last 3 hours. She is otherwise well. *How will you manage this baby?*	*Tip:* Be able to discuss the assessment and management of a febrile child. *(DCH2013 Curriculum-IIA4)*
IIA 4 A 3 month old baby is reported positive for methicillin-resistant Staphylococcus aureus (MRSA) on a skin swab. The swab was performed as part of a screening prior to admission for cardiac surgery. *Consider the implications for the family and child, and also discuss the control of nosocomial infections.*	*Tip:* Understand nosocomial infections and the basic principles of infection control. *(DCH2013 Curriculum-IIA5)*
IIA 4 A 4 month old infant is brought to you with loose stools and excessive crying that is pronounced following bottle-feeds. She has also recently developed a skin rash. *What is the differential diagnosis? Outline a management plan.*	*Tip:* Know the features of cow's milk protein intolerance and its management. *(DCH2013 Curriculum-IIA10)*

Chapter 9.12: The Child with an 'Other' Problem

Other 1 A 2 year old presents with an extensive rash over his arms, legs and trunk. It is very itchy and the skin has areas of lichenification, especially in the creases of the knees and elbows. *Discuss the differential diagnosis and management.*	*Tip:* Be able to diagnose, investigate and manage common skin rashes – *eczema*, acne, impetigo, ammoniacal dermatitis, Staphylococcal scalded syndrome, seborrheic dermatitis, cradle cap, nappy rash, etc. *(DCH2013 Curriculum-Derm1)*
Other 2 A 1 year old has extensive eczema, and the parents have been applying topical steroids to the whole body over the last 2 months. She is admitted to the ward with a chest infection. *What are the potential side effects of long-term topical steroid use? What advice will you give parents?*	*Tip:* Be aware of the different potencies of topical steroids and their side effects. *(DCH2013 Curriculum-Derm2)*
Other 3 A 15 year old girl presents with fever, tiredness and headache. On examination, she has cervical lymphadenopathy, pharyngitis and splenomegaly. She is given amoxicillin and subsequently develops a diffuse erythematous rash. *Consider the differentials and approach to management.*	*Tip:* Know the causes of fever and an erythematous rash, including infectious mononucleosis. *(DCH2013 Curriculum-Derm6)*
Other 4 An 8 year old has developed a fever associated with redness and swelling around both eyes overnight. She has recently had a runny nose. *What is the differential diagnosis and management approach?*	*Tip:* Know the causes and management of cellulitis, including periorbital cellulitis. *(DCH2013 Curriculum-Derm7)*
Other 5 A 6 year old has multiple spots all over the right side of her abdomen and right arm. They are not itchy, but bother her as they sometimes catch on her clothes. Each lesion is about 2-4 mm in size, rounded, and umbilicated at the centre. *What is the diagnosis? What advice will you give the parents?*	*Tip:* Know the causes, clinical features and the management of rashes, including molluscum contagiosum and scabies. *(DCH2013 Curriculum-Derm8)*
Other 6 A 14 year old girl has been losing weight over the last 6 months. She feels she is eating well and exercising normally. On questioning, she feels she is overweight and should go on a 'diet'. Her body mass index is only 13.5 kg/m^2. *Discuss the diagnostic possibilities, and outline a management plan for her.*	*Tip:* Be aware of clinical presentation of adolescents with eating disorders (NICE guidance). *(DCH2013 Curriculum-Adol3)*
Other 7 A 2 year old boy presents with a 6-month history of probable seizures. When he gets upset, he goes blue, seems to lose consciousness and, at times, has brief tonic-clonic movements of his arms and legs, before recovering. *What is the likely diagnosis? How will you counsel the parents? Propose a management plan.*	*Tip:* Understand the principles of managing common behavioural problems such as temper tantrums, *breath-holding attacks*, sleep problems, the crying baby, oppositional behaviour, enuresis and encopresis, school refusal and bullying. *(DCH2013 Curriculum-Beh4)*
Other 8 A 15 year old boy has not shown any evidence of pubertal progress. He is short, does not have any pubic or axillary hair, and he is concerned about his short penis. *What are the diagnostic possibilities? How will you evaluate and manage this boy?*	*Tip:* Know the causes of early and delayed puberty. *(DCH2013 Curriculum-Deve4)*

Other 9 A 14 year old girl has not shown any pubertal growth. She is also noted to have increased carrying angle at the elbows, and a heart murmur. *What are the diagnostic possibilities? How will you evaluate and manage this girl?*	*Tip:* Know about the features of common chromosomal disorders, e.g. Down's syndrome, *Turner syndrome*. *(DCH2013 Curriculum-Gene2)*
Other 10 A 2 year old boy presents with pallor. Clinical examination is normal other than the presence of pallor. *What are the diagnostic possibilities? How will you evaluate and manage this boy?*	*Tip:* Have the knowledge to be able to assess and manage children with anaemia (iron deficiency, haemoglobinopathy and haemolytic anaemia). *(DCH2013 Curriculum-Haem1)*
Other 11 A 7 day old baby is brought with poor feeding and lethargy. His capillary blood gas shows a metabolic acidosis, and serum ammonia performed as part of the investigations is very high: 1,000 mcg/dL (the normal range being 15–45 mcg/dL). *What are the diagnostic possibilities? How will you evaluate and manage this baby?*	*Tip:* Be aware of the common clinical presentations of metabolic disease. *(DCH2013 Curriculum-Met2)*
Other 12 A 4 year old boy presents with a 3-week history of puffy eyes. He feet and abdomen have also become swollen in the last 2 days. A urine dipstick shows 4$^+$ protein and 3$^+$ blood. *What is the differential diagnosis? How will you evaluate and manage this boy?*	*Tip:* Know the causes of haematuria and proteinuria. Recognise features in the presentation that suggest serious or significant pathology (including nephritic and nephrotic syndrome). *(DCH2013 Curriculum-Neph3)*
Other 13 A 14 year old boy presents with shortness of breath and is unable to keep up with his peers during sports. He weighs 90 kg and has a body mass index of 35 kg/m^2. *Outline a full assessment of this obese boy. What practical steps would you advise him to undertake to improve his symptoms?*	*Tip:* Be able to recognise obesity and advise young people and their families about strategies to control or prevent weight gain. *(DCH2013 Curriculum-Nutr3)*
Other 14 A 3 year old boy presents with a squint. Examination shows a non-paralytic convergent squint affecting his left eye. *What further assessments does he require? Outline the management strategy.*	*Tip:* Know the causes, types and the initial management of a squint. *(DCH2013 Curriculum-Ophth3)*
Other 15 One of the babies on the ward received a wrong dose of gentamicin. There is an ongoing investigation into this incident. The parents have come to you and would like to discuss this incident. *Educate yourself on prescribing standards and prescribing errors before meeting the parents. Also be aware of the clinical incident reporting structure within your organisation.*	*Tip:* Know how to find out information necessary for safe prescribing through the use of paediatric formularies and pharmacy liaison. *(DCH2013 Curriculum-PPA1)*
Other 16 There has been an outbreak of an E. coli infection in your catchment area, and a couple of children have been admitted to the hospital with renal failure. *Read about and discuss the outbreak of infectious diseases and control measures.*	*Tip:* Be aware of the causes of outbreaks of infection, their investigation and control. *(DCH2013 Curriculum-CPH3)*

SECTION 10:
CLINICAL SKILLS LOGBOOK

Chapter 10.1: Introduction
Dr Anna Mathew, Dr P Venugopalan

This section has been created to help with the development of clinical examination skills. Examining patients in a fluid, systematic and organised manner, and interpreting your findings accurately to determine a path for further management are the fundamental skills required of a doctor. Communicating these findings to the child or carer and the examiner is another skill that can be honed over time.

In each section of the clinical assessment chapters in this book, video links have been noted at the end of each chapter. These links connect you to sites where clinical examination skills are demonstrated. The RCPCH has not endorsed these sites officially, and candidates could quite possibly find other similar links that are freely accessible. We would advise candidates to watch the structured clinical examination of all systems on their preferred site and then use the clinical skills lists provided in this section to practise with a partner. This can also be done in small groups. The advantage of learning in groups is that it allows collaborative learning, which can empower the individual and generate positive self-reflection.

This logbook contains details of the clinical examination structure that should be undertaken when examining a system. Many doctors would have been trained to undertake a structured and systematic examination of children in medical school, but reinforcing and improving these skills can continue throughout a career. For doctors preparing for postgraduate examinations, the mantra is practice, practice and practice.

There is only 1 clinical assessment station in the DCH clinical examination, which means that a candidate could be required to examine any system of the body. Candidates should be prepared for this and have appropriate skills in all areas. In any 1 system, it is likely that the examiner will ask you to undertake the examination of only a focused area. This is particularly true in the neurological examination, where it is unlikely that candidates will need to demonstrate 'sensation' when examining the peripheral nervous system.

This logbook contains neonatal examination skills. It is unlikely this will be required for the DCH clinical examination, but it has been included here for completeness, as it is an important skill for any doctor looking after babies. There is also a skills list for developmental assessment. As this is complex and varied, a brief outline has been provided, and candidates would benefit from using a developmental assessment textbook alongside this list when practising this area.

By using this logbook, individually, with a partner or even with the help of a tutor/supervisor, you will be able to develop evidence that you have learnt these essential skills and achieved competence.

The following chapters will address the examination of the following systems:

- ENT examination
- Cardiovascular examination
- Respiratory examination
- Gastrointestinal examination
- Neurology: cranial nerve examination
- Neurology: peripheral nervous system examination
- Musculoskeletal examination
- Neonatal examination
- Developmental assessment

Chapter 10.2: ENT Examination
Dr Anna Mathew, Dr P Venugopalan

Examining the ear

Name of the candidate ....Date..................................

Approach	Competent	Needs to improve
Uses *auroscope* with appropriate ear piece		
Introduces self, explains procedure to child and carer		
Positions child appropriately, restraining head and body sideways		
Undertakes *examination*		
Interprets accurately		
Counsels child/carer		

Supervisor/Tutor signature ....Print name..

Examining the throat

Name of the candidate ....Date..................................

Approach	Competent	Needs to improve
Uses *auroscope* and *tongue* depressor		
Introduces self, explains procedure to child and carer		
Positions child, restraining head and body facing forward		
Undertakes *examination* using tongue depressor if required		
Interprets accurately		
Counsels child/carer		

Supervisor/Tutor signature ....Print name..

Chapter 10.3: Cardiovascular Examination
Dr Anna Mathew, Dr P Venugopalan

Examining the cardiovascular system

Name of the candidate ....Date..

Approach	Competent	Needs to improve
Uses *stethoscope* Considers *BP/saturation measurement*		
Introduces self, explains procedure to child and carer		
Position and *appropriate exposure* of the chest, depending on the age		
General examination: Well child or not, cyanosis, pallor, clubbing, dysmorphism, general growth *Pulses:* Palpates radial, brachial, femoral and carotid pulses, looks for radio-femoral delay *Inspection:* Chest deformity, recessions, scars, visible pulses *Palpation:* Cardiac apex, left parasternal heave, thrills over chest, thrill over the carotid arteries *Percussion:* Not usually indicated *Auscultation:* For heart sounds and murmurs over the mitral area, tricuspid area, pulmonary area, aortic area, neck and back of the chest		
Interprets accurately: Able to enumerate the findings, know their significance and synthesise the findings to a logical conclusion		

Supervisor/Tutor signature ....Print name..

Chapter 10.4: Respiratory Examination
Dr Anna Mathew, Dr P Venugopalan

Examining the respiratory system

Name of the candidate ....Date..................................

Approach	Competent	Needs to improve
Uses *stethoscope, pulse oximeter* (where available)		
Introduces self, explains procedure to child and carer		
Position and *appropriate exposure* of the chest, depending on age		
General examination: Well child or not, cyanosis, pallor, clubbing, general growth		
Inspection: Chest shape (Harrison's sulcus, barrel chest), chest deformity, recessions, scars		
Palpation: Trachea, cardiac apex, chest expansion, vocal fremitus		
Percussion: Note over the chest comparing the 2 sides (resonant or not), upper border of the liver		
Auscultation: Air entry, quality of breath sounds comparing the 2 sides, added sounds, vocal resonance		
Interprets accurately: Able to enumerate the findings, know their significance and synthesise the findings to a logical conclusion		

Supervisor/Tutor signature ....Print name..

Chapter 10.5: Gastrointestinal Examination
Dr Anna Mathew, Dr P Venugopalan

Examining the gastrointestinal system

Name of the candidate ....Date...

Approach	Competent	Needs to improve
Uses *stethoscope*		
Introduces self, explains procedure to child and carer		
Position (lie flat) and *appropriate exposure* of the abdomen, depending on age		
General examination: Well child or not, jaundice, pallor, clubbing, general growth, peripheral signs of chronic liver disease *Inspection:* Shape of abdomen, distended veins, visible masses, visible peristalsis, scars *Palpation:* Superficial palpation (tenderness), deep palpation for liver, spleen, kidneys and other masses, fluid thrill (in suspected ascites) *Percussion:* Note over the abdomen (tympanic or not), liver edges (span), shifting dullness *Auscultation:* Bowel sounds, renal bruit Consider genital and perianal examinations where relevant (not usually required in exam settings)		
Interprets accurately: Able to enumerate the findings, know their significance and synthesise the findings to a logical conclusion		

Supervisor/Tutor signature ....Print name..

Chapter 10.6: Neurology: Cranial Nerve Examination
Dr Anna Mathew, Dr P Venugopalan

Examining the cranial nerves

Name of the candidate ....Date...

Approach	Competent	Needs to improve
Uses *ophthalmoscope, tools for visual acuity*		
Introduces self, explains procedure to child and carer		
Positions appropriately (sitting or standing) depending on age		
Cranial nerves: **1st** Smell (rarely done) **2nd** Visual acuity, visual fields, light and accommodation, fundal examination **3rd, 4th, 6th** Ocular movements, ptosis, nystagmus **5th** Sensation, corneal reflex, jaw muscles **7th** Muscles of the face **8th** Whisper in each ear, tuning fork for sensorineural hearing **9th, 10th, 11th** Gag reflex, swallowing, sternomastoids, trapezius **12th** Tongue movements		
Interprets accurately: Able to enumerate the findings, know their significance and synthesise the findings to a logical conclusion		

Supervisor/Tutor signature ....Print name...

Chapter 10.7: Neurology: Peripheral Nervous System Examination

Dr Anna Mathew, Dr P Venugopalan

Examining the peripheral nervous system

Name of the candidate ....Date..................................

Approach	Competent	Needs to improve
Uses *patella hammer*		
Introduces self, explains procedure to child and carer		
Positions appropriately (sitting or standing) depending on age		
General inspection: Dysmorphism, neurocutaneous features, posture, tremor, muscle wasting, fasciculation, gait *Arms:* Motor – Muscle tone, power and reflexes Sensory – Light-touch, pinprick, position and vibration sense *Legs:* Motor – Muscle tone, power and reflexes. Includes plantars and clonus Sensory – Light-touch, pinprick, position and vibration sense *Cerebellar:* Nystagmus, speech, coordination, Romberg, intention tremor, dysdiadochokinesia		
Interprets accurately: Able to enumerate the findings, know their significance and synthesise the findings to a logical conclusion		

Supervisor/Tutor signature ....Print name...

Chapter 10.8: Musculoskeletal System Examination
Dr Anna Mathew, Dr P Venugopalan

Examining the musculoskeletal system

Name of the candidate ....Date...

Approach	Competent	Needs to improve
Uses equipment as relevant		
Introduces self, explains procedure to child and carer		
Positions appropriate to the child and joint examined		
General examination: Well child or not, pallor, clubbing, general growth, skin rashes *Individual joint examination:* Ask for pain/soreness Look – Symmetry, skin changes, muscle bulk, swelling, deformity, posture Feel – Warmth, swelling, tenderness Move – Active and passive, look for hypermobility Assess function – Bring hands to mouth, button clothes, gait, get out of a chair *Video resource:* Appropriate use of pGALS (web link given below), modifying as required http://www.arthritisresearchuk.org/health-professionals-and-students/video-resources/pgals.aspx Please also refer to the 'other systems' chapter in the clinical assessment section.		
Interprets accurately: Able to enumerate the findings, know their significance and synthesise the findings to a logical conclusion		

Supervisor/Tutor signature ....Print name...

Chapter 10.9: The Neonatal Examination
Dr Anna Mathew, Dr P Venugopalan

Examining the neonate

Name of the candidate ....Date..

Approach	Competent	Needs to improve
Uses *stethoscope, ophthalmoscope*		
Introduces self, explains procedure to carer		
Positions appropriately, undresses appropriately		
General examination: Response – Tone, primitive reflexes Growth – Weight, length, head circumference Features – Dysmorphism, birthmarks Colour – Pallor, jaundice, cyanosis Head – Shape, anterior fontanelle Eyes – Red reflex Mouth – Cleft lip and palate Chest – Observe as for system examination; listen to breath and heart sounds. Palpate femoral pulses. Abdomen – Shape and size, palpate for organomegaly Genitalia – Normal male/female, anus patent Back – No defects, no pits, hairy naevi or lipomas over the spinal cord Hips – Stable Limbs – Normal length, talipes		
Interprets accurately: Able to enumerate the findings, know their significance and synthesise the findings to a logical conclusion		

Supervisor/Tutor signature ....Print name..

Chapter 10.10: Developmental Assessment
Dr Anna Mathew, Dr P Venugopalan

Developmental assessment

In the examination, candidates will be expected to undertake a focused developmental assessment, frequently covering only 1 or (at most) 2 domains – for example, gross motor assessment, fine motor assessment, or speech and language assessment. The following pages list skills that children of varying age ranges should achieve in the different domains, and are meant only as a guide to learning.

Name of the candidate ....Date..................................

Approach	Competent	Needs to improve
Equipment depends on task. *Standard developmental assessment pack* should be available		
Introduces self, explains procedure to child and carer		
Positions appropriately depending on age		
Dependant on age and task set (please refer to the chapter on child development, and augment with a standard developmental assessment textbook) *Gross motor* *Fine motor and vision* *Speech and language* *Social skills*		
Interprets accurately: Able to enumerate the findings, know their significance and synthesise the findings to a logical conclusion		

Supervisor/Tutor signature ....Print name..

Developmental assessment (Age 0-12 months - unlikely in the exam)

Name of the candidate ....Date..................................

Approach	Competent	Needs to improve
Equipment depends on task. *Standard developmental assessment pack* should be available		
Introduces self, explains procedure to child and carer		
Positions appropriately depending on age		
Gross motor Ventral suspension Head drops below the plane of the body Head held in same plane as body Prone Attempts to lift head Raises head and chest, propping on forearms Lifts head and chest, extended arms Rolling - Front to back/back to front Sitting Held in sitting, curved back Supported with straight back and head Steadily unsupported Stands alone Primitive reflexes, e.g. Moro, asymmetric tonic neck Reflex, palmer (grasp) reflex Protective reflexes Downward parachute Sideward protective reflex Forward parachute/protective reflex **Fine motor and vision** Hands together Palmar grasp Transfers the object from hand to hand Rakes a raisin Pincer grip Scribbles Vision fixes Follows objects **Speech and language** Babbles Two words without/with meaning **Social skills** Eye contact Stranger anxiety Social interaction		
Interprets accurately: Able to enumerate the findings, know their significance and synthesise the findings to a logical conclusion		

Supervisor/Tutor signature ....Print name...

Developmental assessment (Age 12–18 months)

Name of the candidate .... Date ....

Approach	Competent	Needs to improve
Equipment depends on task. *Standard developmental assessment pack* should be available		
Introduces self, explains procedure to child and carer		
Positions appropriately depending on age		
Gross motor Sitting Sits well on the floor for an indefinite period of time Pulls to standing and lets himself down Crawls upstairs Kneels unaided Standing Walks alone Wide-based gait Runs carefully Climbs into adults' chair Walks upstairs **Fine motor and vision** Picks up fine objects with a neat pincer grasp Drops and throws toys forward Points with index finger at objects Holds 2 cubes Builds tower of – cubes Stands at windows and watches outside Holds a crayon and scribbles Enjoys simple picture books **Speech and language** Knows and turns to their own name Vocalises most vowels Vocalises consonants Speaks 2–20 words Hands objects on request Obeys simple instructions Enjoys nursery rhymes **Social skills** Drinks from cup Uses spoon Plays simple games Indicates wet or soiled pants Imitates everyday activities		
Interprets accurately: Able to enumerate the findings, know their significance and synthesise the findings to a logical conclusion		

Supervisor/Tutor signature .... Print name ....

Developmental assessment (Age 18 months–3 years)

Name of the candidate ....Date..

Approach	Competent	Needs to improve
Equipment depends on task. *Standard developmental assessment pack* should be available		
Introduces self, explains procedure to child and carer		
Positions appropriately depending on age		
Gross motor Runs safely, stopping and starting with ease Climbs on furniture with ease Walks up and down stairs – 1 to 2 steps at a time Throws/kicks ball Jumps with 2 feet together Rides tricycle **Fine motor and vision** Builds tower of 6–9 cubes Imitates/draws line/circle Hand preference obvious Threads large wooden beads Draws man with 2 parts Cuts with scissors **Speech and language** Uses 50–200 recognisable words Interested in general talk Joins in nursery rhymes Continually asking questions Gives full name and sex Counts by rote up to 10 Stycar test performance **Social skills** Spoon feeds/chews Uses fork Simple/sustained role plays Enjoys play with bricks/boxes/toy trains Throws tantrums Washes hands – Needs supervision to dry Dry throughout the night		
Interprets accurately: Able to enumerate the findings, know their significance and synthesise the findings to a logical conclusion		

Supervisor/Tutor signature ....Print name..

Developmental assessment (Age 3-5 years)

Name of the candidate ....Date..

Approach	Competent	Needs to improve
Equipment depends on task. *Standard developmental assessment pack* should be available		
Introduces self, explains procedure to child and carer		
Positions appropriately depending on age		
Gross motor Runs up and down stairs – 1 step at a time Climbs ladders and trees Increasing skill in ball games Walks on a narrow line Skips on alternate feet **Fine motor and vision** Builds bridge/steps Draws a man with 3-5 parts Matches and names colours Good control in writing and drawing Counts fingers Stycar vision tests **Speech and language** Speaks grammatically correctly and intelligibly Tells stories Enjoys jokes and riddles Gives full name, age, birthday **Social skills** Eats with spoon and fork Washes and dries hands Brushes teeth Undresses and dresses alone Appreciates past, present, future		
Interprets accurately: Able to enumerate the findings, know their significance and synthesise the findings to a logical conclusion		

Supervisor/Tutor signature ....Print name...

PAGE INTENTIONALLY BLANK

INDEX

Symbols
22q deletion 144

A
Abdominal migraine 58, 202
Abdominal pain 42, 48, 57, 58, 59, 60, 61, 69, 72, 108, 162, 193, 199, 202, 284, 286
Absence seizure 282
Absent testis 104
Achondroplasia 29
Acidaemia 78
Acidosis 78, 79, 80, 83, 173, 191, 193, 194, 195, 196, 286, 290
Acne 266, 281, 289
Acrocyanosis 279
Active immunity 115
Acutely ill child 4
Adalimumab 59
Adenovirus 79
ADHD (Attention Deficit Hyperactivity Disorder) 21, 22, 23, 24, 25, 26, 187, 232
Adolescent 17, 23, 25, 31, 32, 39, 41, 45, 49, 60, 61, 65, 66, 121, 139, 170, 174, 175, 186, 189, 191, 196, 197, 199, 200, 203, 204, 232, 236, 289
Adrenal hyperplasia 286
Adverse event 111, 112, 113
Aerochamber 272
Airway obstruction 82, 172
Alagille syndrome 144
Alkalaemia 78
Alkalosis 78, 79, 82, 83
Allergen 72, 73, 74
Allergic rhinitis 72, 170, 171, 173, 264, 277
Allergies 71, 73, 74, 76, 114, 170, 173
Alpha-1 antitrypsin 135
Ambiguous genitalia 286
Amblyopia 92
Anaemia 58, 59, 63, 82, 107, 126, 134, 137, 139, 290
Anaphylaxis 72, 73, 74, 75, 76, 114
Anchor statement 9, 15, 20, 53, 56, 87, 90, 120, 124, 164, 165, 168, 208, 212, 238, 242, 249, 262
Angioedema 72, 75, 256
Anopheles mosquito 252
Anti-inflammatory 107, 109, 203, 255, 256, 260
Anti-malarial 2, 249
Anti-thyroid 64, 65
Anticholinergic 98
Antihistamine 71, 73
Anxiety 16, 24, 37, 62, 64, 82, 92, 96, 170, 187, 191, 192, 199, 202, 302,
Apert syndrome 92
Appendicitis 58, 108
Arachnodactyly 155, 157
Arthritis 29, 59, 106, 107, 108, 109, 110, 135, 160, 285, 299
Ascites 135, 296
Asperger syndrome 185
Asphyxia 150
Aspiration 173, 192
Asthma 71, 72, 73, 74, 75, 79, 82, 126, 128, 162, 169, 170, 171, 172, 173, 174, 236, 256, 264, 268, 269, 270, 271, 272, 273, 274, 277
Ataxia 217
Athetosis 213
Atlantoaxial 224
Atopy 72, 170, 171, 173, 268

Atovaquone 249
Atrial septal defect 143, 144
Atrioventricular 143, 144, 224
Auroscope 293
Auscultation 79, 120, 125, 128, 135, 141, 143, 157, 278, 294, 295, 296
Autism 185, 186, 187, 188, 230, 231, 232, 233, 283
Autoimmune 64, 65, 66, 135, 191
Avascular necrosis 107, 110

B
Back to sleep 91, 282
Baclofen 152
Barrel chest 126, 295
Base excess 77, 78, 79
Basic life support 73, 279
BCG (Bacillus Calmette Guerin) 112, 115
Becker muscular dystrophy 148
Beclometasone 171, 172, 270
Bed-wetting 69, 95, 96, 97, 98, 99, 193
Behaviour 5, 8, 22, 23, 24, 25, 26, 30, 37, 39, 49, 64, 66, 96, 97, 99, 179, 180, 183, 184, 185, 187, 188, 191, 198, 200, 216, 230, 231, 232, 246, 287, 289
Beighton score 158, 159, 160
Beta-blocker 64
Beta-agonist 172, 270, 277
Betamethasone 265
Betnovate 265
Biliary atresia 134, 135, 280
Bisacodyl 181
Bladder dysfunction 96
Bleeding per rectum 59, 284
BNFC (British National Formulary for Children) 10, 11, 236, 237, 239, 242, 243, 245, 246, 248, 249, 251, 253, 254, 256, 260, 261, 262, 263, 268, 270, 276
Botulinum toxin 152
Brachycephalic 91, 93, 222
Breastfeed 48
Breast milk jaundice 280, 284
Breath-holding 75, 99, 289
Bristol stool chart 178, 180, 181
BTS (British Thoracic Society) 172, 174, 270, 273, 274, 277
Bronchiectasis 127, 128, 130, 173
Bronchiolitis 79, 80, 81, 82, 83, 278
Bronchodilator 81, 131
Bronchomalacia 139
Bronchospasm 75, 256
Bruising 69, 108, 172, 179
Bruit 135, 296
Bullying 96, 97, 99, 176, 289

C
CAF (Common Assessment Framework) 35
Cafe-au-lait 283
Calprotectin, faecal 60
CAMHS (Child and Adolescent Mental Health Service) 23, 25
Candidiasis 172, 271
Carbimazole 64
Cardiac compromise 64
Cardiomegaly 140
Cataract 172
CDGP (constitutional delay in growth and puberty) 27, 28, 29, 30
Cerebellar 147, 149, 298
Cerebral palsy 97, 150, 151, 152, 179, 180, 215, 216, 217, 219, 220, 222, 227, 230, 281

Cervical spine 200
CFTR (cystic fibrosis transmembrane conductance regulator) 129, 130
Chemoprophylaxis 251, 252
Chemotherapy 114
Child abuse 37, 38, 180
Child development 5, 6, 7, 152, 205, 206, 207, 209, 210, 212, 213, 218, 220, 223, 225, 232, 301
Child in need 35, 36
Child protection 35, 36, 39, 43, 191, 209, 218, 225, 232
Children Act 35, 36, 39
Chlamydia 43, 45, 46, 47, 48, 49
Chloride channel 129
Chromosomal 118, 216, 220, 231, 290
Ciliary dyskinesia 129, 173
Cirrhosis, liver 135
Cleft lip 230, 300
Clicky hip 280
Clonus 147, 149, 150, 282, 298
Clostridium difficile 60
Clubbing 59, 60, 126, 128, 129, 133, 139, 141, 155, 173, 294, 295, 296, 299
Clumsiness 282
Cluster headache 200, 201
CMV (cytomegalovirus) 288
Coarctation, aorta 140, 143
Codeine 258
Coeliac disease 29, 31, 58, 190, 284
Cognition 206, 216
Coma 194, 243, 245, 246
Combination vaccine 115
Compliance 37, 93, 97, 98, 170, 177, 180, 190, 191, 246, 247, 263
Concordance 172, 192
Confidentiality 17, 42, 47
Conjunctivitis 46, 48, 49
Connor's questionnaires 23, 26
Conn's syndrome 82
Consent 14, 17, 43, 44, 97, 120, 163, 164, 185, 208
Constipation 58, 96, 97, 131, 162, 175, 176, 177, 178, 179, 180, 182, 217, 284, 286
Constitutional delay 27, 28
Contraception 41, 42, 43, 44, 45
Contractures 147, 148, 218
Convulsion 277
Coordination 92, 148, 149, 150, 152, 202, 217, 223, 232, 298
Corticosteroids 59, 172, 263, 265, 270, 271, 272, 274
Cot death 91
Cough 77, 79, 101, 126, 128, 130, 170, 171, 172, 173, 202, 272, 277, 278, 279
COX (cyclooxygenase) 256, 257
CPAP (continuous positive airway pressure) 81
Cradle cap 33, 266, 289
Cranial suture 92
Craniosynostosis 91, 92, 93, 94
Critical incident 14
Crohn's disease 58, 59, 60, 61, 256, 284
Crouzon syndrome 92
Cryptorchidism 101, 105
Cultural 17, 120
Curriculum 9, 10, 276, 277, 278, 279, 280, 281, 282, 283, 284, 285, 286, 287, 288, 289, 290
Cyanosis 75, 126, 138, 139, 141, 143, 279, 294, 295, 300
Cyclical vomiting 202
Cystic fibrosis 29, 125, 126, 129, 130, 131, 132, 139, 173

D

DEET (diethyltoluamide) 252
Deformity 92, 93, 94, 126, 139, 155, 179, 258, 294, 295, 299
Dermatitis 93, 264, 266, 289
Dermatologist 263, 266, 267
Dermatomyositis 148
DesmoMelt 98
Desmopressin 98
Detrusor instability 96, 99
Developmental 9, 10, 22, 23, 35, 36, 38, 52, 92, 94, 96, 97, 107, 109, 147, 154, 179, 180, 186, 187, 206, 207, 208, 209, 212, 213, 214, 215, 218, 219, 220, 221, 222, 223, 225, 227, 230, 231, 232, 233, 280, 281, 292, 301, 302, 303, 304, 305
Dextrocardia 127, 139, 141
Diabetes 64, 65, 66, 68, 96, 97, 162, 189, 190, 191, 192, 193, 195, 196, 245, 246, 247, 248, 286
Diaphragmatic hernia 134, 284
Diarrhoea 59, 60, 61, 69, 82, 178, 180, 256, 284
Diastolic 141, 143
Diphtheria 113
Diplegia 147, 151, 150
Disability 38, 110, 131, 152, 187, 188, 204, 209, 210, 215, 218, 219, 222, 223, 224, 225, 226, 231, 232, 233
Disimpaction 181
Dislocation 109, 158
Diuretic 82
Diurnal 96
Dizziness 72, 251
DLA (Disability Living Allowance) 131, 152, 218, 224
DNase (deoxyribonuclease) 131
Docusate sodium 181
Dolichocephaly 157
Domains 206, 213, 220, 227, 230, 301
Domestic violence 37
Dominant 136, 158, 283
Domperidone 203
Dorsiflexion 147
Down's syndrome 138, 144, 154, 220, 223, 224, 225, 279, 283, 287, 290
Drooling 152, 217, 278
Drowsiness 72, 246
DSM-V 231, 232
Duchenne muscular dystrophy 148, 214
Dysdiadochokinesia 298
Dyskinetic 150
Dysmorphic 30, 92, 94, 97, 133, 138, 147, 154, 155, 156, 157, 180, 188, 213, 220, 227, 229
Dysmotility 180
Dysplasia 29, 30, 107, 109, 147, 280
Dyspraxia 230
Dysraphism 179
Dystonia 213
Dysuria 43, 67, 69, 96

E

E. coli 69, 290
Earache 277
Ear discharge 277
Eating disorder 191, 289,
EBV (Epstein Barr Virus) 135
ECG (electrocardiogram) 52, 62, 75, 142
Echocardiogram 142, 224
Echolalia 184, 231
ECMO (extracorporeal membrane oxygenation) 139
Ectopia lentis 157, 158
Ectopic pregnancy 42, 48
Eczema 34, 72, 73, 162, 170, 171, 173, 261, 262, 263, 264, 265, 266, 267, 289
EEG (electroencephalogram) 52, 188
Effusion 108, 109, 127, 128, 141, 258
Egg allergy 114
EHCP (education, health care plan) 223
Ehlers-Danlos syndrome 157
Eisenmenger's syndrome 143
Elastase, stool 130
Elemental formula 59
Emollient 261, 263, 265
Emphysema 127
Encephalopathy 187, 216
Encopresis 70, 99, 179, 180, 289
Endocarditis 139, 142, 279
Endoscopy 61
Enophthalmos 157
Enterocolitis 179, 180
Enuresis 70, 95, 96, 97, 98, 99, 162, 289
Epiglottitis 278
Epilepsy 151, 152, 162, 188, 216, 218, 236, 281, 282, 283
EpiPen 72, 73, 74
Erythema 34, 59, 60, 71, 75, 133, 135, 136, 264, 289
Ethics 14
Eumovate 265
Eustachian 225
Evidence base 17, 52, 54, 56, 86, 88, 110, 203, 251, 267
Exomphalos 134
Exophthalmos 64, 66

F

Fabricated illness 39, 287
Failure to thrive 173, 180, 283, 284, 287, 288
Falciparum, Plasmodium 252
Familial short stature 28, 29
Fasciculation 298
Fatty acid 246
FBN1 (Fibrillin 1) gene 158
Fertility 48, 59, 101
Fine motor 206, 207, 220, 221, 222, 223, 301, 302, 303, 304, 305
Finger-nose test 149
Fissure 59, 157, 178, 179, 222, 283
Fistula 59, 60, 135, 179, 284
Fits 282, 287
Fluctuation 103
Fluid thrill 135, 296
Folic acid 136
Fontanelle 92, 93, 285, 300
Foot arch 155, 156, 157
Forced expiratory volume 273
Foreign body 128, 129, 173, 278
Formoterol 172
FP10 237, 238, 249
Fracture 107, 258, 259
Fragile X 283
Fraser guidelines 41, 43, 44
Frog-like posture 281
Fundoplication 134
Funny head 91
Funny turn 282

G

Gag reflex 297
Gait 107, 147, 149, 150, 151, 216, 298, 299, 303
Gallstone 136
Gastro-oesophageal 129, 151, 173, 281, 284
Gastroschisis 134
Gastrostomy 131, 133, 152, 214
Genetic 24, 29, 30, 60, 93, 96, 97, 154, 157, 158, 180, 184, 187, 188, 206, 229, 264, 281, 283
Gesture 221
Gigantism 157
Gillick competence 43, 44, 45
Glandular fever 135
Glargine 195
Glucagon 244, 245, 246
Glucogel 245
Glucose 68, 77, 137, 192, 194, 195, 245, 246, 247
Glue ear 225, 277
Gluteal 109, 110, 179
Glycogen storage 135, 245, 246
Glycopyrronium 152
Glycosylated haemoglobin 189
GMFCS (Gross Motor Function Classification System) 217
Goitre 64, 65, 66
Gower's sign 148, 149, 214
Graves disease 65, 66
Green book 112, 116
Groin pain 110
Gross motor 152, 206, 207, 213, 214, 215, 216, 223, 301, 302, 304, 305
Growth 27, 28, 29, 30, 31, 32, 36, 38, 52, 58, 59, 60, 64, 65, 73, 93, 94, 97, 125, 129, 133, 136, 138, 139, 142, 146, 154, 160, 172, 176, 178, 179, 180, 187, 202, 215, 222, 271, 280, 284, 285, 287, 290, 294, 295, 296, 299, 300
Guillain-Barre syndrome 82
GUM clinic (genitourinary) 41, 43, 44, 46, 47

H

Haemangioma 280
Haematuria 68, 290
Haemoglobin 60, 137, 189, 285, 290
Haemolytic anaemia 134, 136, 137, 290
Haemophilus influenzae 69, 113, 136
Haemorrhage 65, 216, 256, 281
Hand dominance 151, 221
Hand flapping 232
Hand washing 120, 208
Harrison's sulcus 126, 139, 295
Hashimoto's thyroiditis 65, 66
Hay fever 170, 171
Hazelnut 71, 72, 74
HbA1C (glycosylated haemoglobin) 189, 190, 191, 192
Headache 42, 92, 112, 197, 198, 199, 200, 201, 202, 203, 204, 247, 251, 252, 289
Health visitor 34, 98, 230
Hearing 24, 151, 152, 185, 186, 206, 209, 213, 214, 215, 217, 218, 220, 222, 223, 224, 225, 227, 229, 230, 233, 281, 297
Heart failure 138, 139, 257, 279
Heel-prick 130
Helmet 92, 93
Hemiplegia 97, 150, 151, 216
Hepatitis 49, 115, 135, 253, 280, 288
Hereditary spherocytosis 135, 136, 137
Hernia 100, 101, 102, 103, 104, 105, 108, 134, 135, 284
Hickman line 126, 149
High stepping 147, 150

309

Hip 107, 108, 109, 110, 147, 216, 280, 285
Hirschsprung's disease 177, 178, 179, 180, 284
HIV (human immunodeficiency virus) 40, 43, 45, 49, 114, 253, 277, 288
Hives 72, 75
Hoarseness 172
Hoarse voice 75, 271
Holt-Oram syndrome 144
Hospital admission 131, 199, 270, 272
Hospitalisation 80, 81, 170, 190
Humidified oxygen 81
Hydrocele 101, 102, 103, 104
Hydrocortisone 265
Hyperactivity 21, 22, 23, 26
Hyperbilirubinaemia 150
Hyper-extendable 155
Hyperinflation 126
Hypermobility 155, 157, 158, 159, 160, 299
Hypersensitivity 74, 112, 114, 256
Hypertelorism 283
Hypertension 25, 135, 136, 140, 143, 199, 200
Hyperthyroidism 63, 64, 65, 66, 286
Hypertonia 149
Hypertonic saline 81, 131, 194
Hyperventilation 82, 173
Hypoglycaemia 190, 191, 192, 193, 195, 243, 245, 246, 247, 248, 286
Hyponatremia 98
Hypopigmented 281
Hypoplastic left heart 143
Hypospadias 101
Hypotension 72, 74
Hypothyroidism 29, 63, 65, 107, 179, 190, 224, 286
Hypotonia 149, 281, 283

I
ICD-10 (International Classification of Diseases) 231, 232
Ichthammol 266
IgE 71, 72, 73
Ileus 130
Immunisation 38, 81, 111, 112, 113, 114, 115, 116, 164, 170, 191
Immunodeficiency 40, 80, 114, 173
Immunodeficient 80
Immunoglobulin 65, 114, 115
Immunosuppressive 114
Impetigo 266, 289
Impulsivity 22, 37
Inactive vaccine 115
Incontinence 175
Infection 40, 41, 43, 45, 46, 47, 48, 49, 58, 64, 65, 68, 69, 70, 76, 77, 79, 81, 82, 96, 97, 98, 99, 101, 103, 104, 105, 107, 108, 109, 115, 116, 119, 120, 125, 127, 129, 130, 135, 136, 150, 171, 193, 200, 208, 216, 217, 225, 236, 253, 265, 277, 278, 288, 289, 290
Infectious 49, 60, 66, 112, 116, 289, 290
Inflammatory 29, 30, 48, 58, 60, 61, 104, 107, 108, 109, 113, 126, 133, 134, 139, 203, 255, 256, 257, 260, 264, 272, 284, 285
Infliximab 59, 60
Influenza virus 79
Inguinal hernia 100, 101, 102, 103, 105, 108, 134
Inhaler 125, 170, 171, 172, 174, 268, 269, 271, 272, 273, 274

Innocent murmur 144
Insecticide 252
Insect repellent 252
Inspection 97, 120, 125, 133, 138, 146, 148, 154, 229, 294, 295, 296, 298
Insulin 31, 189, 190, 191, 192, 193, 194, 195, 196, 243, 245, 246, 247, 286
Intention tremor 149, 298
Interval symptom 170, 172, 173
Intussusception 284
Irritable hip 109
Irritability 92, 112, 178, 200, 246
IRT (immunoreactive trypsinogen) 130

J
Jaundice 133, 134, 136, 137, 280, 284, 286, 296, 300
Jendrassik manoeuvre 147, 149
Joint 59, 107, 108, 109, 110, 112, 147, 148, 155, 156, 157, 158, 160, 193, 217, 229, 231, 257, 258, 259, 285, 299
Juvenile 29, 66, 106, 108, 109, 135, 148, 282, 285

K
Kernicterus 150
Ketoacidosis 82, 173, 190, 191, 193, 194, 195, 196, 286
Klinefelter syndrome 157
Kocher 110, 134
Kyphoscoliosis 82, 151, 155
Kyphosis 155

L
Language 18, 20, 152, 184, 185, 186, 187, 206, 207, 209, 217, 223, 227, 228, 229, 230, 231, 232, 233, 301, 302, 303, 304, 305
Learning difficulty 150, 223
Learning disability 38, 231
Lens dislocation 158
Leuconychia 133
Leukaemia 106, 107, 135
Leukotriene receptor 172, 270
Levonorgestrel 41, 42
Lid lag 64, 66
Limb length 30, 155
Limp 106, 107, 108, 109, 110, 119, 146, 150, 285
Lipohypertrophy 195
Live vaccine 112, 114, 115
Local tutor 276
Logbook 291, 292
Long acting insulin 44, 172, 194, 195, 245, 270, 277
Loose stools 60, 178, 288
Lordosis 155
Lower motor neurone 147, 149
Lycra splint 216
Lymphadenopathy 104, 134, 289
Lymph node 101, 103, 134, 277

M
Malabsorption 129, 130, 284
Malarone 249, 251
Malignancy 29, 101, 104, 108, 114, 135, 277, 285
Malnutrition 29, 30
Malrotation 284
Maltreatment 36, 96, 97, 187
Manikin 14
Manometry 178
Marfan's syndrome 157, 158

Mark sheets 9, 14, 18, 21, 52, 53, 54, 86, 87, 88, 119, 120, 122, 164, 166, 170, 176, 184, 190, 198, 207, 208, 210, 237, 238, 240, 250, 254, 261, 268
MASTA (travel health clinic) 251
Maternal alcohol 280
MDI (metered dose inhaler) 271, 272
Measles 112, 113, 114, 115, 188
Mebendazole 70
Meconium 130, 176, 178, 179, 180
Mediastinal 127, 173
Medical devices 14
Medication overuse 171, 199, 200, 202
Megarectum 177, 180
Menarche 283
Meningitis 82, 113, 136, 150, 216
Menisci 257
Mental health 23, 25, 37, 44
Metabolic disease 290
Metatarsal 259
Methylphenidate 25
Microarray 188
Micturition 67
Migraine 58, 162, 199, 200, 201, 202, 203, 204
Milk protein 288
Mite 34, 35
Mitral stenosis 141, 143
Mitral valve prolapse 158
MMR vaccine (measles, mumps, rubella) 112, 113, 114, 115, 188
Molluscum contagiosum 289
Monoclonal antibodies 81
Montelukast 172, 270
Morning-after pill 41
Moro 214, 302
Morphine 258
Mosquito 252
Motor delay 92, 179, 185, 213, 216, 223
Mouth ulcer 59, 60
Movicol 176, 177, 181
MRSA (methicillin-resistant staphylococcus aureus) 288
Mucopolysaccharidoses 135
Multidisciplinary 17, 30, 99, 130, 152, 186, 209, 215, 217, 218, 222, 223, 225, 232, 281
Mumps 112, 113, 188, 277
Murmur 119, 141, 142, 143, 144, 145, 156, 157, 279, 290, 294
Muscle tone 213, 281, 286, 298
Muscular dystrophy 82, 148, 214, 281
Mutation 129, 130, 158, 283
Myalgia 112, 252
Myoclonus 282
Myopathy 148
Myopia 158

N
Nappy rash 266, 289
Nasogastric 81, 152, 214
Navicular bone 259
Neck swelling 277
Neglect 24, 29, 30, 35, 36, 37, 38, 39, 178, 179, 180, 187, 230, 287
Neomycin 114
Neonatal 37, 48, 93, 100, 130, 136, 137, 150, 173, 185, 216, 219, 224, 280, 283, 284, 292, 300
Nephritis 68, 257, 290
Nephrotic syndrome 68, 290
Neural tube 134
Neuroblastoma 107

Neurodisability 152, 204, 209, 215, 218, 219, 222, 225, 232
Neurofibromatosis 231, 283
Neuromuscular 97, 109, 173, 179, 281
NICE guidelines (National Institute of Care and Excellence) 22, 26, 52, 56, 58, 61, 68, 70, 73, 76, 81, 83, 86, 95, 98, 99, 101, 105, 179, 181, 182, 185, 186, 188, 200, 201, 203, 204, 233, 248, 263, 264, 267, 285, 289
Night terror 282
Nissen fundoplication 134
Nitrites 68
Non-accidental 39, 108, 287
Non-judgemental 48
Non-steroidal 107, 200, 203, 255
Non-verbal 16, 19, 20, 124, 164, 166, 168, 176, 184, 206, 210, 212, 217, 218
Noonan syndrome 29
Nosebleed 287
Notifiable 253
NSAID (non-steroidal anti-inflammatory drug) 203, 255, 256, 257, 258, 259, 260
Nutritional 38, 125, 131, 133, 152, 285
Nystagmus 149, 220, 297, 298

O
Obesity 82, 107, 283, 290
Obstructive sleep apnoea 199, 200
Occupational therapist 152, 217, 223, 232
Oedema 74, 75, 80, 82, 128, 139, 144, 155, 194
Oligohydramnios 92, 109
Omeprazole 256
Ophthalmia neonatorum 48
Ophthalmology 49, 215, 222
Ophthalmoscope 297, 300
Opiate 82
Opioid 256, 257, 258
Orbital cellulitis 198, 289
Orchidopexy 103, 104, 105
Orthopaedic 152, 218, 257, 258
Orthoses 214
Orthotic 147, 213, 217, 220
Osgood-Schlatter disease 107
Osler's node 139
Osteosarcoma 107
Otitis media 48, 277
Ottawa rule 259
Oxygen 80, 81, 82, 125, 138, 139, 142, 256, 280

P
Pacing wire 140
Pain 24, 42, 43, 44, 48, 57, 58, 59, 60, 61, 67, 68, 69, 72, 82, 96, 104, 107, 108, 109, 110, 111, 112, 120, 135, 144, 147, 162, 176, 177, 178, 179, 180, 181, 193, 198, 199, 200, 201, 202, 224, 254, 256, 257, 258, 259, 260, 277, 278, 279, 284, 285, 286, 299
Palate 155, 156, 157, 230, 300
Palivizumab 81
Pallor 72, 79, 108, 126, 134, 136, 139, 202, 246, 285, 290, 294, 295, 296, 299, 300
Palmar 133, 221, 222, 223, 302
Palpation 120, 127, 135, 140, 147, 148, 294, 295, 296
Palpitation 62, 65, 144, 279, 286
Panic attacks 75, 173

Pansystolic 141, 142, 144, 156, 157
Papillary necrosis 257
Paracetamol 112, 200, 203, 254, 256, 257, 258, 259
Parachute 214, 302
Parainfluenza virus 79
Parasternal 127, 140, 141, 142, 143, 294
Parenteral therapy 246
Parotid 112
Parotitis 277
Parvovirus 136
Passive immunity 81, 115
Patella hammer 298
Patent ductus 140, 143
Pavlik harness 109
Peak flow meter 125, 173, 273
Peanut 71, 72, 74
PEF (peak expiratory flow) 273
PEG (percutaneous endoscopic gastrostomy) 133, 152
Penicillin 136
Periodic syndrome 199, 202
Periorbital cellulitis 289
Permethrin 35
Personality 202
Perthes disease 106, 107, 110, 285
Pertussis 113
pGALS (paediatric gait, arms, legs, spine) 156, 160, 299
Phobia 177, 179, 191, 193, 198, 200, 201, 263
Phonology 230
Phonophobia 200, 201
Photophobia 198, 200, 201
Physiotherapy 130, 131, 152, 217, 223
Picosulfate, sodium 181
Picture book 228, 303
Pigmentation 134, 286
Pincer grasp 221, 222, 303
Piperazine 70
Plagiocephaly 91, 92, 93, 94
Plantar flexion 147
Plasmodium, falciparum 252
Plaster cast 110
Platelet 57, 58, 62, 256, 260, 285
Pleurisy 278
Pneumococcal 113
Pneumonia 48, 58, 79, 82, 136, 173, 278
Pneumothorax 127, 128, 158
Polio 49, 113, 115, 253, 288
Polycythaemia 139
Polydipsia 96, 193, 286
Polymyxin B 114
Polyuria 96, 193, 286
Poor feeding 79, 144, 279, 286, 290
Portacath 126, 128, 129, 131, 139
Portage 224, 226
Portal hypertension 135, 136
Postnatal 37, 105, 216, 284, 286
Posture 18, 20, 122, 124, 144, 147, 148, 150, 152, 164, 166, 168, 210, 212, 213, 216, 217, 281, 298, 299
Posturing 151
PPI (proton pump inhibitor) 256
Prader-Willi syndrome 29, 283
Pragmatics 230
Pregnancy 37, 40, 41, 42, 48, 101
Pregnant 40, 41, 42, 65
Premature 37, 81, 92, 93, 116, 119, 146, 150, 216, 281
Prematurity 24, 81, 92, 93, 101, 109, 150, 170, 173, 280

Prescription 10, 72, 74, 170, 189, 190, 192, 194, 236, 237, 238, 239, 240, 242, 243, 244, 245, 247, 249, 250, 251, 252, 253, 254, 255, 256, 258, 259, 261, 262, 263, 266, 268, 269, 270, 274
Pretend play 184, 227, 231
Primary care 4, 8, 28, 76, 114, 236, 264, 279, 287
Primitive reflex 151, 214, 300, 302
Processus vaginalis 101, 102
Prochlorperazine 203
Proguanil 249
Prolapse, rectal 130, 158
Prolonged fever 142
Prone 94, 214, 302
Prophylaxis 45, 81, 142, 203, 249, 251, 252, 279
Prostaglandin 256, 257
Protein-losing enteropathy 58
Proteinuria 58, 65, 67, 68, 81, 106, 108, 129, 130, 137, 192, 264, 288, 290
Pruritus 69, 251
Pseudomonas 130
Psychiatrist 4, 7, 25, 26, 37, 180, 186, 188, 232
Psychological 17, 22, 24, 93, 177, 179, 181, 193, 200, 263
Psychologist 130, 185, 186, 192, 223, 232
Ptosis 297
Puberty 27, 28, 29, 30, 31, 32, 59, 64, 103, 289
Pulse oximeter 83, 138, 139, 142, 295
Pyloromyotomy 134
Pyuria 68

Q
Quadriplegia 97, 150, 151

R
Radioiodine 65
Ramstedt pyloromyotomy 134
Ranitidine 256
Red flag 107, 108, 178, 179, 181, 201, 202, 203, 215, 222, 252
Reflexes 147, 149, 150, 151, 214, 216, 298, 300, 302
Reflux 129, 134, 151, 173, 217, 281, 284
Refractive error 200, 225
Regression 108, 187, 231
Rehabilitation 152, 218
Reinforcement 24, 147, 149, 181
Renal 29, 68, 70, 82, 97, 99, 134, 135, 172, 173, 199, 200, 251, 257, 286, 290, 296
Respiratory 47, 48, 74, 75, 77, 78, 79, 80, 81, 82, 101, 107, 109, 118, 119, 125, 126, 128, 129, 130, 131, 139, 158, 172, 173, 174, 194, 218, 270, 273, 274, 277, 278, 280, 292, 295
Respite 209, 218, 225, 232
Retinal detachment 158
Retrognathia 157
Rett syndrome 187
Reward system 97, 98
Rhinitis 48, 72, 170, 171, 173, 256, 264, 277
Rickets 285
Role player 14, 15, 16, 21, 22, 27, 28, 33, 34, 40, 41, 46, 47, 162, 164, 169, 175, 183, 189, 197
Romberg sign 149, 298
Rotavirus 113
Rubella 112, 113, 188
Russell-Silver syndrome 29

311

S

Sacral agenesis 179
Sacral dimple 97
Safeguarding 34, 35, 36, 37, 39, 43, 70, 86, 99, 287
Safe sex 41, 42
Salbutamol 73, 74, 81, 126, 170, 171, 268, 270, 273, 277
Salicylate 59, 81, 82, 131, 194
Saline nebuliser 81
Salmeterol 172, 270
Sarcoptes scabiei 34
Scabies 33, 34, 289
Scalded skin 38, 266, 289
Scalp swelling 280
Scaphocephaly 150
Scoliosis 82, 92, 151, 155, 156, 157, 179, 218
Screening programme 49, 224, 225, 286, 288
Seborrhoeic dermatitis 266, 289
Sedation 258
Seizure 151, 152, 187, 190, 202, 243, 245, 246, 252, 282, 289
Sellotape test 69
SENCO (Special Educational Needs Coordinator) 24
Senna 181
Sensory sensitivity 184, 185, 186
Sepsis 136, 180, 280
Septic arthritis 106, 107, 108, 109, 110
Sexually transmitted 41, 47, 49
Shared care 25, 130
Shifting dullness 135, 296
Shock 47, 75, 82
Shortness of breath 75, 138, 272, 290
Short stature 27, 28, 29, 30, 31, 32
Sickle cell disease 108, 137
SIGN guideline (Scottish Intercollegiate Guideline Network) 174, 277
Sinding-Larsen disease 107
SLE (Systemic Lupus Erythematosis) 135
Slipped femoral epiphysis 107
Smoker 170
Soiling 96, 176, 177, 178, 180
Space occupying lesion 281
Spacer 125, 170, 171, 172, 174, 268, 271, 272, 273
Spastic 147, 150, 151, 152, 179, 217
Specialist 21, 22, 25, 64, 72, 73, 74, 98, 99, 104, 109, 114, 115, 130, 173, 181, 209, 217, 218, 232, 236, 243, 245, 258, 265, 266, 273
Speech 16, 152, 184, 185, 186, 201, 206, 207, 209, 215, 217, 222, 223, 227, 228, 229, 230, 231, 232, 233, 277, 298, 301, 302, 303, 304, 305
Spherocytosis 135, 136, 137
Spider naevi 134, 136
Spirometry 273
Splenectomy 134, 136, 137
Splint 147, 214, 216, 217
Sprain 256, 257, 258
Squint 155, 202, 213, 220, 225, 281, 290
Standard setting 7, 15, 53, 87, 119, 120, 162, 164, 165, 207, 208, 237
Staphylococcus 69, 130, 265, 266, 288, 289
Step-wise approach 172, 254, 257, 262, 269, 273
Stereotyped 232
Stereotypic 184, 185, 187, 232
Sternberg sign 155, 156, 157
Sternomastoid tumour 92, 297
Sternotomy 126, 140, 141, 142
Steroid phobia 263
Stethoscope 128, 141, 294, 295, 296, 300
STI (sexually transmitted infection) 42, 43, 47, 48
Sticky eye 46, 47
Storage disorder 133, 134, 135, 246
Strabismus 225
Strangulation, hernia 101
Streptococcus 69, 136, 265
Streptomycin 114
Stridor 75, 126, 173, 278
Sturge-Weber syndrome 281
Substance misuse 37
Sumatriptan 203
Suppurative 66, 129
Supravalvular 144
Syncope 144, 279
Synovitis 106, 107, 109, 110

T

Tachycardia 25, 62, 63, 64, 65, 74
Tacrolimus 266
Tactile fremitus 127
Tall stature 64, 65, 154, 157, 160
Tapping apex 140
Target height 27, 29, 31
Teenager 28, 41, 42, 44, 65, 107, 164
Temper tantrum 99, 289
Tenderness 103, 107, 135, 258, 259, 296, 299
Tension headache 200, 201
Testicular torsion 58, 104, 108
Tetanus 112, 113
Tetralogy of Fallot 142, 143
Thalassaemia 134, 135, 137
Thick blood film 253
Thoracotomy 126, 140
Threadworm 69, 70
Thrombocytopenia 107, 256
Thromboxane 256
Thrush 69, 193
Thyroid 31, 63, 64, 65, 66, 224
Thyroidectomy 65
Thyroiditis 64, 65, 66
Thyrotoxicosis 63, 64, 66
Tiptoes 215, 222
Toddler 103, 107, 208, 236
Toileting 97, 98, 177, 181, 217, 223
Tongue depressor 293
Tonic neck reflex 214, 302
Tonsillitis 277
Torsion 58, 101, 104, 108
Torticollis 92, 93
Toxic trio 37
Tracheoesophageal fistula 284
Tracheostomy 126, 139
Tramadol 258
Trampolining 224
Transfer factor 65, 221, 302
Transillumination 103
Transplant 114, 131, 134
Transposition 143, 213
Trauma 24, 37, 68, 106, 107, 109, 150, 178, 257, 258
TRAVAX (travel health information website for professionals) 251, 253
Tremor 64, 126, 133, 149, 298
Trendelenburg 107
Triceps 149, 216
Tricuspid atresia 143
Tricuspid regurgitation 142, 143,
Tripod grasp 221
Triptan 203
Trisomy 21 144, 180, 279
Truncus arteriosus 143
TSH (thyroid stimulating hormone) 63, 64, 65, 66
Tuberculosis 173, 278
Tuberous sclerosis 231, 281
Tummy time 93, 94
Tunica vaginalis 101, 102
Turner syndrome 283, 290
Twin pregnancy 92
Typhoid 115
Tyrosinaemia 135

U

Ulcerative colitis 58, 60, 256
Ultra-long-acting insulin 194, 195
Undescended testis 100, 101, 102, 103, 104, 105
Unlicensed medication 236, 239
Unprotected sex 40, 41, 42
Unsteadiness 224
Upper motor neurone 147, 148, 149
Urticaria 72, 75
Uveitis 285

V

Vacant spell 282
Vaccines 112, 113, 114, 115, 116, 170, 188, 191
Vaginal swab 69
Varicocele 101
Vas deferens 103, 130
Vascular lesion 200
Venous hum 143, 144
Ventral suspension 214, 302
Ventricular septal defect 140, 142, 143, 144, 224
Vertebral anomaly 97
Vibration sense 298
Video links 292
Visible peristalsis 296
VOCA (voice output communication aid) 217
Vocal fremitus 295
Volumatic 272
Vomiting 42, 59, 61, 68, 69, 72, 81, 82, 92, 173, 178, 179, 180, 193, 194, 199, 200, 201, 202, 203, 258, 281, 284, 286
Vulvitis 69
Vulvovaginitis 68, 69, 70

W

Waddling 107, 147, 149, 150
Wasting 110, 147, 148, 149, 298
Weakness 82, 151, 214, 246, 252
Weight loss 57, 58, 59, 60, 64, 65, 69, 96, 108, 193, 278
Wet wrap 266
Wheelchair 147, 214
Wheeze 77, 79, 126, 128, 170, 171, 172, 173, 268, 272, 277, 278
WHO (World Health Organisation) 246, 260
William's syndrome 138, 144, 154
Wilson's disease 135

Y

Yellow fever 114, 115

Z

Zinc 266